Essentials of Planning and Evaluation for Public Health

Karen (Kay) M. Perrin, PhD, MPH

Associate Professor, Assistant Dean of Undergraduate Studies

College of Public Health

University of South Florida

Tampa, Florida

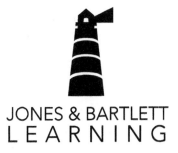

JONES & BARTLETT
LEARNING

World Headquarters
Jones & Bartlett Learning
5 Wall Street
Burlington, MA 01803
978-443-5000
info@jblearning.com
www.jblearning.com

Jones & Bartlett Learning books and products are available through most bookstores and online booksellers. To contact Jones & Bartlett Learning directly, call 800-832-0034, fax 978-443-8000, or visit our website, www.jblearning.com.

Substantial discounts on bulk quantities of Jones & Bartlett Learning publications are available to corporations, professional associations, and other qualified organizations. For details and specific discount information, contact the special sales department at Jones & Bartlett Learning via the above contact information or send an email to specialsales@jblearning.com.

Production Credits

Publisher: Michael Brown
Associate Editor: Lindsey Mawhiney
Editorial Assistant: Nicholas Alakel
Production Manager: Tracey McCrea
Senior Marketing Manager: Sophie Fleck Teague
Manufacturing and Inventory Control Supervisor:
  Amy Bacus
Composition: Cenveo Publisher Services

Cover Design: Kristin E. Parker
Manager of Photo Research, Rights & Permissions:
  Amy Rathburn
Cover, Title Page, and Chapter Opener Image:
  © Vladitto/Shutterstock, Inc.
Box Image: © iStockphoto.com/mediaphotos
Printing and Binding: Edwards Brothers Malloy
Cover Printing: Edwards Brothers Malloy

To order this product, use ISBN: 978-1-284-05019-6

Library of Congress Cataloging-in-Publication Data
Perrin, Karen M., author.
  Essentials of planning and evaluation for public health / Karen Perrin.
    p. ; cm.
  Includes bibliographical references and index.
  ISBN 978-1-4496-7434-2 (pbk.)
  I. Title.
  [DNLM: 1. Health Care Evaluation Mechanisms. 2. Program Evaluation–methods. WA 525]
  RA427
  362.1–dc23
                          2014024921
6048

Printed in the United States of America
18 17 16 15 14   10 9 8 7 6 5 4 3

Dedication

Kevin
My husband
1950–2014

Contents

Preface

This text was written for undergraduate public health students enrolled in an introductory course related to program planning and evaluation. The chapters are divided into a sequential order that forms the foundation for the knowledge needed to understand basic evaluation projects. This text is not intended to achieve complete understanding or proficiency in the complex subject of program planning and evaluation and research needed in the field of public health. However, the chapters provide an overview of topics needed to review published literature, collect primary data, analyze data using basic statistics, and present results in written or verbal formats for intended audiences.

The first three chapters set the stage for program planning and evaluation. Chapter 1 explains the differences and similarities between evaluation and research along with how to review literature and develop measureable goals and objectives. Chapter 2 introduces ethics, which is a core element in program planning and evaluation and needs consideration during the development phase. Chapter 3 explores determinants of health, such as health disparities and access to health care. Without attention to social determinants, evaluators miss the key elements in the lives of their target audience that influence health outcomes.

The next several chapters define terms and concepts that should be understood prior to planning an evaluation. Chapter 4 introduces various types of theories and models along with examples from current literature on how the theories and models have been used as the framework for project development. The list of theories and models is not intended to be comprehensive, but rather an introduction to examples. Chapter 5 defines the concepts of reliability and validity as well as random and systematic errors. The chapter ends with a detailed description of how to conduct a pilot test and why pilot testing is essential. Chapter 6 explains the similarities and differences between qualitative and quantitative data, then goes on to provide a more detailed discussion related to types and methods utilized in qualitative data.

The next two chapters provide information about study design and survey development. Chapter 7 presents some basic tools for study design, including types of variables, group assignment, constructs, and operational definitions. After these concepts are explained, the three basic types of study design (true experimental, quasi-experimental, and nonexperimental) are defined and examples are provided to enhance understanding. Chapter 8 focuses on survey design, including types of surveys and how to select them. Various tests, inventories, and scales are introduced along with examples and reasons for selecting one survey type over another. A discussion of how culture and diversity influence data collection is included near the end of the chapter.

Chapters 9, 10, and 11 focus on basic skills related to data analysis. Chapter 9 introduces how data are classified as categorical or continuous and then organized using frequency distributions. Building on this knowledge, the concepts of measures of central tendency, the normal curve, standard deviation, and variance are explained in detail. This chapter serves as the foundation for understanding the next two chapters. Chapter 10 describes terms related to population and samples. There are three main topics covered: sample size considerations, probability and nonprobability samples, and sampling bias. Each topic deserves substantial consideration when determining the sample size needed for any evaluation or research project. Chapter

11 introduces inferential statistics and defines the terms *scientific hypothesis*, *research questions*, *null hypothesis*, and *alternative hypothesis*. The next section presents basic statistical tests (e.g., chi-square, *t*-tests, and correlation coefficients). The chapter ends with a discussion of type I and type II errors.

The last four chapters provide skills related to budgets, reports, and presentations, culminating in a case study. Chapter 12 is divided into two sections. The first section describes various types of budgets and budget justifications. The second section defines the types of cost analyses and how each type is used. Chapter 13 illustrates several ways to present results, including abstracts, executive summaries, reports, manuscripts, posters, and verbal presentations. Chapter 14 is a lengthy case study covering all aspects of program planning and evaluation presented in this text.

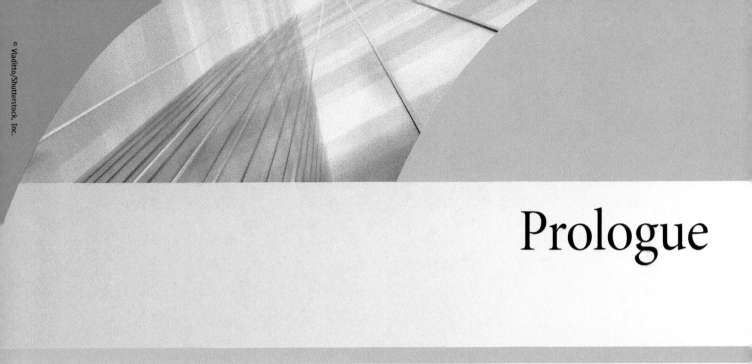

Prologue

Essentials of Planning and Evaluation for Public Health by Kay Perrin, PhD, MPH is an important addition to our *Essential Public Health* series. It provides the ideal text for an undergraduate course in program planning and evaluation, which is an increasingly important part of public health education at all levels.

The Recommended Critical Component Elements of an Undergraduate Major in Public Health expect that all undergraduate public health majors, including those in health education, will "know the fundamental features of project implementation and evaluation."[1] These "critical component elements" are now being used by the Council on Education for Public Health (CEPH) as part of the criteria for accreditation of undergraduate public health majors. The *Essentials of Planning and Evaluation for Public Health* will aid in accomplishing this objective.

Dr. Perrin's book includes many important features that will appeal to a wide range of students. Dr. Perrin provides an accessible, engaging, and active participation text. As she describes in the Preface, it is organized in a step-by-step process that introduces undergraduates to all of the key elements of program planning and evaluation. The text makes extensive use of case studies for public health applications. Her treatment of quantitative methods is accessible, requiring only a minimum of mathematics. Overall, Dr. Perrin's text is clear, easy to read, and has a personalized style of writing that makes learning both productive and enjoyable.

Dr. Perrin is widely recognized for developing new styles of teaching that engage students inside and outside the classroom. Her extensive and creative teaching experience is evident in every chapter of the text. Dr. Perrin brings to her writing extensive experience teaching and applying principles of program planning and evaluation. Her clinical and public health research background provides the perfect combination to understand the roles and goals of program planning and evaluation.

Finally, on a personal note, Kay Perrin was recently presented the Riegelman Award for Excellence in Undergraduate Public Health from the Association of Schools of Public Health. I was delighted that she was chosen, especially knowing that I had nothing to do with the selection process. Dr. Perrin's nominator wrote that she "continues to foster excitement about the field of public health in the undergraduate arena . . . and most importantly nurture future public health leaders through her unwavering commitment to undergraduate public health education." I couldn't agree more.

I'm delighted that Kay Perrin's work is now a part of our *Essential Public Health* series. I'm confident that you will find it to be an important addition.

Richard Riegelman, MD, MPH, PhD
Editor, *Essential Public Health* series

1. Association of Schools of Public Health. *Recommended Critical Component Elements of an Undergraduate Major in Public Health*. Available at: http://www.asph.org/UserFiles/CCE_2012-08-03-FINAL.pdf. Accessed February 4, 2014.

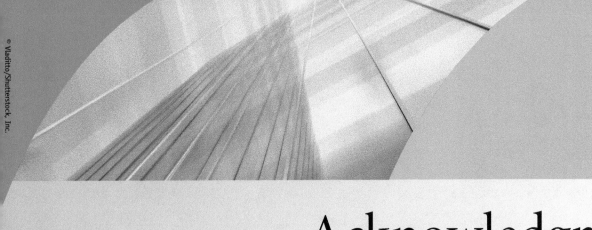

Acknowledgments

During process of writing this book, I received assistance and support from numerous family, friends, and colleagues.

Kevin, my husband, supported me through the many weekends that were consumed with writing. He allowed me the opportunity to fulfill my dream.

Laura Merrell, public health doctoral student, edited each chapter with great attention to detail. Her superb skills greatly contributed to the quality of this text.

Dr. Richard Riegelman provided guidance and mentoring as I embarked on writing this text. His constructive comments improved the overall quality of this text.

Dr. R. Clifford Blair offered valuable advice throughout the process. As a biostatistician and author, he offered humor and encouragement whenever I was exhausted.

After decades of teaching courses and engaging in community service, hundreds of public health students have taught me the skills and expertise needed to write this text.

University of South Florida, College of Public Health granted me time to complete this public health text.

Most educators say that the best way to learn a subject is to teach it. After writing two textbooks, I have revised this advice to say:

"The best way to learn a subject is not to teach it, but rather to write a book about it."

CHAPTER 1

Introduction

By the end of this chapter, the student will be able to:

1. Define program planning and evaluation.
2. Review the literature.
3. Discuss how to conduct a needs assessment.
4. Evaluate goal statements and objectives.
5. Create a logic model.
6. Evaluate the positive and adverse influences of stakeholders.
7. Differentiate the various types of evaluations.

KEY TERMS

goals and objectives
logic model
program planning
stakeholders
types of evaluations

INTRODUCTION

This chapter begins by defining program planning and evaluation. The next topic of discussion is an overview of how to conduct a needs assessment. Program planning involves identification of the type and design of program needed to address a health issue; achieving consensus from individuals providing or participating in the program; securing essential financial, personnel, and location resources; and sustained program implementation by staying true to the original design, which is also called program fidelity. Program evaluation is used for determining the day-to-day program management, short-term results, and long-term program impact. Program evaluations involve data collection and analysis to influence changes to improve program effectiveness.[1] When planning a program or conducting an evaluation, once the goal and objectives are in place, the investigation begins to take shape.

If you are wondering why you need to know about program planning, let's explore the practical side of these skills. If you decide to attend graduate school to obtain your master's in public health (MPH) degree, you will conduct an evaluation by asking a few questions prior to making your final decision:

1. What resources do you have available for graduate education? (Needs assessment)
2. Which universities offer a master's in public health degree with your specialization of interest? (Review of available information)
3. Why do you want to obtain an MPH degree? (Goal)
4. What specific knowledge, skills, or training do you wish to gain during an MPH program? (Objectives)
5. How will you map out your strategy for making the final decision? (Logic model)
6. What type of numerical data (e.g., cost, length of program, required courses) is available on the university website? (Quantitative data)
7. During the university visit, what information do you hope to obtain by talking to currently enrolled MPH students? (Qualitative data)
8. What are the budget constraints influencing your decision? (Budget)
9. What criteria will you use to make your final decision? (Evaluation)

10. How will you interpret the data? (Data analysis)
11. What is your final decision? (Final report)

Once you realize the usefulness of program planning and evaluation skills in daily life, this text will become more practical and beneficial. You will learn skills and methods to assist with a wide range of program planning and evaluation methods in your personal and professional life.

OVERVIEW OF PROGRAM PLANNING AND EVALUATION

Let's begin with a little historical background related to program planning and evaluation. In the 1960s, health education programs were implemented with little planning and limited evaluation. For example, in 1962, Kennedy became the first president to sponsor studies on smoking and public health.[2] By 1964, the landmark report entitled "Smoking and Health: Report of the Advisory Committee to the Surgeon General of the Public Health Service" revealed the negative health effects of smoking.[3] The health messages in this report were simple and straightforward, and merely told people to stop smoking because it is not good for their health. These messages were not targeted to a particular audience or population, so the messages were generally ignored. Over the years, evaluators learned that targeted messages are most effective. For example, test this concept the next time that you watch a television commercial. Are you more likely to watch an advertisement for a new product if the individuals on the screen are similar to your age, gender, and ethnicity? On the other hand, if the individuals are older with gray hair, are you less likely to show interest in the message? The next few paragraphs show how targeted messages evolved over time.

In the 1970s, during her husband's presidency, First Lady Nancy Reagan started the "Just Say No" advertising campaign as part of the U.S. War on Drugs.[4] This health message illustrates the next step in health education messages. This message was targeted to adolescents rather than to the entire U.S. population, and the message was focused on reducing peer pressure.[5]

By the 1980s, the health messages were carefully planned and implemented by involving the target audience in planning the methods. For example, the U.S. Office on Smoking and Health, a federal government agency, led strategic efforts aimed at preventing tobacco use and promoting smoking cessation among adolescents. They designed anti-smoking public service announcements featuring popular movie stars of the time, such as Brooke Shields. In 1986, the American Lung Association (ALA) started another similar campaign focused on smoking cessation targeted at pregnant women. Joan Lunden, the popular host of the television news program *Good Morning America*, was pregnant at the time and became the National Chairman of ALA's Smoking and Pregnancy Education Campaign. The slogan of this focused campaign was "Quit smoking . . . you're breathing for two."[6]

In the 1990s, health messages added evaluation components to the targeted program planning and implementation. In California, the anti-smoking media campaign added a targeted message that helped smokers to learn how to stop smoking. This health message was targeted at smokers, provided tools to quit smoking, and was rigorously evaluated to determine the effectiveness of the media campaign.[7]

By 2000, health programs were meticulously planned, implemented, and evaluated. The planning stage used input from the targeted audience, but also used valuable data from previous health program evaluation to determine the effectiveness. For example, the U.S. Department of Health and Human Services and the Centers for Disease Control and Prevention published numerous studies related to the link between smoking and morbidity and mortality.[8–12]

Using the anti-smoking health messages in the previous examples, it can be seen that current health programs are designed by conducting a thorough review of the literature to determine the best practices and effectiveness data from previous studies. In addition to a health program being carefully planned, implemented, and evaluated, the cost effectiveness of a health program has become vitally important. Funders no longer have the money to initiate health programs without knowing the cost effectiveness or the "bang for their buck." In other words, funders want to know how many individuals will gain an improved quality of health if they provide money for a specific, high-quality health program.

Although it might seem reasonable to start any program with the planning phase and end with the evaluation, this logic is not correct. It is essential to design the program plan and its implementation parallel with the evaluation. It is not possible to implement a program that has not been fully planned, nor is it possible to create an evaluation after the implementation phase is complete. Each phase is intertwined with the other program components.

The best way to show how program planning and evaluation are merged is to review the basic steps in the process. Each step involves a series of questions that must be addressed prior to moving forward. If any of the steps are skipped, it is unlikely that the program plan or evaluation will succeed. **Table 1-1** describes a brief overview of the process. Each step is described in detail throughout the remainder of this chapter.

Now's let's explore each step in greater detail. The final phase in program evaluation is analyzing the data (information) you have gathered and reporting (sharing) the results.

TABLE 1-1 Overview of Program Planning and Evaluation

Step	Topic	Questions	Examples
One	Stakeholders	Who are the stakeholders and community partners? Were they invited to the pre-planning stage? What is their common interest for change?	Community members Staff Board of Directors
Two	Needs Assessment	How was the need for the proposed program and evaluation determined?	Baseline data Needs assessment
		Are there adequate resources available for the proposed program?	Funding Time Location Staff
Three	Review of the Literature	What are the best practices reported from similar evaluations?	Best practices
Four	Goals and Objectives	What are the goals and objectives of the program and evaluation?	Change behavior Increase awareness Seek opinions Measure effects
		How will the planners know that the goal or outcome objectives were met?	Attendance Satisfaction surveys Change in baseline data over time
		Who is expected to participate?	Stakeholders Community members Employees of the organization
		How will expected audience be invited?	Print media Social media Radio and television ads Billboards
Five	Implementation	What is the format?	1-day event 6-week seminar series Health fair Tabletop display Online education modules
		What is the budget? What is the funding source? Is the program plan complete?	Grant Donation Internal funding from organization
Six	Evaluation	What data will be gathered? What protections are in place for human subject compliance? How will data be gathered? What research methods will be used for analyses? What are the roles of the evaluators?	Demographics Sign-in sheets Satisfaction surveys Secondary data from existing records Newspaper articles Public access data
Seven	Results	Who will analyze the data? Will the stakeholders be involved in interpretation of findings? How will the results be disseminated?	Evaluator Statistical consultant Final reports posted online Paper copies distributed to stakeholders

Data from Centers for Disease Control Evaluation Working Group. Steps in Program Evaluation. Available at: http://www.cdc.gov/healthyyouth/evaluation/applied/steps.htm. Accessed April 17, 2014.

The rest of this chapter describes in detail the concepts of stakeholders, needs assessment, goals and objectives, types of evaluation, and logic models.

ROLE OF STAKEHOLDERS

At times, it is difficult to determine which comes first, the needs assessment or the stakeholders. Sometimes a community issue, such as the rising crime rate, is identified first, and then a group of stakeholders comes together to try to address the issue, perhaps by coming up with a plan of action. Other times, a group of community partners gathers together, such as a local ecological Sierra Club, with the main purpose of planning how to solve a problem that they perceive. Because stakeholders, such as staff members, community leaders, neighborhood organization members, and political leaders, shape how a program is planned, implemented, and evaluated, team members consider the level of influence and power held by stakeholders.[13] Stakeholders have specific roles. By learning these roles, each phase of the program design meets diverse needs. Traditionally in program planning and evaluation, stakeholders were viewed as policymakers, program sponsors, program management, evaluation staff, or program staff. Even though target participants were often included in the list of stakeholders, they were not necessarily viewed as equal partners. Over time, the target audience has gained status and equal partnership. Now these stakeholders are viewed as having the empowerment to sustain community development projects by embracing disenfranchised groups.[14] As shown in **Table 1-2**, stakeholders with low power and high legitimacy (or trustworthiness) represent service recipients or frontline staff. When the high-power and low-legitimacy stakeholders omit the less empowered individuals from the program design, there is less utilization and sustainability.[15]

TABLE 1-2 Stakeholders and Power

Low Power/High Legitimacy	High Power/Low Legitimacy
Recipients	Policymakers
Frontline staff	Funding agencies
Disenfranchised individuals	Evaluation staff
Target population	Program sponsors
Program staff	Program competitors

Data from Mark MM, Shotland RL. Stakeholder-based evaluation and value judgments. *Evaluation Rev.* 1985; 9:605–626.

Over the past few decades, evaluators have recognized the importance of stakeholder involvement. When stakeholders participate from the first program planning meeting through the evaluation, they are more likely to anticipate problems, provide legitimacy to community partners, share data resources, and assist with final decisions.[14] Along with the advantages they bring, stakeholder participation may pose some challenges. For example, a program funding sponsor (high power) stakeholder's opinions may differ from neighborhood homeowner (high legitimacy) stakeholders' opinions. According to Guba and Lincoln,[15] the team should not avoid such conflict, but rather welcome dissimilar opinions and encourage open dialogue for greater understanding of perspectives.

The following are some questions to consider when determining the role of the stakeholders:

- What is the common interest among all of the stakeholders?
- How will the low-power, high-legitimacy stakeholders be assured of equal power throughout the planning and evaluation process?
- How and when will stakeholders be invited to participate in the planning phase?
- Are meetings held at convenient times and locations for low-power, high-legitimacy stakeholders who have less flexible work schedules?
- Is the program methodology flexible and open to change based on stakeholder opinion?

Stakeholders with various roles and power are critical to the success and sustainability of programs whether in an organization, neighborhood, or community. However, different perspectives and vested interests cause clashing viewpoints for most programs. To overcome this potential conflict, it is essential to find some common ground among all members. Until all stakeholders agree on the goal statements, there is no purpose in moving forward. Once agreement is achieved on the goal statements, the specific objectives are modified to include diverse views on how to reach the goal. For example, a community-based ecological group may wish to ban the use of pesticide lawn fertilizers, because water running off the lawns causes increased algae blooms in the local bay water. When the discussion centers on whether lawn fertilizers should or should not be banned, no agreement is reached. However, once the stakeholders agree that incentives should be given to local homeowners that convert their lawns from green grass to xeroscape (use of natural, draught-resistant plants that do not need watering, fertilizer, and monthly maintenance), the stakeholders find common ground for agreement.

NEEDS ASSESSMENT

Now that common ground has been identified, it is important for the stakeholders and community members to form a partnership or coalition. At the introductory meeting, it is important that every member is treated equally and with respect. For example, the neighborhood housing member's opinion and contribution is given the same weight as the city council member's. The stakeholders decide on two or three broad target areas that will serve as the framework for planning the needs assessment. See **Table 1-3**.

REVIEW OF THE LITERATURE

The next step is to review the current published literature. Evaluators need to know what other information is published and discover the best practices on their topic. Best practices are methods or techniques that have consistently shown to be more effective than others and may be considered a benchmark within a field. For example, evaluators may discover a publication that describes a best practice initiative that uses specialized air filters to improve indoor air quality at an auto shop that repairs and paints vehicles. At this point, it may be

TABLE 1-3 Planning a Needs Assessment

Step One	Involve Community Partners and Stakeholders	The involvement of community partners is an ongoing activity due to changes in personnel and agencies. Stakeholders work together to identify needs, outcomes, mandates, measure strengths, choose priorities, find resources, set performance objectives, develop action plans, determine resources, and check progress for impact on outcomes.
Step Two	Identify Needs and Desired Outcomes	The anticipated needs and outcomes are identified by the community partners/ stakeholders. In some cases, the needs and outcomes are mandated by legislative, financial, or community-driven requirements.
Step Three	Examine Strengths and Capacity	Using the needs and outcome goals, baseline data are obtained to understand the strengths of the relationship between existing programs and the identified needs.
Step Four	Set Priorities	After examining the baseline data, it is possible to match the current strengths of the community with the identified needs and desired outcomes. Following this matching process, the members rank the goals in order of priority needs and available funding and existing resources. Stakeholders also consider how long a program can exist given the available resources.
Step Five	Seek Resources	Depending upon the selected priorities and available funding and existing resources, the members may determine the necessity of seeking additional resources.
Step Six	Set Performance Objectives	For each of the selected priorities, the members determine a matching anticipated outcome.
Step Seven	Create an Action Plan	A plan is created that shows exactly what will be done, in an order that reflects the identified priorities based on baseline data, strengths, needs, and resources.
Step Eight	Allocate Resources	Using the priorities and action plan, a budget is developed including current and anticipated resources (e.g., funding, donations, volunteers, community support).
Step Nine	Oversee Progress of Goals and Objectives	Throughout the implementation, it is important to track the objectives and provide feedback where necessary as soon as possible to address performance levels and resources.
Step Ten	Report Back to Community Members and Stakeholders	Results of the needs assessment are shared with community members and stakeholders. Such accountability assures further buy-in as the process moves into the implementation phase.

Data from U.S. Department of Health and Human Services. Health Resources and Services Administration, Maternal and Child Health Bureau. Title V Maternal & Child Health Block Grant Program Needs Assessment. Available at: http://mchb.hrsa.gov/programs/needsassessment/. Accessed April 17, 2014.

tempting to easily enter your topic into an Internet search engine. Although this technique yields hundreds of websites related to the topic, it does not produce material suitable for a review of the literature. Keep in mind that the constant expansion of information available on the Internet does not mean that it is reliable, because anyone can post information. The posted information may serve as an infomercial to sell a product, service, or even one individual's opinion on a topic. Generally, a quick way to discern if a website offers valuable information is to glance at the ending of the web address, or uniform resource locator (URL). If the URL ends with .gov, .edu, or .org, chances are the site presents reliable information. However, if the URL ends in .com or .net, you need to proceed with caution when incorporating the information into your literature review.

Rather than entering the topic into a search engine, it is important to read reliable publications that professionals and researchers have written on the topic of interest. This process yields a peer-reviewed literature review. The term *peer-reviewed journal* can be defined as follows: Academic and scholarly colleagues write a manuscript about their research and submit the manuscript to a professional journal whose editor reviews the manuscript and sends it to several other professionals with expertise on the topic. The peer experts examine the manuscript, review the content, inspect for wrong or erroneous information, edit, and decide if the manuscript is suitable to the specific journal. They write comments back to the editor. The editor shares the reviewer comments with the manuscript's authors. If the manuscript is accepted with revisions, the suggested changes are made and the manuscript is resubmitted, reviewed again, and published. This process allows scholarly peers to review the research of their colleagues prior to publication, thus academic journals are called refereed or peer-reviewed journals. In contrast, documents posted on Internet sites are not typically reviewed through a peer-reviewed process and therefore frequently lack academic rigor, consistency, and attention to detail.

A compelling literature review involves delving into a variety of credible professional reference materials. This process is best accomplished by visiting a university campus library and gaining access to the professional sources through online databases as well as assessing printed materials at the library. If you are not familiar with using databases that house peer-reviewed journals, it is recommended that you review the available tutorial modules or ask the librarian for assistance. As previously described when conducting a peer-reviewed literature review, it is not acceptable to enter the topic into an Internet search engine and use whatever information appears on the screen. This technique yields unreliable information.

To begin a literature review, you need to become familiar with the databases used in health including, but not limited to, MedLine, CINAHL, FirstSearch, Ovid, and PsychINFO. After you access the appropriate database, you may use the "keyword" option to begin your search. This type of search may be limited further by choosing from the following search forms: "Any of the words," "at least one of the words," or "must contain all of these words." For example, suppose you are interested in knowing what has been written about the global efforts to eradicate malaria over the last 10 years. You may wish to use "must contain all of these words." If you do not know much about your selected topic, use the "any of the words" option, and cast a wide net related to the topic. Let's say that you are interested in prevention of back injuries among childcare workers. This option will be voluminous and not provide the exact information for your search, but it allows you to explore a wide variety of publications. By reading through a wide variety of publications, you gain knowledge about what research has been done on the topic previously.[16]

Besides the keyword option, databases provide the opportunity to limit your search, such as by years, language, subjects, and reviews. For example, you may limit your search to recent publications between 2002 and the present, written in English, and limited to human subject research. In addition, you have the choice of selecting review publications. The review publications are useful when starting your search, because such publications provide an overview of the literature written on a specific topic. When you find a few specific recently published peer-reviewed publications, you learn how other researchers investigated the same issue, methods used for the investigation, limitations and challenges, results, conclusions, and suggestions for further research. Although the literature review process is time-consuming initially, it saves time later by avoiding the mistakes learned by other researchers. If you find a peer-reviewed publication of particular interest, you may contact the author to discuss the publication in greater detail. Generally, authors are pleased to discuss their research findings.

To further limit the scope of your search to the most recent publications, it is useful to conduct a Boolean search. This time-saving technique allows you to limit your search efficiently by using three logical operations: OR, AND, and NOT. See **Box 1-1**. Keep in mind that some database search engines offer simpler, but not identical, forms of search statements. It is useful to try a few different search statements until you become accustomed to the database that you are using. If you get confused, refer to the help pages provided by the search engines.[17]

In addition to using the peer-reviewed journal databases, it is also helpful to use the other library resources for

BOX 1-1 Examples of Publication Searches Using Boolean Search Terms

Boolean Search:
   Example One
      Topic: Malaria rates
      Boolean logic: AND
      Search: global AND international malaria rates
   Example Two
      Topic: Air quality

Boolean logic: NOT
   Search: Indoor NOT outdoor air quality
Example Three
   Topic: Sports medicine
   Boolean logic: OR
   Search: adolescent OR teen sports medicine

your review of the literature. The following discussion provides the advantages and disadvantages of printed materials.

Books

Books provide a good starting point for a review of the literature, because they offer a valuable general overview on specific subjects. Even though the information is less up to date due to publishing time, books should be included in any thorough literature review.

Government Documents

Depending on your field of study, many government documents are posted online through specific agency websites. These documents are extremely useful for a wide variety of topics. If you are not familiar with various government databases related to your topic, the reference librarian will offer valuable assistance.

Nongovernmental Organization (NGO) Documents

These organizations post valuable trend data and information related to specific topics. If you are not familiar with nongovernmental organizations, it is best to seek the advice of a reference librarian.

Newspapers

Although newspapers are written for a general audience, the information provides the public perception on current events and summaries of recent trend data, such as political polls. It is useful to contrast newspaper articles with other sources for a comparative review of the literature.

Magazines

Like newspapers, magazines are intended for a general audience, with the purpose of selling advertisements. Unless the topic involves investigating how a specific topic is portrayed in magazines, generally this information is not useful for scholarly literature reviews.

Theses and Dissertations

Because these documents are not published, they are usually only available from the library or through interlibrary loan. Keep in mind that this type of research was conducted by students, so the findings need to be viewed with caution.

Completing the Literature Review

Once you have completed your literature research, it is time to compile the information into an organized document. One common mistake is confusing the terms *annotated bibliography* and *a review of the literature*. An annotated bibliography contains a brief summary of each citation followed by a short evaluation. The document includes the strengths or weaknesses of the material presented in the citation. For an annotated bibliography, the source citations are presented in alphabetical order and each citation is presented as a new paragraph. Because citations are provided with each summary, there is no need for a reference page at the end of the document. A review of the literature is a compilation of the multiple resources presented in narrative format. The literature review presents all sides of an argument to avoid bias, and areas of dispute are emphasized for the reader. Literature reviews are usually organized around topics rather than presented in chronological order by year of publication, and the citations are presented at the end of the paper.

DEVELOPMENT OF GOALS AND OBJECTIVES

Once the needs assessment and the review of the literature are complete, the next step involves development of the goals and objectives of the program planning and evaluation. For most community organizations, this is the time in program planning and evaluation to hire a professional evaluator to assist with planning evaluation activities right from the time the goals and objectives are developed through the final report. The evaluator's expertise keeps the program on track. Keep in mind that evaluators ask questions with the purpose of

TABLE 1-4 Decision Box

	Important	Not Important
Changeable	A	B
Not Changeable	C	D

A = Strong: Important and changeable
B = Weak: Not important, but changeable
C = Weak: Important, but not changeable
D = Very Weak: Not important and not changeable

improving an existing program or initiating a new program. It is common for evaluators with limited experience to propose goals that are broad and implausible. After narrowing the topic, it is useful to stop and critically evaluate the proposed program. To assist with this process, refer to **Table 1-4**, and read the descriptions for A, B, C, and D. For your topic, place an X in the box that best defines your evaluation.

If the X is in B, C, or D, the proposed program needs reconsideration and modification. With limited resources and time, programs need to concentrate on important and changeable issues. Regardless of the location of X, it is useful to reconvene the needs assessment committee to confirm, change, or refute the goals prior to moving forward with the program planning. It is not unusual for team members to refine goals several times.

Another way to develop the goals is to use results of the needs assessment and the best practices from the literature review to answer the questions in **Table 1-5**.

Let's look at a few examples of focused goal statements:

- *Goal Statement One*: Within the next 6 months, 100% of the factory workers in the assembly-line division of the manufacturing plant will participate in three worker safety classes in the format of their choice (group class, one-on-one education, self-paced workbook, Internet education modules).

  Who: Factory workers

TABLE 1-5 Questions to Focus the Goal Statements

Who?	Identify the target population.
What?	Describe the main purpose of the program.
When?	Ascertain the time frame or length of the program.
Where?	Describe the specific location of the program.

What: Preferred method of health education: Group class, one-on-one education, self-paced workbook, Internet education modules
When: In the next 6 months
Where: Assembly-line division of the manufacturing plant

- *Goal Statement Two*: In the next 6 months, the incidence of employees with allergic reactions due to carpet mold in the lobby area of a building will decrease by 100% due to the use of the new cleaning solution and technique.

  Who: Employees
  What: Allergic reaction due to carpet mold
  When: 6 months
  Where: Lobby area

- *Goal Statement Three*: Over the next 12 months, the local grocery store chain will decrease the use of paper and plastic bags by 50% by charging $0.02 per bag starting on January 1.

  Who: Local grocery store chain
  What: Decrease use of paper and plastic bags by 50% by charging $0.02 per bag
  When: Starting January 1
  Where: Local grocery store chain

The process of writing excellent goal statements involves numerous drafts and discussion with team members. Because team members may not have time to physically meet to write the goal statements, it is advisable to send drafts via email to receive comments during the process. Once everyone agrees on the wording, it is valuable to schedule a meeting to revisit the results of the needs assessment, refine the goals, finalize goal statements, and begin to write measureable objectives. See **Box 1-2** to test your skills.

Now that the team members have identified the stakeholders, conducted the needs assessment, reviewed the literature, and finalized the goal statements and objectives, it is time to explore the process of implementation.

BOX 1-2 Test Your Skills

Write two goal statements for a program related to increasing the number of people working at a local large retail store who join the community-wide weight-loss/fitness program.

IMPLEMENTATION

After the planning phase is complete, it is time to begin the implementation process. Implementation is defined as the execution of the plan or simply doing what was planned. The implementation entails a detailed step-by-step process. Think of the implementation with the same level of detail needed for a computer program. Each line of the computer code must be correctly executed before the next line of code is read by the computer. The same process is true for implementing a program plan.

To ensure that each step of the plan is considered and implemented, it is useful to develop a timeline. Timelines are developed as a team process, so everyone shares their thoughts, ideas, and concerns. It is essential that team members take responsibility for action items; otherwise, the implementation is delayed. Once the timeline is finalized, it is posted as a visual cue. However, after a timeline is finalized, it is typically expanded and modified throughout the entire implementation process. Some teams use a whiteboard to post the timelines, so it can be easily changed as needed. Depending on the implementation size, timelines are displayed by month, week, day, or even hour, if necessary. In addition, teams may develop a timeline for each phase of the implementation. **Table 1-6** illustrates an example of a timeline for staff training.

As shown in Table 1-6, the implementation timeline includes every possible detail, so team members know the expectations for each week. Once one phase has been

TABLE 1-6 Work Safety Training Timeline

Month/Week		Action Item	Details	Person Responsible
July	7/3	Team meeting	Finalize implementation timeline	Team leader: JL
	7/10	Curriculum	Order adequate number of curriculum copies	Clerk: SA
	7/17	Discussion of worker safety training	Meet with eight designated worker safety trainers to discuss training sessions	Team member: FC
	7/24	Finalization of worker safety training	Finalize 16 worker safety training sessions: 2 per month in each designated divisions	Team member: DE
	7/31	Design observation checklist	Three team members meet to design observation checklist for use while observing trainings	Team members: BR, CD, LR
August	8/7	Practice training sessions	Eight trainers schedule practice training sessions with other team members to finalize timing and quality; receive feedback	Designated team members: BR, CD
	8/14	Worker safety training	Eight team members complete 16 worker safety training sessions; ensure fidelity in training by following protocol	Designated team members: BR, CD
		Track data	Log how many workers attend each training session	Designated team members: BR, CD
		Workers not trained	Schedule additional training dates as desired by each designated division; provide additional training dates and times	Clerk: SA
	8/21	Observations	Using the checklist, assign four team members each randomly to observe two trainings	Designated team members: LR, DE
		Additional worker safety training sessions	Conduct make-up training for workers unable to attend previously scheduled trainings	Designated team members: BR, CD
	8/28	Fidelity	Team members review results of observation checklists for fidelity	Designated team members: BR, CD

completed, it would be necessary to develop a new timeline for the next phase. Even for large, multi-year programs, it is advisable to develop a timeline for the entire project, and then break each segment into workable components for managing daily and weekly activities.

Besides a timeline, the implementation phase entails a method to ensure program fidelity. This method involves the development of all written policies and procedures. For example, as mentioned in Table 1-6, checklist observation documents program implementation. Other written policies include, but are not limited to, procedures for obtaining informed consent documents and specific instructions for any procedure that requires adherence to a step-by-step implementation for program fidelity. Once the policies and procedures are in place, the implementation process continues throughout the duration of the program. In parallel to the implementation data–collection process, evaluation data are collected at each step of the program. The following discussion introduces the types of evaluation used to assess each phase of programs.

INTERNAL AND EXTERNAL EVALUATORS

Before discussing types of evaluations, it is useful to describe the two types of evaluators: internal and external. The basic difference is that internal evaluators are employees of the organization that is being evaluated. External evaluators are not directly employed by the organization being evaluated, but have expertise and experience not available within the organization. See **Table 1-7**.

TYPES OF EVALUATIONS

The main purpose of any evaluation is to address whether the goals and objectives of a program or intervention were achieved. The complexity of the program and the evaluation determines the type and quality of the decisions. Whether the evaluation is simple or complex, each one requires rigorous and detailed design for success.[18] Although there are numerous types of evaluations, this chapter focuses on the most common types of evaluations: formative, summative, process, outcome, and impact.

Formative Evaluation

Formative evaluation, also called exploratory evaluation, focuses on the elements of the program and is conducted during the planning and implementation phase. Think of a formative evaluation as ensuring that the program is "formed" correctly. The issues of concern are related to the appropriateness and feasibility of the program materials, messages, and methods used to conduct the program for the target audience. Formative evaluation includes qualitative (e.g., interviews, focus groups, print media) or quantitative (numbers, rates, percentages, ratios, etc.) data or a mix of both kinds of data. At each point throughout the planning, implementation, and evaluation phases, data are collected from the target audience (see **Box 1-3**). For example, during the needs assessment and planning phase, surveys are pilot-tested, revised, and completed by a small sample of participants. Such preliminary data determine what changes are

TABLE 1-7 Comparison of Internal and External Evaluators

Internal Evaluators	External Evaluators
Directly employed by the organization	Employed as a consultant
Easy access to the staff employed by the program under review	Staff may or may not be willing to talk to an outsider
Greater awareness of the operations and nuances of the organization	Free of internal politics and personalities
Credibility and trust among the staff; may find that staff do not wish to share personal information with a colleague	Must build trust; staff may be more willing to confide in an external evaluator
Less costly unless organization has to pay to cover for any additional duties of the evaluation; may involve hidden costs	Cost determined by assigned contract; no hidden fees
May or may not have technological experience	All skills are known at the onset of the project
May unknowingly bias other workers to sway evaluation in one direction	May bring a fresh perspective from the results and recommendations of evaluation
Other workers may not find results to be credible from an insider's viewpoint	Perceived as more objective

needed to improve the readability and understanding of the final survey. Later, during the implementation phase, interviews or focus groups are conducted to confirm the usefulness of the messages and materials. Throughout the program, formative data are collected, and portions of the program are modified as needed to address identified concerns.[19]

BOX 1-3 Formative Evaluation Questions

Questions for leaders where the program will be implemented:
 What do you know about this program?
 What are the benefits to your organization for agreeing to implement this program?
 What problems do you foresee with the implementation of this program in this organization?
 What will the organization need to implement this program?
 What are the costs associated with the implementation?
Questions for organization members:
 What do you know about this program?
 What have you heard about this program?
 What are the benefits of this program to the organization?
 What are the program barriers experienced by the organizations?
 What are the benefits of this program to the organization members?
Questions for potential participants in organizations:
 What made you decide to attend this program?
 What is most appealing about this program?
 What do you think that you will gain by participating in this program?
 Why did you decide to attend this program?

Summative Evaluation

Summative evaluation determines if the program met any combination of measurement about impact, outcome, or benefits. Think of summative evaluations as a cumulative or comprehensive evaluation. This type of evaluation is frequently conducted by external evaluators. Generally, quantitative data are used for summative evaluations, because standardized surveys are best suited for measuring specific objectives. For example, a local seafood packing factory noticed an increase in worker injuries due to wet floors and moving heavy boxes. The factory administrators plan to institute a new safety

program to ensure that all employees receive education about worker safety procedures. Because the factory is open 24 hours, 7 days per week, they decided to make a safety education video. Employees are given a 90-minute break during work hours to view the 30-minute video followed by a 60-minute interactive workshop with a physical therapy technician to practice skills presented in the video. Three days after an employee completed the safety training, a satisfaction survey was mailed to their home address along with a self-addressed stamped envelope to return the completed survey. The survey is limited to specific questions about the employee's level of satisfaction related to knowledge and skills about their safety training. These data provide a summary of the impact, outcome, and benefits of the factory's new safety training program (see **Box 1-4**).

BOX 1-4 Summative Evaluation Questions

What goal and objectives were answered by the summative evaluation?
 What type of statistical test was used to analyze the satisfaction survey data?
 Were statistically significant results found? If so, explain.

Process Evaluation

Process evaluation examines all aspects of program implementation. In some situations, this evaluation investigates the organizational and administrative aspects of the program. During a process evaluation, the evaluation monitors the feedback of the program by investigating the issues that influence the implementation and the environment surrounding the implementation (see **Box 1-5**).[20]

BOX 1-5 Process Evaluation Questions

Is the program staying true to the original design, also called program fidelity in the implementation process?
 Are the quality and quantity of the services and products maintained at the capacity level expected?
 Is the level of satisfaction sustained across participating groups?
 Is there any identified reason that one group of participants is no longer participating?

Outcome Evaluation

Outcome evaluation obtains program data to document short-term results. These descriptive data define output activities, such as number of individuals calling the toll-free number following a local public service tobacco-cessation advertisement campaign. Also, these data make it possible to assess the short-term program results for the target audience—for example, change in the percentage of factory worker injuries 6 months after every employee attended the worker safety training. Other information obtained from outcome evaluation includes knowledge, attitude or behavioral changes, and institutional policy changes (see **Box 1-6**). According to Stead, Hastings, and Eadie,[21] health literacy, social influence, and health policy are the types of action needed for health promotion outcomes. Health literacy relates to an individual's knowledge and understanding of a health issue or concern. Social influence explores the availability of personal support and community empowerment. Health policy relates to how strategies are incorporated into organizational practice.

BOX 1-6 Outcome Evaluation Questions

Were the short-term goals achieved by the program?
    What was the stakeholder's level of satisfaction in the program implementation?
    Did specific health knowledge and motivation increase participation among the target population?
    Did availability of social support positively impact the participant's health outcome?

Impact Evaluation

Due to excessive costs and lengthy time commitment, impact evaluations are rarely possible. When feasible, impact evaluation is the most inclusive type of evaluation due to the focus on outcome objectives. Because of external influences, the results are not always attributable directly to the program. Impact evaluation provides results related to long-term data such as recidivism rates, changes in morbidity and mortality data, or long-term maintenance of a behavioral change (see **Box 1-7**).

BOX 1-7 Impact Evaluation Questions

What external influences impacted the results?
    What percentage of participants was lost to follow-up over the longitudinal study?
    Was the expected behavior change sustained over the expected period of time?
    How did the expected cost compare to the actual cost of the impact evaluation?

LOGIC MODELS

Now that the team members have completed the previously discussed tasks, it is time to organize the data and information onto one spreadsheet. Even though there are numerous types and designs, all logic models are a graphic depiction of a program from the planning phase through the evaluation. Logic models link the goal statements and objectives to interventions and outcomes. Such models are an excellent way to communicate the big picture to others. This type of communication facilitates buy-in from stakeholders, personnel, and the target audience. Keep in mind that there are books written about logic models. The information in this section is merely intended to introduce the concept of logic models. While looking at three sample logic models, review the definitions provided for each term. Although each logic model is slightly different, the choice of which one to use is up to the evaluators. See **Tables 1-8** and **1-9**, and **Figure 1-1**.

Goal Statements and Objectives

The goal statements and objectives provide the program overview. Each goal statement is listed and followed by the measureable objectives.

Inputs

The inputs are defined as the resources available for the program including human resources and stakeholders, such as funders, community partners, program staff, collaborators, and volunteers. Fiscal resources are funding, donations, and special grants. Physical resources provide office space and equipment, office and storage space, computers and software, and other special tools, such as cameras and recording devices. Knowledge resources encompass teaching materials, curriculum, learning

TABLE 1-8 Logic Model Example

Program: Community Garden Goal: Within 12 months, the Terrace Community will establish one community garden for growing vegetables and fruit.					
Inputs	**Activities**		**Outcomes**		
What we invest	What we do	Who we reach	Why this project: Short-term results	Why this project: Intermediate results	Why this project: Long-term results
Master gardeners Volunteers Materials Plot of land Equipment	Conduct workshops Prepare the soil Plant garden Promote activities Work with media	Community Grocery stores Local restaurants Juice bars City council	Awareness Knowledge Skills Motivation Involvement	Planting Growing plants Social action Excitement Decision making	Healthier Fresh food Social asset Civic engagement Environmental

Data from The National Network of Libraries of Medicine, National Library of Medicine. Including Evaluation in Outreach Project Planning. Planning and Evaluating Health Information Outreach Projects. Outreach Evaluation Resource Center. Available at: http://nnlm.gov/evaluation/booklets/booklet2/booklet2_blank_worksheet1_form.pdf. Accessed September 13, 2013.

competencies, and certification requirements. By listing every resource under inputs, it is easy to determine what is missing and needs to be obtained for the program to begin.

Activities

Activities involve what needs to be accomplished to achieve the objectives. For example, if an objective requires the development of a community coalition, the activity describes a detailed plan for forming a community coalition. If the objective involves teaching a health course, the activity explains how the resources are used to advertise the course, schedule the date and time, recruit and enroll students, collect fees, invite guest speakers, and so forth for the course to be a success.

Outputs

Outputs link the research questions, goal statements, and objectives to the short-term, intermediate, and long-term outcomes. Outputs may also be viewed as the process evaluation.

TABLE 1-9 Logic Model Example

Questions						
Goal Statements	Inputs and Resources	Activities	Outputs/ Process Evaluation	Outcomes/Impact and Outcome Evaluation		
				Short-term	Intermediate	Long-term
Objectives	Resources	Needs assessment	Products	Baseline data	Tracking	Documentation
	Human Fiscal Physical Educational	Baseline data Recruitment Focus groups Surveys Interviews Number of training sessions	Services pro- vided Themes Profits Number of persons trained	Knowledge, atti- tudes, behaviors, and beliefs Income generated Knowledge gained	Retention and follow-up rates Implementation strategies for future events	Decreased costs due to improved conditions Policy changes due to intervention Strategies for institutional changes
External Influences: social media, environment effects, political impact						

Modified from McCawley P. University of Idaho Extension. Logic Models. Available at: http://www.uiweb.uidaho.edu/extension/LogicModel.pdf. Accessed January 12, 2012.

FIGURE 1-1 Logic model example.

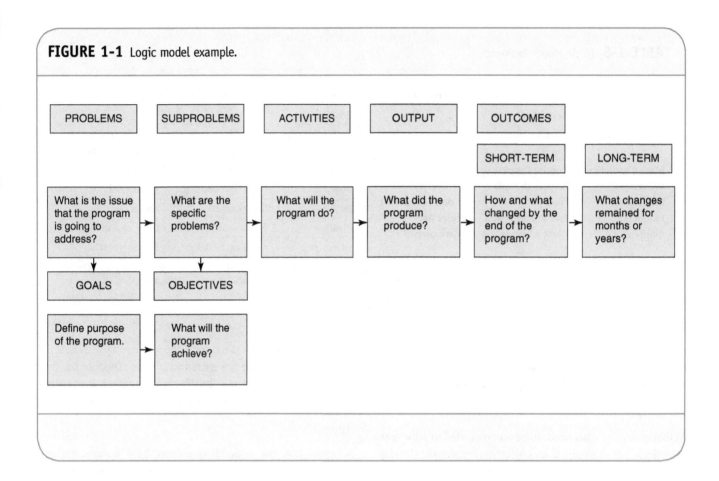

While outputs include products, goods, services, and the people served by the program, process evaluation monitors the overall implementation activities. Products, goods, and services include web pages, fact sheets, publications, software, curriculum handbooks, community events, courses, and demonstrations. The people served are described by their demographics and characteristics; percentage of target population reached; change in knowledge, attitude, beliefs, and behavior achieved; and overall level of satisfaction expressed.

Outcomes

Outcomes are expressed as short-term, intermediate, or long-term. Each phase communicates the impact of the program thus far. Short-term outcomes reflect awareness of the issue, motivation to change, and the knowledge, attitudes, skills, beliefs, and behaviors needed to make the desired change. Intermediate outcomes build on short-term outcomes and track participation and practices of target audience; changes in policies within institutions, businesses, and government agencies; and implementation of strategies by individuals and groups. Long-term outcomes or program impacts follow intermediate outcomes by documenting improved economic, health, educational, social, environmental, or political conditions that relate back to the goal statement. Impact determines permanent change beyond the end of the program. It is the lasting effect of change of institutional policies. For example, over time the smoke-free indoor air quality goal statement produced a permanent nationwide ban of smoking in restaurants, bars, and domestic air flights.

External influences either support or oppose the goals. Due to the level of institutional, community, and participant opinion of the goal statement, the program planning process changes to better match the baseline opinion of the community. For example, if the community supports building a walk-in free clinic for the homeless population, the inputs, activities, outputs, and outcomes will differ from those of a community that opposes a free clinic. However, if the community has the opinion that a free homeless clinic will increase the number of homeless people, then the program starts at a completely different place. Other types of external influences include similar and competing programs or services, socioeconomic conditions, governmental policies, and so forth.

SUMMARY

This chapter provided an overview of similarities and differences between research and evaluation starting with the development of questions. The basic difference is that research generates new knowledge, while evaluation seeks to improve existing programs. Following a discussion about needs assessments and how to review existing published literature, the remainder of the chapter focused on the identification of the program type and design; consensus building among individuals participating in the program; and resources needed such as funding, personnel, and location resources. Program evaluation was defined as day-to-day program management, short-term results, and long-term program impact. Program evaluations include data collection and analysis.

CASE STUDY: HEALTHY FOOD/HEALTHY STUDENTS (HFHS)

Dr. Johnson, the school board administrator of a large urban school district, wanted to offer healthier food options in the cafeteria but was not sure what changes needed to occur in the cafeteria. She is aware of the federally subsidized school lunch programs, but at this point she is gathering information from a number of resources about the quality of subsidized food provided, amount of food that is consumed and amount that is thrown away each day, the amount of snack food and sodas purchased from school vending machines, and so forth. She decided to start the process by conducting a pilot test needs assessment in six schools (two elementary, two middle, and two high schools) evenly distributed across the county. Volunteers were recruited from the students, teachers, staff, and parents to serve on the committee overseeing the needs assessment. After writing a few broad goal statements, the committee conducted focus groups with each group represented. The focus group results showed some general themes that the committee used to develop a short survey. The survey was printed on postcards and made available in several locations (cafeteria, main office, teacher/staff lounge, and homerooms). Drop boxes were available at various locations. The survey was also made available online on the school websites.

While the survey data were collected over a 3-week period, the committee worked with the cafeteria manager. The committee requested secondary data about the most popular and least popular food choices, sodium and sugar content of popular items, and availability of fresh fruit and vegetables. They ranked the current purchased food choices by popularity, cost, and health factors. This grid was compared to the focus group and survey results. After analyzing the needs assessment data, the committee wrote a goal statement and three measureable objectives.

Goal Statement

The school cafeteria team will investigate how to improve the quality of available food and drink choices in the school cafeterias to encourage healthy eating.

Objectives

1. By the end of November, the school cafeteria team will collect 3 weeks' worth of baseline data in the pilot test schools regarding what cafeteria foods served are eaten and what foods are thrown away.
2. By the end of November, in the pilot schools, the school cafeteria team will collect baseline data about the fat, sodium, and sugar content of 100% of foods and drinks served in the cafeteria.
3. By the end of November, the school cafeteria team will investigate how to modify the school district soft drink company contract to exchange the purchase of high-sugar drinks to lower sugar or sugar-free flavored water drinks or pure water.

The committee collected data from students, teachers, staff, and parents throughout the assessment phase. The baseline pilot study data were presented in the final report to the school board administrator as the first step in modifying the cafeteria food choices. From this report, the school board could move forward in further modifying school cafeteria food offerings toward healthier foods.

Case Study Discussion Questions

1. Discuss other options that might have been used for the data collection.
2. What other types of data could be collected to address the objectives?
3. Now that the baseline data have been collected, what might be the next steps for the committee?

STUDENT ACTIVITIES

Cubing is an activity that involves exploring one issue from six different directions.[22] For this exercise, divide the class into equal groups of six students per group. Allow each group to select a health science topic of their choice. For the example, the topic is "bachelor of science in health science (BSHS) degree." Each student is assigned one of the following six questions:

1. Describe: What is the bachelor of science in health science degree?
2. Compare: How does the BSHS compare to other undergraduate degrees?

3. Associate: What does the BSHS degree make you think of?

4. Analyze: What should we look for in the ideal BSHS degree?

5. Apply: Apply what we know about undergraduate college degrees to the BSHS degree.

Argue for and against it: Identify arguments for and against the BSHS degree.

REFERENCES

1. The Centers for Disease Control and Prevention. IPOM: Immunization Program Operations Manual. Available at: http://www.cdc.gov/vaccines/imz-managers/guides-pubs/ipom/index.html. Accessed April 17, 2014.

2. The History Channel. Nixon signs legislation banning cigarette ads on TV and radio. *This Day in History*. Available at: http://www.history.com/this-day-in-history/nixon-signs-legislation-banning-cigarette-ads-on-tv-and-radio. Accessed September 13, 2013.

3. U.S. Department of Health and Human Services. Smoking and Health. Report of the Advisory Committee to the Surgeon General of the Public Health Service. Available at: http://profiles.nlm.nih.gov/ps/retrieve/ResourceMetadata/NNBBMQ. Accessed September 13, 2013.

4. The First Ladies. Nancy Reagan. Available at: http://www.firstladies.org/biographies/firstladies.aspx?biography=41. Accessed September 13, 2013.

5. Evans RI. (1998). An historical perspective on effective prevention. In Bukoski WJ and Evans RI, Eds. *National Institute on Drug Abuse Research Monograph Series No. 176, Cost-Benefit/Cost-Effectiveness Research on Drug Abuse Prevention: Implications for Programming and Policy*. NIH Publication No. 98-4021 (pp. 37–58). Washington, DC: U. S. Department of Health and Human Services, National Institutes of Health, Superintendent of Documents, U.S. Government Printing Office; 1998.

6. U.S. National Library of Medicine. Visual Culture and Public Health Posters. Available at: http://www.nlm.nih.gov/exhibition/visualculture/celebrity.html. Accessed September 13, 2013.

7. Popham WJ, Potter LD, Bal DG, Johnson MD, Duerr JM, Quinn V. Do anti-smoking campaigns help smokers quit? *Public Health Rep*. 1993;108(04):510–513.

8. Centers for Disease Control and Prevention. Smoking-Attributable Mortality, Years of Potential Life Lost, and Productivity Losses—United States, 2000–2004. *MMWR*. 2008;57(45):1226–1228.

9. Centers for Disease Control and Prevention. Cigarette Smoking-Attributable Morbidity—United States, 2000. *MMWR*. 2003;52(35):842–844.

10. Centers for Disease Control and Prevention. Smoking-Attributable Mortality, Years of Potential Life Lost, and Productivity Losses—United States, 2000–2004. *MMWR*. 2008;57(45):1226–1228.

11. U.S. Department of Health and Human Services. A Report of the Surgeon General: How Tobacco Smoke Causes Disease: What It Means to You. Atlanta, GA: U.S. Department of Health and Human Services, Centers for Disease Control and Prevention, National Center for Chronic Disease Prevention and Health Promotion, Office on Smoking and Health; 2010.

12. Centers for Disease Control and Prevention. Cigarette smoking among adults—United States, 2004. *MMWR*. 2005;54(44):1121–1214.

13. Azzam T. Evaluators' responsiveness to stakeholders. *Am J Eval*. 2010;3(1):45–65.

14. Mark MM, Shotland RL. Stakeholder-based evaluation and value judgments. *Evaluation Rev*. 1985;9:605–626.

15. Guba EG, Lincoln YS. *Fourth Generation Evaluation*. Newbury Park, CA: Sage; 1989.

16. Shuttleworth M. Experiment Resources. What is a Literature Review? Available at: http://www.experiment-resources.com/what-is-a-literature-review.html. Accessed January 12, 2012.

17. Barker J. Basic Search Tips and Advanced Boolean Explained. Teaching Library University of California, Berkeley. Available at: http://www.lib.berkeley.edu/TeachingLib/Guides/Internet/Boolean.pdf. Accessed January 12, 2012.

18. McCawley P. University of Idaho Extension. Logic Models. Available at: http://www.uiweb.uidaho.edu/extension/LogicModel.pdf. Accessed January 12, 2012.

19. Posavac EJ, Carey RG. *Program Evaluation: Methods and Case Studies*. Upper Saddle River, NJ: Pearson Education, Inc.; 2007.

20. Habicht JP, Victora CG, Vaughan JP. Evaluation designs for adequacy, plausibility and probability of public health programme performance and impact. *Int J Epidemiol*. 1999;28:10–18.

21. Stead M, Hastings G, Eadie D. The challenge of evaluating complex interventions: a framework for evaluating media advocacy. *Health Educ Res*. 2002;17(3):351–364.

22. Orr SK. Exploring stakeholder values and interests in evaluation. *Am J Eval*. 2010;31(4):557–569.

CHAPTER **2**

Ethics

By the end of this chapter, the student will be able to:

1. Define the basic ethical principles.
2. Summarize the ethical violations of the U.S. Public Health Service Syphilis Study at Tuskegee.
3. Examine ways to maintain confidentiality of medical records and research data.
4. Explain the function of the institutional review board.

KEY TERMS

beneficence
institutional review board
justice
respect for persons

INTRODUCTION

This chapter provides an overview of ethics. After providing a brief historical background of ethical issues, the historical landmark case of the U.S. Public Health Service Syphilis Study at Tuskegee, which involved unethical practices in public health research, is described. Then the basic principles of scientific research ethics are defined. This discussion is followed by how these principles are applied to the role of the institutional review board (IRB), development of informed consent documents, and consideration of special populations. The chapter ends with a discussion of the ethical principles and challenges as applied to evaluations.

HISTORICAL BACKGROUND OF ETHICAL PRINCIPLES

In 1949, following the Nazi Nuremberg Trial in Germany after World War II, the U.S. National Institutes of Health, Office of Human Subjects Research issued the Nuremberg Code: Directives for Human Experimentation. The following bullets summarize the Nuremberg Code:[1]

- Voluntary consent is required.
- Research must be of societal value.
- Previous studies justify the need of the research.
- Research must avoid physical and mental suffering and injury.
- No research may be conducted if prior knowledge suggests the occurrence of death or disability.
- Risk must not exceed humanitarian benefits.
- Research planning must protect subjects from injury, disability, or death.
- Research may only be conducted by qualified researchers.
- Individuals participating in research may withdraw at any time.
- Researchers must end the research if there is cause for concern of subjects regarding their safety.

Later, the U.S. Department of Health and Human Services' Office for Human Research Protections (OHRP) was created for the protection of the rights of individuals involved in research, to provide clarification, guidance, and advice; distribute educational information; and maintain regulatory oversight.[2] In 1979, the U.S. National Commission for the Protection of Human Subjects of Biomedical and Behavioral Research wrote the Belmont Report to describe the ethical principles that apply to human subject research. In 1981, the U.S. Department of Health and Human Services and the Food and Drug Administration revised the Belmont Report to be compatible with current statutes.[3]

It is important to review the U.S. Public Health Service Syphilis Study at Tuskegee. This historical landmark case involved unethical practices in public health research that have shaped scientific medical practices in the United States.

Syphilis is a sexually transmitted infection of great importance to public health as it may not present symptoms for years, increasing chances of it being spread among people before being treated. Syphilis causes many health problems, including painful lesions and sores, and, if left untreated, dementia in later life. Syphilis may also be passed from an infected mother to her newborn child. In 1932, the U.S. Public Health Service started a research study about the progression of syphilis in Macon County, Alabama near Tuskegee. Of the 600 impoverished African American males in the study, 399 had syphilis and 201 did not have syphilis. The men were never told that they were involved in a research study, and they did not receive proper medical care to treat syphilis. For study participation, the men received free medical exams, meals, and burial insurance; however, they were never allowed to quit participating in the study. In 1936, the study's first clinical report was published. In 1947, penicillin was available to effectively treat syphilis, yet the men never received treatment. During World War II, 250 men in the study registered for military service, were diagnosed with syphilis, and obtained treatment for syphilis. After 40 years, in 1972, the Assistant Secretary for Health and Scientific Affairs announced the end of the Tuskegee Study, and an advisory panel declared the study to be unethical. By the time the study ended, 74 men were alive. Of the original 399 men, 28 had died of syphilis, 100 had died of related complications, 40 wives had been infected, and 19 children had been born with congenital syphilis. In 1973, a class action lawsuit was filed on behalf of the men and their families. In 1974, an out-of-court settlement was reached for $10 million plus lifetime medical benefits and burial services to all living participants. In 1975, the benefits were extended to wives, widows, and children. The last study participant died in January 2004, and in 2009 the last widow receiving benefits died. There are 15 remaining children receiving medical and health benefits. The Tuskegee Study left a legacy of mistrust among the African American community of the medical establishment and many public health efforts.[4] On May 16, 1997, after 65 years, President Clinton apologized for the government's syphilis study in Tuskegee, Alabama.[5]

BASIC ETHICAL PRINCIPLES

From this historical background, let's move into a discussion of basic ethical principles. Regardless of the discipline or field of study, ethics can be defined as a system of moral principles and values applied to all aspects of evaluation and research that involve contact with human subjects. To understand ethics, it is important to learn basic terminology. The basic ethical principles are respect for persons, beneficence, and justice. After learning the definitions, it becomes apparent that each principle is understandable on its own. However, when several ethical principles are considered jointly, the overlap leads to contradiction.

Respect for persons or autonomy

Respect for persons or autonomy is divided into two sections. First, each individual is treated with respect and given adequate information to make an informed decision, including having no treatment or alternative treatments. Informed decisions should be made without excessive influence of others. Second, individuals with diminished decision-making capacity require extra protection, depending on the risk of harm and the likelihood of benefit. Throughout the process of participatory involvement, autonomy should be reassessed to ensure that participating individuals maintain their self-determination and understand risks and benefits. All participants are shown respect, and no reasonable information is withheld.[3] For example, when recruiting low-income individuals for an evaluation project, their participation remains voluntary, and their poverty status should not lead to coercion or undue influence over the protocol. Questions of respect for persons or autonomy include the following:

- Does each potential participant have the personal capacity to willfully choose to participate in the evaluation?
- Is anyone feeling internal or external pressure to participate?
- Are the incentives for participation appropriate?
- Do the participating individuals understand that they are free to withdraw from the program or evaluation at any time?

Beneficence

Beneficence is aligned with the Hippocratic Oath, "do no harm," by protecting individuals from harm by maximizing possible benefits and minimizing possible risks of harm. In other words, beneficence is when the chance of possible benefit outweighs the risk of possible harm. Beneficence assumes that risks are minimized as individuals and society benefit from participation. Beneficence is often ambiguous, particularly when there is minimal risk with no definitive and measurable benefits. At this point, the participant's choice must be free of coercion and be given all possible choices to make a completely informed decision. The evaluator is required to stop the process at any time when it becomes clear that there is a possibility that participants could be harmed.[6] Questions of beneficence include the following:

- Is the health program or evaluation providing benefits to the participants?
- Is it possible that the evaluators stand to gain more from the evaluation than the participants, such as data collection for academic publications and future grant applications to promote their personal careers?
- Are the participants protected from possible risks of harm or reprisal for participating in the evaluation process?

Justice

Justice requires a fair distribution of burden and benefits, so that every individual with the same condition, job description, geographical location, and so forth has an equal chance of being selected to participate.[7] When evaluators recruit volunteers, it is essential to justify the selection process. Volunteer participants may not be chosen simply because of their availability or compromised position in society but rather for reasons directly related to the goals and objectives of the evaluation. Justice requires that every individual have equal access to the benefits. For example, if the evaluation is conducted within a large organization, each employee should have an equal chance to participate in a focus group (burden) and receive the gift card incentive (benefit). Questions of justice include the following:

- Is there a fair distribution of burden and benefits?
- Does every individual in the target audience have the same chance of being selected to participate?
- Is random assignment being used appropriately?

Although respect for persons, beneficence, and justice are the main ethical principles, additional ethical principles of nonmaleficence, paternalism, and utilitarianism should be defined.[3]

Nonmaleficence

Nonmaleficence is defined as refraining from causing harm or from acting with malice toward a person. Questions of nonmaleficence include the following:

- Even if the participant signed the informed consent paperwork, does the participant experience anxiety when responding to personal questions?
- If an individual is involved in a longitudinal study for several years, do constant reminders to remain involved in the study feel like an invasion of their privacy over time?

Paternalism

Paternalism involves a relationship of uneven power between the recruiter and individuals being recruited. For example, it is paternalistic for an administrator to insist that all employees participate in the evaluation being conducted within their facility. In this case, the administrator is assuming a parental role while placing the employees in the role of children. Questions of paternalism include the following:

- Did the administrator treat the employee as a child?
- Was information withheld from the employee because the administrator did not think that the employee should be told about potential closing of the clinic?

Utilitarianism

Utilitarianism is the decision, behavior, or action that achieves the greatest good for the greatest number of people.[7] For example, the evaluator recruits individuals who smoke at least two packs of cigarettes per day to participate in a new smoking cessation program. Because the evaluation is funded by a pharmaceutical company, the true purpose of the program is to determine the time and place where heavy smokers are able to smoke in states with strict indoor air quality laws. By participating in this program, the evaluator is deceitful and violates utilitarianism. Although the smokers receive some information about smoking cessation, the pharmaceutical company is researching how to market a new smoking cessation nicotine product to heavy smokers. Although the evaluator argues that the end product is a new smoking cessation tool to help smokers to stop smoking (the greatest good for greatest number), the truth is that this evaluation is deceptive when participants do not know what the immediate goals of the evaluation are. The goal of this evaluation was not designed to help these current participants, but rather to design advertising materials for future smokers. This type of research design involves questionable ethics. Questions of utilitarianism include the following:

- Is the program designed to assist current or future participants?
- Is only one specific group, such as participants with low health literacy, recruited for this study?

ETHICAL LINKS BETWEEN RESEARCH AND EVALUATION

Building on the historical background and basic ethical principles, let's explore the ethical links between research and evaluations. Keep in mind that the purpose of research is to create new knowledge, whereas the purpose of evaluation is to improve programs. While many types of public health research do not involve human subjects (e.g., soil and water sampling, air pollution levels), most public health research is focused on creating new knowledge for humans. Any type of research that involves collecting any type of data (interviews, tissue samples, survey completion, etc.) from human subjects must involve an ethical review to ensure safety of the human subjects. This review process is conducted by the institutional review board that is described in the next section. Now let's discuss evaluations. Even though evaluations are not creating new knowledge, like research, most evaluations involve collecting data from human subjects. Although there are differences between the purpose of research and the purpose of evaluation, the need to protect human subjects remains the same. That being said, there can sometimes be some blurring between research and evaluation on certain projects. It is possible for one project to involve both research and evaluation. For example, a funded project conducts research to develop an innovative teen pregnancy prevention curriculum for after-school programs. The same team implements the innovative curriculum and conducts the evaluation to determine if teen pregnancy rates have dropped over the 5-year longitudinal evaluation.

INSTITUTIONAL REVIEW BOARD

An institutional review board (IRB) is a committee that serves to formally approve, monitor, and review every type of biomedical and behavioral research and evaluation that involves human subjects. The purpose of the IRB is to protect the rights and welfare of the human subjects. At the national level, the U.S. Food and Drug Administration (FDA) and the U.S. Department of Health and Human Services (HHS) oversee IRB regulations including approval, required modifications of research, and disapproval of research.[8] Keep in mind that each agency or division under the FDA and HHS has its own rules and regulations for biomedical and behavioral research. At the local level, institutions have their own IRB committees, such as universities, hospitals, clinics, health departments, and school districts. Every IRB committee performs oversight functions of all research and evaluations conducted on human subjects within its institution. In some situations, researchers and evaluators must obtain IRB approval from more than one committee. For example, if a university professor receives state funding to conduct an evaluation at a local health department clinic, the professor must receive IRB approval from the university IRB and also from the local health department IRB committee.[3]

To accomplish the purpose of the IRB, the committee members review research or evaluation protocols, informed consent documents, recruitment brochures, surveys, interview and focus group question guides, and all other materials related to the research. The IRB also reviews procedures involving previously collected personal data or secondary data, such as medical charts, lab and medical test results, prescription drug data, satisfaction surveys, financial information, and any other type of outcome data. The main objective is to assess the ethics and methods to ensure that participation is informed and voluntary and that all individuals are capable of making personal decisions. The IRB committee approves research and evaluations that provide informed consent for participants, show that the risks to the participants are balanced with potential societal benefits, and have undergone participant selection that is fair with equal distribution of risks and benefits to eligible participants.[9] Each IRB committee requires a written application the with following required components:[3]

- Research protocols and amendments/evaluation goals and objectives
- Written informed consent forms
- Participant recruitment procedures and advertisements
- Written information provided to participants
- Evaluation/research plan
- Information about availability of compensation and schedule of payments
- Safety information to accommodate any adverse conditions resulting from the research/evaluation including name and contact information of principal investigator, lead researcher, or evaluator; evidence of his or her qualifications; and names of all personnel involved with any aspect of research

Depending on the type of research, IRB committees request additional information and multiple document revisions prior to making a final approval decision. Applications of the general principles to the conduct of research or evaluation lead to consideration of the following requirements: informed consent, risk–benefit assessment, and selection of individuals.

Informed Consent

Informed consent is the hallmark of human subject research, because it reflects the individual's right to respect and autonomy. Informed consent is not a one-time encounter to obtain an individual's signature, but rather an ongoing process to assure that human subjects continue to understand that their involvement is voluntary. According to the U.S. Department of Health and Human Services,[9] the informed consent document must include the following components: full disclosure, comprehension, adequate compensation, and voluntary choice.

Full Disclosure

Full disclosure involves revealing the purpose and expected duration of the subject's participation, procedures involved, description of potential risks and benefits, appropriate alternative procedures or treatments, confidentiality of records, and a statement affirming that participation is voluntary and refusal or withdrawal will not result in a penalty or loss of entitled benefits. All informed consent forms must be written using layperson's words with simple sentence structure and presented in the preferred language of each potential human subject for maximum comprehension. In addition, informed consent documents include information on the principal investigator's name and how to contact him or her to answer questions and to explain the research participant's ability to withdraw from the study or evaluation at any time without penalty. It is important that participants understand that their participation is not required and the range of risks and benefits involved. The written informed consent document is given to each participant and orally discussed by the principal investigator. In some situations, there must be a third party present to witness the process, including the participant's and researcher's signatures.[9]

Informed consent problems arise when the data collection is likely to change the response or behavior of the participants. For example, suppose the purpose of the evaluation is to streamline the flow of patients at a local clinic by using a new computerized check-in system. One aspect of the evaluation involves observing the clinic employees as they assist patients with the new system when checking in. Because the employees know that they are being watched, their behavior is affected. Whenever data collection involves incomplete disclosure, it is essential to explain this situation in the IRB application, make sure that undisclosed risks are no more than minimal, and plan debriefing sessions along with dissemination of results. Full disclosure may never be withheld to increase recruitment or cooperation.[3]

Comprehension

When explaining the informed consent document, it is important that participants understand every aspect of the research. This understanding means that the document must be written in the preferred language of the individual and at an appropriate written and verbal literacy level. The time and location of obtaining consent is considered. Consent is obtained during normal business hours in a quiet location. Individuals may wish to have family members present to hear the explanation and ask questions, although the participating individual retains the final decision. For example, if the document is explained quickly in a noisy hospital waiting room, chances are that the individual will not be allowed sufficient time to make an informed choice. Obtaining the informed consent is viewed as an educational process. It is the evaluator's responsibility to ensure that participants understand and comprehend the information. As potential risks increase, so does the obligation of complete understanding prior to giving consent. Sometimes an added safeguard is used, such as asking the individual to repeat the explanation to verify understanding and comprehension. IRB committees need to make every effort to enhance the subject's comprehension. Even with the best intentions, an evaluator may communicate every aspect of the informed consent document, but the participant may fail to fully understand his or her participation. The reasons for lack of understanding may be due, but not limited to, his or her mental capability being diminished by age; physical or mental disabilities; being under the influence of medications, alcohol, or other substances; fear of reduced services; need for monetary compensation; or real or imaginary feelings of coercion. When research involves a specific medical condition, such as dementia, an individual's legal guardian is assigned to sign the informed consent, make surrogate decisions, and protect the participant from harm.[9]

Adequate Compensation

Adequate compensation for participation in research is not specifically stated in the federal regulations. The IRB committee determines the risk of possible coercion and reasonable compensation for each situation. Incentives must neither be so attractive that potential participants are blinded to the risks nor conceal accurate information for admission into the lucrative research. Compensation does not need to be a cash payment. Other types of compensation include bus tokens, travel reimbursement, babysitting services, movie tickets, or gift cards.[9]

Voluntary Choice

Voluntary choice involves an agreement to participate in research or an evaluation after individuals understand every aspect of the study. In addition, conditions must be free of coercion and undue influence. Coercion occurs when a person in power threatens harm if individuals do not agree to participate in the research or evaluation and sign the consent form. For example, a prisoner would experience coercion if the warden announces that all prisoners must participate in a study or else special privileges will be evoked. Undue influence happens when an excessive incentive is offered for participation. For example, a tobacco company is developing a new e-cigarette and wants to test their product with current low-income smokers. They expedite recruitment of current low-income smokers by offering $1000 to every current low-income smoker who is willing to use their new e-cigarette for 7 days. Because current low-income smokers need $1000, they would sign consent forms without asking questions to receive the excessive cash payment. Undue influence also occurs when a family member is persuaded to convince the patient to participate in the study, thus removing the patient's choice. Threatening to revoke healthcare services is also a threat of undue influence.[3] Other considerations of informed consent involve observational research, active and passive consents, secondary data, and cultural diversity concerns.

Observational Research

When human behavior is observed, researchers request an informed consent waiver because subjects may act differently when observed. For example, evaluators are evaluating a bullying prevention curriculum in a high school. They gather baseline data by staging a student bullying scene in a parking lot of one of the two high schools that will receive the bullying prevention curriculum over the next 9 months. At the end of the intervention, the evaluators stage another bullying scene in the other high school parking lot to determine the change after the intervention. For this type of research, IRB committees apply common sense and consider the degree of risk for the subjects involved without their consent.

Active Consent and Passive Consent

These terms are commonly used in a school setting when a study involves noninvasive research with students under age 18 years. When a passive consent form is used, the researcher gives the students a document to take home to their parents or guardian. With passive consent, the parent or guardian may read about the noninvasive research. If the document is not returned to school, the student will participate in the research. If the parent or guardian does not wish the student to participate, the signed form must be returned to school. Because it is common that students do not give such forms to their parents, the parents are never made aware of the research. In this case, if the parent never responds for numerous reasons, the student is allowed to participate in the research. To clarify, passive consent means the student participates due to "passive" parental consent. For active consent, the researcher sends the document home with the students. The student is unable to participate unless the document is signed by the parent and returned by the student. Parents need to be "active" for their child to participate. In this case, the researchers offer incentives for students to return the signed form in a short period of time. For example, the class with the greatest number of returned signed forms by Friday receives a pizza party, or each student who returns a signed form receives a school t-shirt.

Secondary Data

Common examples of secondary data include patient medical charts, birth and death certificates, traffic violations, motor vehicle records, medical billing records, school attendance records, and insurance company vehicular claims data. Most secondary data research and evaluations use aggregate data, which are defined as records that do not contain any personal or identifying information that could be linked back to a specific individual. For example, school administrators use secondary data to evaluate the impact on elementary students who change schools more than one time during any given school year by linking the data to the number of days absent and their test scores. Secondary aggregate data provide specific information about the students who changed schools more than one time during one academic year. Data are de-identified and do not include student names, addresses, or contact information. By linking the elementary students who have changed schools more than one time with their number of days absent and test scores, school administrators are able to determine the impact of changing schools. The research questions for this study are based on the health effects and stress caused by adjusting to new schools and the impact on the students' test scores. Biased data would result if the students were lost because they moved to a school outside of the county or the students were not included in the study because they moved into the county after moving several previous times elsewhere.

Cultural and Diversity Issues

IRB committees verify if the evaluation staff has appropriate cultural and diversity sensitivity training so that participating individuals are treated with respect. If participating individuals feel comfortable, they are more likely to respond honestly to personal questions. For example, even though the evaluator from one culture views the interview question as routine, the responding person from another culture may view the identical question as intrusive. Topics that may be considered sensitive in various cultures include diverse marriage and parenting attitudes, sexual behaviors, employment loyalty, loyalty to healthcare practitioners, religious beliefs and practices, use of traditional medical treatments, and so on. Researchers need to be comfortable with not only the topic, but also the potential ethical issues that may arise when recruiting individuals from various cultural backgrounds.[6]

Risk–Benefit Assessment

The risks and benefits are carefully weighed by the IRB committee, investigator, and participating individuals. Based on known data, risk is defined as the chance that harm may occur. Risk is usually viewed as high, moderate, or low. Risks may include psychological, physical, legal, social, and economic harm. Benefit is viewed as the value of positive health or welfare gained through the study. The risk–benefit ratio assessment is the probability and extent of possible harm versus anticipated benefits. In the IRB application, it is essential to clearly state known risks according to the published literature and available alternative choices. For the IRB committee, any potential risks must be justified and offset by benefits when feasible. For participating individuals, they must understand the risk–benefit ratio, have the opportunity to ask questions, and be able to withdraw their participation at any time.

Selection of Individuals and Special Populations

When IRB committees review an application, particular attention is paid to special populations that may be recruited for participation. Each category of special populations poses unique considerations related to informed consent. Special populations include individuals who are dependent on public healthcare services due to low socioeconomic status, individuals with limited English language skills, children, individuals with mental health disabilities, prisoners or institutionalized individuals, hospitalized and very sick patients with diminished comprehension due to medications or emergency treatment, the elderly population, and pregnant women. Any of these individuals may concede their rights to gain additional or faster medical benefits or to please their healthcare practitioners. If there

is any doubt about consent being truly voluntary, the individual should be removed from the selection. Such individuals need protection against recruitment selection due to convenience, medical diagnosis, or socioeconomic status.[9] Overall, the researcher or evaluator and the IRB committee must be aware of the unique ethical concerns when recruiting individuals from special populations.

ETHICAL GUIDELINES FOR EVALUATORS

From the previous discussion, you learned about the importance of the institutional review board and the informed consent process. This section focuses on the ethical integrity of the profession of evaluation. The following three tables illustrate ethical guideline summaries from several professional evaluation associations. It is apparent that all three examples are similar and closely parallel the same concepts used by IRBs. For example, in 2004 the American Evaluation Association ratified their ethical principles to guide professional evaluators. See **Table 2-1**.

A second example is from the Joint Committee on Standards for Educational Evaluation. See **Table 2-2**. A third example is taken from the United Nations Development Program Norms for Evaluation. See **Table 2-3**.

CHALLENGES FACED BY EVALUATORS

After reading through the guidelines, the ethical issues seem straightforward and easy to follow. However, it is not uncommon for evaluators to find themselves in situations where the ethical guidelines become blurred. Let's explore some possible situations that illustrate some of the potential ethical challenges.

First, although it may seem like there are different ethical issues for internal and external evaluators, they face the same

TABLE 2-1 American Evaluation Association

Topic	Definition
Systematic inquiry	Conduct systematic, data-based inquiries related to the evaluation.
Competence	Present accurate and knowledgeable information to stakeholders.
Integrity and honesty	Safeguard the honesty and integrity of the entire evaluation process.
Respect for people	Respect the security, dignity, and self-worth of all individuals participating in the evaluation.
Responsibilities for general and public welfare	Ensure the diversity of interests and values to represent participating individuals and the general public.

Data from the American Evaluation Association's Guiding Principles for Evaluators. Available at: http://www.eval.org/p/cm/ld/fid=51.

TABLE 2-2 Joint Committee on Standards for Educational Evaluation

Topic	Definition	Questions
Utility	Provide practical information needed by the given audience.	Is the purpose of your evaluation clear? Who needs the information and what information do they need? Will the evaluation provide relevant, useful information in a timely manner?
Feasibility	Evaluations take place in the field and should be realistic, prudent, diplomatic, and frugal.	How practical is your evaluation? How much money, time, and effort can you invest? Is the planned evaluation realistic, given the time, resources, and expertise available?
Propriety	The rights of individuals affected by evaluations should be protected.	What steps need to be taken for your evaluation to be ethical and legal? Do these steps protect the rights and welfare of the individuals involved? Do they engage those affected by the program and the evaluation?
Accuracy	Evaluations should produce and convey accurate information about a program's merit and value.	Have you documented your program clearly and accurately? What design will provide accurate, valid, and reliable information? Have you demonstrated that your measures are valid and reliable? Have you used appropriate analyses, and are your conclusions justified? Is your report impartial?

Data from Joint Committee on Standards for Educational Evaluation. Program Evaluation Standards. Available at: http://www.jcsee.org/program-evaluation-standards. Accessed September 2, 2013; and National Institute of General Medical Science. How-To Guide: Standards and Ethics for Evaluation. Available at: http://www.nigms .nih.gov/Research/Evaluation/standards_ethics.htm. Accessed September 2, 2013.

issues but differ in how they are resolved.[10] For example, an internal evaluator, Jackie, uncovers that the Department Head of Medical Records, Mr. Smith, is stealing prescription pads and is forging the physician's signature to acquire pain medications for resale. As an evaluator, Jackie has the ethical and legal obligation to report the information. However, she knows that Mr. Smith's house was recently foreclosed due to his wife being laid off as a corporate attorney. She also knows that Mr. Smith has a child with disabilities and the medical bills are quickly becoming overwhelming. If Jackie reports the evidence to the Board of Directors, Mr. Smith will lose his job. As an internal evaluator who is aware of Mr. Smith's personal circumstances, Jackie may be tempted to ignore her findings. On the other hand, the external evaluator, Ken, uncovers the same information and reports the findings immediately without regard for Mr. Smith's personal situation. In the end, both evaluators report the finding and Mr. Smith is fired; however, Jackie experiences many sleepless nights over the situation, and Ken sleeps fine without ever knowing the outcome of his reported findings.

TABLE 2-3 United Nations Development Program Norms for Evaluation

Topic	Definition
Independent	Evaluators are free from conflict of interest related to the scope, content, and recommendations of their evaluation reports.
Intentional	Purpose of the evaluation is clear and understood between all individuals at the onset.
Transparent	The credibility of evaluators is essential for the stakeholders.
Ethical	Evaluators convey personal and professional integrity, respect of institutions, keep all information confidential, maintain confidentiality of information, and value for customs, beliefs, and cultures of individuals.
Impartial	Evaluators attempt to remove potential bias and maximize objectivity to increase credibility of the final evaluation report.
Timely	Evaluators design evaluations within specific timelines and agree to deliver final reports in a timely manner.
Used	Evaluations provide information to improve quality of evidence-based decision making.

Data from Better Evaluation. Define Ethical and Quality Standards. Available at: http://betterevaluation.org/plan/manage_evaluation/ethical_evaluation. Accessed September 2, 2013.

Second, evaluators attempt to conduct evaluations that are free from political interference, but sometimes they are not shielded from the political side of the organization. For example, the administration may arrange personal interviews under the pretext of convenience for the evaluators. However, in reality, the scheduled interviews are with specific and targeted individuals, so the truth is not discovered by the evaluators. On the other hand, some key stakeholders may seek out interviews with the evaluators to press their specific agenda for the evaluation. It is not the job of evaluators to become investigative detectives, but they do need to be aware of any underlying politics that may be present. Evaluators can decrease the political discord by increasing the number and diversity of individuals at the table when designing the evaluation. In addition, if evaluators suspect that the evaluation has the potential of political overtones, the evaluators may wish to add detailed language in the contract related to how the evaluation is to be conducted. Lastly, if the evaluators question the integrity or purpose of the evaluation, it is within the rights of the evaluator to deny the opportunity to work on the evaluation process. Most importantly, evaluators never wish to obtain the reputation of conducting questionable evaluations loaded with political connotations.

Third, evaluators need to determine if and when individuals participating in the evaluation will be paid. There are times when an incentive is viewed as a bribe for participation and other times when an incentive is appropriate. For example, if the evaluator is conducting a 60-minute focus group with pregnant women regarding their satisfaction with their prenatal care, it is appropriate to provide bus tokens or taxi fare and a $10 gift card for their time. However, it is not appropriate to pay homeless individuals $300 per interview regarding their opinion of a city council vote on the need to build more shelter space. This incentive would be viewed as a bribe.[10]

Fourth, evaluators have an obligation to the individuals participating in any aspect of the evaluation. Participants need to be aware of the limits of confidentiality of the data they provide. Evaluators must guarantee that confidential data cannot be traced back to one individual.[11] Also, evaluators need to be respectful of the diversity of all participating individuals (e.g., age, gender, cultural background, disability, personal interactions, and customs). The problem with bias is that it is difficult to recognize it in your own work and writing. Therefore, it is advantageous to have several colleagues read final reports in search of potential biases that were not recognized by the author. For example, if the evaluator is not familiar with local customs common to the geographic region in which the evaluation was conducted, the final report may include some bias unknown to the evaluator. This situation could be viewed as positive (truly an external viewpoint with limited bias) or negative (lack of understanding of the acceptable practice).

CONFIDENTIALITY OF PERSONAL INFORMATION

In all disciplines, it is essential to maintain the confidentiality of personal information. After obtaining informed consent from an individual, investigators are responsible for protecting every aspect of the participant's personal information, including contact information, survey responses, medical data, test results, and interview responses. The investigators are responsible for maintaining this protection according to the institutional or organization policies after the completion of the evaluation or research. It cannot be emphasized enough that all data must be secured, either through being stored in locked cabinets or in password-protected databases. More elaborate procedures are necessary when the collected data involve sensitive information such as criminal activities or sexual behaviors. When the evaluation involves assigning codes for identifiers, the evaluator must separate the actual names from the assigned codes to maintain confidentiality. For example, an evaluator working in a local high school could use a three-step process. First, the high school students are given a paper with a graphic of a telephone keypad. The evaluator would ask the students to create a 6-digit code using the first letter of their first name and the first five letters of their last name, which will become their numeric signature. The student, Kevin Williams, would select 594554 (K = 5, W = 9, I = 4, 5 = L, 5 = L, I = 4). See **Box 2-1**.

Second, the high school students are given the informed consent documents to sign with only their numeric signature. And third, the high school students that signed and returned

BOX 2-1 Creating a Confidential Identification Code

1	ABC 2	DEF 3
GHI 4	JKL 5	MNO 6
PQRS 7	TUV 8	WXYZ 9
TONE *	OPER 0	#

the informed consent are given the survey to complete. The first line of the survey asks the high school students to enter the numeric signature created by writing the keypad graphic numbers in the boxes provided on the survey.

In all disciplines, the investigators are responsible for ensuring that their staff receives the required training on federal guidelines related to data confidentiality. For example, hospital administrators must ensure confidentiality of patient medical records just as investigators must protect data collected from participants. The most common guideline for patient and data confidentiality is the Health Insurance Portability and Accountability Act (HIPAA), which passed in 1996 under President Bill Clinton. Title I of HIPAA protects the health insurance workers and their families if they change or lose their jobs. Title II of HIPAA is known as *administrative simplification* and establishes the national standards for electronic healthcare transactions and national identifiers for providers, health insurance plans, and employers.[7] For the consumer, HIPAA provides individuals the right to determine who may read or receive a copy their medical records, add corrections to their medical records, give permission for sharing health information, and file a complaint with the healthcare provider, health insurer, or the federal government. Anyone may file a complaint at the HHS website (http://www.hhs .gov/ocr/hipaa/). The type of medical information that is protected includes information added to the individual's medical record, conversations shared between healthcare providers about an individual's care, personal medical information in computer system databases, and billing information.[12]

Whether in health care or research, evaluators, hospital administrators, and principal investigators or head researchers are responsible for ensuring that each person providing health care or working on research or evaluations must be familiar with the details of HIPAA and know how to protect the privacy of patient data, records, conversations, surveys, or any other information that is collected. Several websites offer training for HIPAA and research certification, including:

- http://research.unc.edu/offices/research-compliance -program/privacy/hipaa/
- http://privacy.health.ufl.edu/training/visitors/ instructions.shtml
- http://www.hhs.gov/ocr/privacy/hipaa/understanding/ training/index.html

SUMMARY

This chapter begins with a historical overview of ethics and a discussion of the basic principles of ethics. The next section describes the purpose of the institutional review board (IRB),

including how to design comprehensive informed consent documents including the consideration of special populations. Then ethical guidelines for evaluators and challenges faced by evaluators are presented. Last, it focuses on the necessity of learning the importance of maintaining confidentiality of personal information collected from participating individuals.

CASE STUDY: DIAZ VERSUS HILLSBOUROUGH COUNTY HOSPITAL AUTHORITY

In 1987, Karen Perrin reported to the high-risk perinatal outpatient clinic at Tampa General Hospital with affiliation to University of South Florida in Tampa. She was looking forward to a busy day and the change of pace. Karen had worked at Tampa General since January 1986. Her normal assignment was labor and delivery, but as a part-time nurse, it was not unusual for her to fill in elsewhere. For the next 2 weeks, Karen worked at the outpatient high-risk pregnancy clinic while Sue, the clinic's head nurse, took off time for her wedding. In fact, it turned out that Karen worked in the clinic for 4 weeks. She worked in the clinic for 2 weeks, returned to her regular position for 2 weeks, and then was again temporarily assigned to the clinic for 2 additional weeks, because Sue's daughter became ill.

Among other clinic tasks, Karen cared for high-risk pregnant women who came to the clinic for amniocenteses. Amniocentesis is a procedure in which a needle is inserted through a woman's abdomen to extract amniotic fluid for testing.[13] Karen entered each patient's name, hospital number, and Medicaid or insurance number into the "amnio" record log at the desk. She took the patient's weight and blood pressure, measured her belly, and checked her urine. She set up the tray of amniocentesis needles and test tubes and labels for the tubes. She explained the procedure to the patients, offered reassurance, and asked if they had any questions.[14]

During her clinic assignment, Karen noticed something unusual. The pregnant women did not ask questions about the procedure. Karen noted that, "I kept seeing all these women having amnios. Over and over and over. I'd see them one week, I'd say, 'Why are you back again?' I'm looking in their chart and I'm seeing that this is amnio #5, amnio #6 . . ."[14] When she talked with the pregnant women, it was clear that they did not understand why they were having so many amniocenteses. Their response was always the same, "The doctor told me, if I don't do them, my baby will die," she recalls.[15]

An Inquiry

In late 1987, Karen consulted her supervisor. A meeting was schedule with the Vice President of Nursing and the Director of the Perinatal Unit. They told her that the pregnant women were part of a medical study that had been approved by the university and hospital institutional review boards (IRBs); therefore, they considered the matter closed. Her supervisor told her to drop the issue and not pursue additional investigation into the matter. Karen did not stop because she suspected that the women were unaware of a medical study. She continued to press for further investigation. In February 1988, at a final meeting, the Vice President of Nursing made it clear that she had not taken any action nor did she intend to investigate the matter further.

The Next Step

Karen shared her concerns with a friend who happened to be a civil rights attorney, Stephen Hanlon. Under the advice of Mr. Hanlon and the American Nurses Association, Karen was instructed to gather the evidence. She went to the high-risk clinic, took the "amnio" record log, made a copy, and returned the log to the clinic drawer. She returned a few days later to copy the last few pages only to discover that "Someone had taken a razor blade and cut all the pages out of the book. The pages were gone, and they were never found again. This was our only evidence."[14] She provided the copied "amnio" record log to Stephen Hanlon. She also found the contact information for 10 women in the log who had multiple amniocenteses. She contacted them by mail and stated that their rights may have been violated and invited them to contact her. Only one woman, Flora Diaz, age 16, responded.

The Lawsuit

In January 1990, Stephen Hanlon filed a federal class action lawsuit accusing the university, the hospital, and two physician researchers of ignoring the U.S. Department of Health and Human Services regulations on informed consent. Although the lawsuit was initially filed in response to a fetal-lung study[16] involving approximately 280 women, investigation revealed some 30 studies at Tampa General involving 5000 pregnant women between November 1986 and January 1990. Because none of the women or their babies were harmed, this case is not about malpractice but rather dignitary harm. The women were used as research subjects without their informed consent.

Doctors' Perspective

Walter Morales, MD, one of two physician researchers in the lawsuit, denies any wrongdoing: "I can assure you I would never do anything to a research subject that I wouldn't do to my own wife."[17] Further, he notes that he wishes the case had gone to trial instead of being settled because he does not believe that the facts would show the patients were coerced

into signing the forms.[15] Further, the results of the study were published in the *Journal of Obstetrics and Gynecology* and, as a result, the combined use of corticosteroids and thyrotropin-releasing hormone is now common practice in many hospitals.[18]

The Settlement

After almost 10 years of litigation, the case was settled out of court. Under the agreement, the university and the state of Florida paid $2.7 million, and Tampa General Hospital paid $1.14 million.[19] In addition to the cash payment, the hospital and university agreed to revise record keeping so that information on study participants was easily accessible in a database. Tampa General Hospital and the University of South Florida also agreed to apply a standard readability test to their consent forms before submitting future projects to the IRB.

A Postscript

Karen Perrin, whistle-blower in this case, was removed from patient care and laid off from the hospital in September 1990.[20] The hospital made attempts to revoke her nursing license, but she successfully defended her actions with the assistance of the American Nurses Association.[21] Karen completed her master's in public health in 1990 and her PhD in 1996 from the College of Public Health at the University of South Florida. Currently, she is an associate professor at the University of South Florida and lectures on medical ethics.[14] Dr. Perrin is the author of this text.

Case Study Discussion Questions

1. What other actions could the nurse have taken?
2. What is the role of the medical residents in this case?
3. What is the role of the nurse supervisor?

STUDENT ACTIVITIES

1. Write a 200-word case study describing a violation of an ethical principle related to a proposed program plan design and evaluation.
2. Obtain two examples of IRB applications from a local hospital, health clinic, school district, or university. Compare and contrast the information required on each document.

REFERENCES

1. National Institutes of Health, Office of Human Subjects Research. Regulations and Guidelines, Directives for Human Experimentation, Nuremberg Code. Reprinted from *Trials of War Criminals before the Nuremberg Military Tribunals under Control Council Law*, No. 10, Vol. 2,

pp. 181–182. Washington, DC: U.S. Government Printing Office; 1949. Available at: http://ohsr.od.nih.gov/guidelines/nuremberg.html. Accessed January 12, 2012.

2. U.S. Department of Health and Human Services, Office for Human Research Protections. HHS Announces Proposal to Improve Rules Protecting Human Research Subjects. Available at: http://www.hhs.gov/ohrp/index .html. Accessed January 12, 2012.

3. U.S. Department of Health and Human Services. The Belmont Report. Available at: http://www.hhs.gov/ohrp/humansubjects/guidance/ belmont.html. Accessed January 12, 2012.

4. Centers for Disease Control and Prevention. The U.S. Public Health Service Syphilis Study at Tuskegee—The Tuskegee Timeline. Available at: http://www.cdc.gov/tuskegee/timeline.htm. Accessed January 12, 2012.

5. Centers for Disease Control and Prevention. The U.S. Public Health Service Syphilis Study at Tuskegee—A Presidential Apology. Available at: http://www.cdc.gov/tuskegee/clintonp.htm. Accessed January 12, 2012.

6. Better Evaluation. Define Ethical and Quality Standards. Available at: http://betterevaluation.org/plan/manage_evaluation/ethical_evaluation. Accessed September 2, 2013.

7. Centers for Medicare and Medicaid Services. HIPAA—General Information. Available at: https://www.cms.gov/hipaageninfo/. Accessed January 12, 2012.

8. U.S. Department of Health and Human Services. Regulations. Available at: http://www.hhs.gov/ohrp/humansubjects/index.html. Accessed January 12, 2012.

9. U.S. Department of Health and Human Services, Office for Human Research Protections. IRB Guidebook. Available at: http://www.hhs.gov/ ohrp/archive/irb/irb_guidebook.htm. Accessed January 12, 2012.

10. Church C, Rogers M. Search for Common Ground. *Designing for Results: Integrating Monitoring and Evaluation in Conflict Transformation Programs.* Available at: http://www.sfcg.org/programmes/ilt/ilt_manualpage .html. Accessed September 20, 2013.

11. United Nations Evaluation Group. United Nations Evaluation Group Ethical Guidelines. Available at: http://www.unevaluation.org/ethical guidelines. Accessed September 20, 2013.

12. National Hospice and Palliative Care Organization. Summary of the HIPAA Privacy Rule. Available at: http://www.caringinfo.org/files/public/ ad/HIPPA_Privacy_Rule.pdf. Accessed January 12, 2012.

13. O' Connor TL. *A Patient Guide to Amniocentesis.* Tampa, FL: Tampa General Hospital; 1987.

14. Werner D. Personal communication with Dr. Karen Perrin in preparation for forthcoming book. Donna Werner, PhD, Philosophy Chairperson, Humanities Department, St. Louis Community College, St. Louis, MO.

15. Aronson P. A medical indignity. *National Law Journal.* 2000:A1.

16. Morales WJ, O'Brien WF, Angel JL, Knuppel RA, Sawai S. Fetal lung maturation: the combined use of corticosteroids and thyrotropin-releasing hormone. *Obstet Gyneco.* 1998;73:111-116.

17. Hanlon S. Clinical Research Trials and Tribulations. Presentation, American Bar Association, November 10, 2000.

18. Kaighin A. Physician defends research on fetuses. *Tampa Tribune.* February 3, 1990.

19. Ricks D. Court case mars legacy of helping doctor: research was based in compassion. *Orlando Sentinel.* March 26, 1990.

20. *Diaz v. Florida Board of Regents,* 8:90-cv-00120-HLA (2000).

21. Washington W. Hospital, USF settle "dignity" suit. *St. Petersburg Times.* March 11, 2000.

CHAPTER **3**

Determinants of Health

By the end of the chapter, students will be able to:

1. Describe three historical public health changes that have taken place over the last century.
2. Define the concept of health disparities.
3. Examine how *Healthy People 2020* relates to the social determinants of health.
4. Rate which social determinants of health are most essential for optimal health outcomes.
5. Create a MAP-IT project for a local community health issue.

KEY TERMS

health disparities
Healthy People 2020
social determinants of health

INTRODUCTION

This chapter introduces how evaluators look beyond disease and disability when planning and evaluating health programs. It begins by laying a foundation by presenting a brief overview of historical achievements in public health. It is difficult to plan and evaluate future health programs without knowing some of the past success stories. The historical background is followed by an introduction to a discussion of health disparities and social determinants as defined in the U.S. Department of Health and Human Services *Healthy People 2020* program. At the end of the chapter, using an evaluation tool called MAP-IT (Mobilize, Assess, Plan, Implement, Track), a method to achieve the *Healthy People 2020* objectives in program planning and evaluation is described.

HISTORICAL VIEW OF ACHIEVEMENT IN HEALTH

In the 20th century, individuals in the United States enjoyed improved health and life expectancy due to many public health achievements. See **Table 3-1**. For example, deaths due to motor vehicles decreased after the production of safer vehicles, the introduction of seatbelt laws, and the advocacy of Mothers Against Drunk Driving (MADD). As a result of these and other changes, life expectancy increased by more than 30 years over the century. Not only are people living longer, but *how* people are dying has also changed over the same time period.

OVERVIEW OF THE *HEALTHY PEOPLE* INITIATIVE

Over the years, the leading causes of death in the United States have changed from infectious disease like influenza and enteritis to chronic disease influenced by behavioral choices, such as tobacco usage, poor diet, lack of physical activity, and alcohol consumption.[6] This change in disease patterns is commonly called the *epidemiologic transition*. Building on the shift to chronic disease, in 1979, the U.S. Department of Health and Human Services published the Surgeon General's Report *Healthy People: The Surgeon General's Report on Health Promotion and Disease Prevention*. This document described the current health of the U.S. population and set goals for future health improvements. Every decade since that time, the document is updated with a new health focus.[7] For 2020, the focus moved from disease prevention and health promotion to a focus on eliminating health disparities and promoting health equity.

Building on the four decades of *Healthy People*, it is useful to understand the concept of health measures. The

TABLE 3-1 Ten Great Public Health Achievements in the United States, 1900–1999

Cardiovascular disease[1]	Fewer deaths from stroke and coronary heart disease due to smoking cessation and blood pressure control due to early detection and treatment
Contraceptive and family planning options	Altered social and economic roles of women through smaller family size, longer intervals between pregnancies, fewer maternal and infant deaths
Fluoridation of drinking water[2]	Reduction of childhood tooth decay and tooth loss in adults
Food safety	Less microbial contamination and increase in nutritional content
Healthier mothers and babies	Improved hygiene and nutrition, antibiotics, greater access to health care, and maternal and neonatal medical advances
Highway safety[3]	Safer motor vehicles, improved vehicles and highway engineering, and increased use of seatbelts, child safety seats, and motorcycle helmets
Infectious disease control	Clean water and improved sanitation; antimicrobial therapy for tuberculosis and sexually transmitted diseases
Occupational safety[4]	Fewer injuries in the workplace environment including safer protective equipment, improved ventilation, fewer toxic exposures, shorter work hours
Tobacco control	Recognition of tobacco use as a health hazard: successful anti-smoking campaigns changed social norms to reduce initiation of tobacco use, increase cessation, and reduce environmental tobacco smoke exposure
Vaccinations[5]	Reduced number of childhood diseases: measles, mumps, rubella, chickenpox; latest HPV vaccine to reduce cervical cancer

Data from the Centers for Disease Control and Prevention. Morbidity and Mortality Weekly Report. Ten great public health achievements—United States, 1900–1999. *MMWR.* 1999; 48(12) 241–243.

Healthy People databases monitor four cross-cutting measures: general health status, health-related quality of life and well-being, determinants of health, and health disparities. See **Table 3-2** for brief definitions of each health measure.

After reviewing the four cross-cutting measures, the discussion moves to the specific goals and objectives for each of the health measures. Keep in mind that the *Healthy People* website (http://www.healthypeople.gov) is very useful for

TABLE 3-2 Foundation of the Four Health Measures and Definitions

Health Measures	Definition
General Health Status	Life expectancy: Life expectancy at birth and life expectancy at age 65.
	Healthy life expectancy: The average number of healthy years a person can expect to live if age-specific death rates and age-specific morbidity rates remain the same throughout lifetime.
	Years of potential life lost: A summary measure of premature mortality (early death) that represents the total number of years not lived by people who die before reaching a given age.
	Physically and mentally unhealthy days: The number of days in the past 30 days that individuals rated their physical or mental health as not good.
	Self-assessed health status: A measure of how an individual perceives his or her health—rating it as excellent, very good, good, fair, or poor.
	Limitation of activity: A measure of long-term reduction in a person's ability to do the usual activities of daily living (bathing/showering, dressing, eating, getting in and out of bed, walking, using the toilet), instrumental activities of daily living (using the telephone, doing light housework, preparing meals, shopping, managing money), play, school, or work.
	Chronic disease: A measure of the prevalence the leading causes of death and disability in the United States including heart disease, cancer, and stroke.

TABLE 3-2 Foundation of the Four Health Measures and Definitions (Continued)

Health Measures	Definition
Health-Related Quality of Life and Well-being (HRQoL)	HRQoL is a multidimensional concept that includes domains related to physical, mental, emotional, and social functioning that goes beyond direct measures of population health like life expectancy and causes of death, and instead focuses on the impact health status has on quality of life. HRQoL assesses positive aspects of a person's life like their positive emotions and life satisfaction.

Determinants of Health	Determinants of health are those factors that make some people healthy and others unhealthy. They include:
	Policies: Local, state, and federal policies affect individual and population health.
	Social determinants:
	  Availability of resources needed to meet daily needs (quality education, employment, living wages, transportation, and healthy food)
	  Social norms and attitudes (discrimination, exposure to crime, violence, and social disorder)
	  Social support, social interactions, and socioeconomic conditions
	Physical determinants:
	  Natural environment (plants, weather, or climate change)
	  Built environment (buildings or transportation)
	  Worksites, schools, and recreational settings
	  Housing, homes, and neighborhoods
	  Exposure to toxic substances and other physical hazards
	  Physical barriers (ramps for people with disabilities, good lighting, trees, or benches)
	Health services:
	  Adequate or lack of access to health services, lack of availability of specific services, high costs, lack of insurance coverage, and limited language access
	Individual behavior:
	  Many public health and healthcare interventions focus on changing individual behaviors such as substance abuse, diet, and physical activity.
	Biology and genetics:
	  Age; sex; HIV status; inherited conditions, such as sickle cell anemia, hemophilia, cystic fibrosis, and carrying the BRCA1 or BRCA2 gene, which increases risk for breast and ovarian cancer; and family history of heart disease

Disparities	Disparities and inequity measures include measures of the differences in health status based on race/ethnicity, gender, physical and mental ability, and geography. Other influences on health include:
	  High-quality education
	  Nutritious food
	  Decent and safe housing
	  Affordable, reliable public transportation
	  Culturally sensitive healthcare providers
	  Health insurance
	  Clean water and air

Modified from United States Department of Health and Human Services. *Healthy People 2020*. Available at: http://www.healthypeople.gov/2020/about/tracking.aspx.

evaluators. *Healthy People 2020* provides excellent definitions for important public health issues and allows a specific view of the U.S. goals and objectives related to all aspects of health.

USING *HEALTHY PEOPLE 2020:* GOALS AND OBJECTIVES

As previously stated, the four cross-cutting health measures are used as the overarching framework for the specific goals and objectives for federal and state public health activities. As evaluators plan and evaluate health programs, *Healthy People 2020* serves as a valuable resource for the national goals and objectives. For example, if evaluators wish to study oral health, it is beneficial to search *Healthy People 2020* to obtain a national perspective. See **Table 3-3**.

Before moving forward, let's step back and put the pieces together. So far, we have discussed historical public health achievements that moved the leading causes of death from infectious to chronic diseases and the creation of *Healthy People* over the decades. Using these two discussions as the foundation, the four foundations of health measures were introduced followed by an oral health example of how to use *Healthy People 2020* to obtain the national goals and objectives. Next the discussion moves into another layer of *Healthy People 2020* by exploring the overarching concept

TABLE 3-3 Example of a Goal and Objectives from *Healthy People 2020*

	Healthy People 2020
Topic	**Oral Health**
Goal OH-1	Prevent and control oral and craniofacial diseases, conditions, and injuries, and improve access to preventive services and dental care.
Baseline	33.3% of children aged 3 to 5 years had dental caries experience in at least one primary tooth in 1999–2004.
Target	30.0%
Target Setting	10% improvement
Data Source	National Health and Nutrition Examination Survey (NHANES), CDC/NCHS

Courtesy of United States Department of Health and Human Services. Healthy People 2020. Available at: http://www.healthypeople.gov/2020/topicsobjectives2020/overview.aspx?topicId=32.

of determinants of health. This section is later divided into health disparities and health equity. Let's begin with an understanding of determinants of health.

DETERMINANTS OF HEALTH

Healthy People 2020 defines determinants of health as policymaking, social determinants, physical determinants, health services, and individual behavior. This section explores each of the determinants of health in detail, and then moves into health disparities and health equity.

Policymaking

The health of individuals is affected by policies developed at the local, state, and federal levels. Suppose a state developed a law requiring that bars become smoke free. Some states base this no-smoking ordinance on the type and amount of food served to determine if the eating establishment is considered a bar or a restaurant. An evaluation could be conducted to determine the health outcome of the number of sick days of employees in the partially smoke-free establishments versus those in establishments with complete smoking bans.

Social Determinants

Social support, social interactions, and socioeconomic conditions are the basic elements of social determinants of health. If individuals have resources, such as education, employment, transportation, and healthy food, they are also likely to have social networks. Social networks have little to do with the number of friends an individual has on a social media site. Instead, social networks are the people that individuals contact when they need a ride, need help in securing employment, or just want to talk or engage in social activities. How does this affect health? Social networks are the connections between people for social and emotional benefit. For example, when a large corporation opens in a mid-size town, the effects go further than just creating an opportunity for employment. These consequences impact every aspect of the social fabric of the community from the opening of a new local hang-out restaurant to the impact of increased social services, such as lower unemployment; increased community engagement; and improved schools, libraries, social services, and roads due to increased tax revenue. Numerous evaluations are conducted in such circumstances to establish what should be done in order to maintain the population during economic recovery because of the presence of new industries. There are many social determinants of health. However, they are generally thought of in five major categories: neighborhood and built environment, health and health care, social and community context, education, and economic stability. See **Figure 3-1**.

FIGURE 3-1 Social determinants of health.

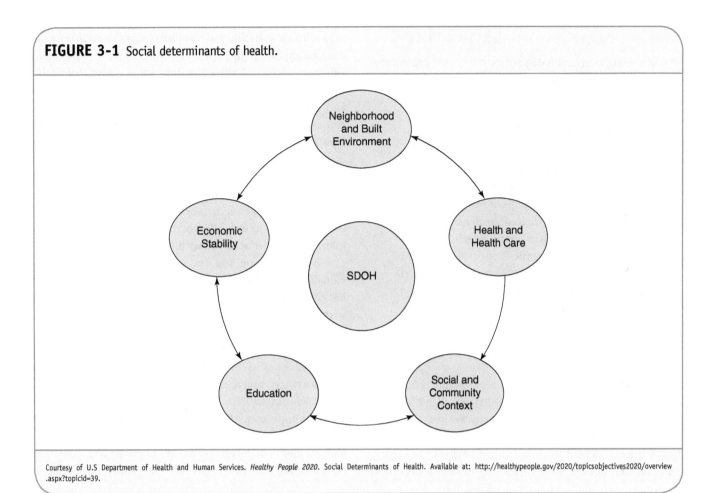

Courtesy of U.S Department of Health and Human Services. *Healthy People 2020*. Social Determinants of Health. Available at: http://healthypeople.gov/2020/topicsobjectives2020/overview.aspx?topicid=39.

Physical Determinants

Physical determinants of health include the natural and manufactured environment, transportation, worksites, schools, recreation facilities, homes, neighborhoods, and exposure to physical hazards (e.g., industrial pollution, vehicle pollution, water pollution from chemical waste) and physical barriers (e.g., lack of bike lanes discourage individuals from riding their bikes for transportation or exercise). For example, the county school district board votes to increase the number of children who attend their local neighborhood school rather than bus children across the county to equalize socioeconomic ratios within all elementary schools. By attending an elementary school close to their homes, the children are able to participate in after-school activities, and the parents are more likely to become involved in school activities due to the close proximity of the evening meeting. Children also make friends in their neighborhood, and more children are able to walk to school, thus increasing their physical activity.

Health Services

The U.S. healthcare system is complex and complicated, even for those individuals who have access to health insurance and regular medical care. For example, a young family has two healthy children. When the third child is born, a genetic mutation, such as Down syndrome, is discovered. The family has health insurance, but the deductible is $2000 per family member. Once the deductible payment is met, the family pays 20% of medical bills and the health insurance pays 80%. This sounds like a reasonable policy for most circumstances. However, if you consider that in this family their new baby's hospital bill is $87,000, this family would be responsible for paying 20% of the medical bill, which amounts to $17,400. Even with adequate health insurance, the family could easily be pushed into serious financial debt after several years of providing medical care for their third child.

Now that you have an understanding of health determinants, the discussion moves to an exploration of health disparities and health equity.

HEALTH DISPARITIES AND HEALTH EQUITY

While investigating health disparities, it becomes evident that there are multiple definitions for the same concepts.[8]

Health Disparities

Healthy People 2020 defines health disparity as:

> a particular type of health difference that is closely linked with social, economic, and/or environmental disadvantage. Health disparities adversely affect groups of people who have systematically experienced greater obstacles to health based on their racial or ethnic group; religion; socioeconomic status; gender; age; mental health; cognitive, sensory, or physical disability; sexual orientation or gender identity; geographic location (rural or urban); inequities in income, education, and access to health care and other characteristics historically linked to discrimination or exclusion.[9]

Other health influences include high-quality education, nutritious food, decent and safe housing, affordable and reliable public transportation, culturally sensitive healthcare providers, health insurance, and clean water and air.[9] In addition, health disparities lead to an individual's inability to achieve and maintain optimal health, resulting in such problems as higher infant mortality and low birth weight rates; shorter life expectancy; and higher rates of chronic disease, stroke, and substance abuse.[9] Health evaluators acknowledge that health disparities are interconnected with biological, environmental, and lifestyle behaviors that negatively impact health outcomes. For example, an elderly Hispanic female living with type 2 diabetes in government housing in a large urban city has multiple health disparities and perhaps limited access to adequate healthcare services. She is likely to experience poor health outcomes with a shorter life expectancy.

A second example is taken from *Healthy People 2020*; see **Table 3-4**. The definition of infant mortality is defined as infant deaths that occurred within the first year of life.

While planning and evaluating health programs, individuals need to take into account the participants' level of health disparities. For example, if county commissioners wish to improve access to reliable public transportation for persons with disabilities, the evaluation team conducts a needs assessment to determine the percentage of persons with disabilities in the county and the availability of public transportation equipped with disability ramps and appropriate wheelchair lifts. After reporting the baseline data to the county commissioners, the evaluation team would suggest conducting focus groups with persons with disabilities and their caregivers as well as public transportation administrators in order to provide viewpoints from multiple

TABLE 3-4 Example of Disparity: Comparison of Education and Infant Mortality Rates

Healthy People 2020 Maternal, Infant, and Child Health (MICH) Goals and Objectives	
MICH-1.3 Reduce the rate of all infant deaths (within 1 year) Baseline: 6.7 infant deaths per 1,000 live births occurred within the first year of life in 2006 Target: 6.0 infant deaths per 1,000 live births Target-Setting Method: 10% improvement	
Education	Infant Mortality Rate
0–8 years	6.6
9–11 years	9.3
12 years	8.1
13–15 years	6.1
16 years or more	4.2
The infant mortality rate for mothers with 9–11 years of education is 5.1 infant deaths per 1000 live births (or 121%) greater than the rate of mothers with 16 or more years of education (9.3 – 4.2 = 5.1).	

Courtesy of Kline R and Huang D. Defining and measuring disparities, inequities, and inequalities in the Healthy People initiative. National Center for Health Statistics. Centers for Disease Control and Prevention. Available at: http://www.cdc.gov/nchs/ppt/nchs2010/41_Klein.pdf; U.S. Department of Health and Human Services. *Healthy People 2020* Available at http://www.healthypeople.gov/2020/topicsobjectives2020/objectiveslist.aspx?topicId=26.

stakeholders. At this point, the county commissioners may determine the annual cost of outfitting all public transportation with adequate equipment for use by persons with disabilities. This change would allow persons with disabilities to travel freely around the county and eliminate the need to pre-arrange their transportation needs by scheduling specialty van service that is currently known to be inadequate and involves long waits.

Health Equity

According to *Healthy People 2020*, health equity is defined as the fair distribution of health determinants, outcomes, and resources within and between segments of the population, regardless of social standing. Health equity is also defined as a desired goal that includes a special effort to improve the health of those who have experienced social or economic disadvantage. Health equity has three components: inequity, inequality, and burden.[8] First, health inequity is the systematic, avoidable, and unjust difference in the distribution or allocation of a resource between groups.[8,10,11] Second, health inequality is the differences, variations, and disparities in the health achievements of individuals and groups of people.[12] Third, burden explores the number of people who are affected in specific groups and in the total population, the number of people benefitting from the environmental or healthcare resources, and the level of fairness in the distribution of resources.[8,10,11]

Let's explore how an evaluator uses each of the four components of health equity to determine how an individual's level of education affects his or her health. In this scenario, it is useful to refer to *Healthy People 2020*. See **Box 3-1**.

Using the information in Box 3-1, respond to the following questions:

- How does a fair distribution of educational resources, regardless of social standing, affect health equity?
- How does unjust distribution of educational resources between groups (health inequity) affect health among groups?
- How is educational attainment affected by a disparity in the health achievements among groups of people?
- How is the educational attainment for the number of people in specific groups affected by the level of fairness in the distribution of resources?

USING *HEALTHY PEOPLE 2020*

Now that you are familiar with *Healthy People 2020*, there are numerous ways for evaluators to use the information. *Healthy People 2020* offers several tools for implementation including DATA2020, evidence-based resources, *Healthy People in*

BOX 3-1 *Healthy People 2020* and Evaluation

Healthy People 2020 Goal: AH-5.1 Increase the proportion of students who graduate with a regular diploma 4 years after starting 9th grade.

Baseline: 74.9% of students attending public schools graduated with a regular diploma in 2007–2008, 4 years after starting 9th grade.

Target: 82.4%

Target-Setting Method: 10% improvement

The following points reflect how high school graduation affects health:

- Positive effects: Longer life expectancy, improved health and quality of life, health-promoting behaviors like getting regular physical activity, not smoking, and going for routine checkups and recommended screenings.
- Negative effects: Discrimination, stigma, or unfair treatment in the workplace can have a profound impact on health; discrimination can increase blood pressure, heart rate, and stress, as well as undermine self-esteem and self-efficacy. Family and community rejection, including bullying of lesbian, gay, bisexual, and transgender youth can have serious and long-term health impacts including depression, use of illegal drugs, and suicidal behavior. Places where people live and eat affect their diet. More than 23 million people, including 6.5 million children, live in "food deserts"—neighborhoods that lack access to stores where affordable, healthy food is readily available (such as full-service supermarkets and grocery stores).

Action, and MAP-IT.[13] Whether the public health program is being planned, implemented, or evaluated, it is useful to employ data tools available in *Healthy People 2020*.

DATA2020

DATA2020 is an interactive tool that allows users to explore data and technical information related to the *Healthy People 2020* objectives. This information is valuable to evaluators who are interested in comparing their local data to national data or objectives. Review **Figures 3-2, 3-3, 3-4,** and **3-5.** Figure 3-2 shows the topics of interest. For this discussion, public health infrastructure was selected for the example.

After hitting "Continue," Figure 3-3 shows that DATA2020 has 46 results related to public health infrastructure. Hit "View Data."

When you view the data, there are several options of data available. Figure 3-4 shows an objective for public health infrastructure, "PHI-4.1 Increase the proportion of 4-year colleges and universities that offer public health or related majors." By clicking on "TOTAL," you are able to open the charts available to PHI-4.1. Figure 3-5 shows the baseline data of 7 in 2008 and that the goal for 2020 is 10.0. **Figure 3-6** shows the specifics of the data used for the bar graph in Figure 3-5. The type of data shown in these examples is

FIGURE 3-2 DATA2020 search.

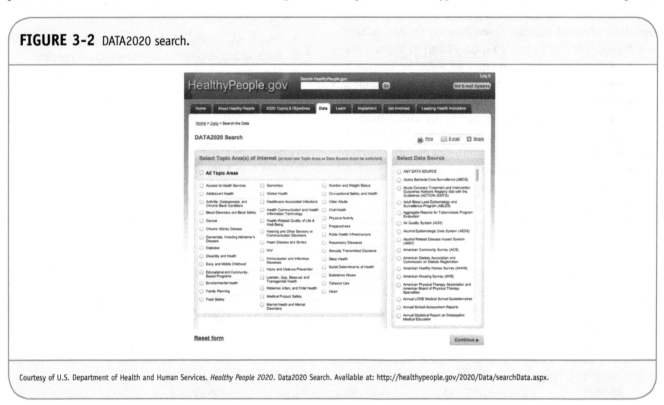

Courtesy of U.S. Department of Health and Human Services. *Healthy People 2020*. Data2020 Search. Available at: http://healthypeople.gov/2020/Data/searchData.aspx.

FIGURE 3-3 DATA2020 interim results.

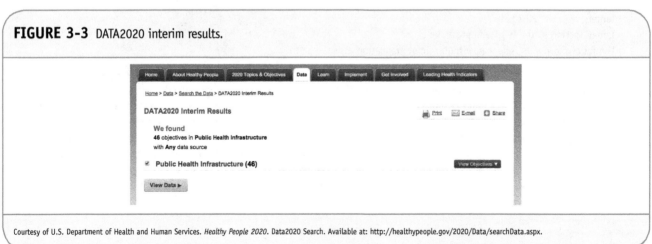

Courtesy of U.S. Department of Health and Human Services. *Healthy People 2020*. Data2020 Search. Available at: http://healthypeople.gov/2020/Data/searchData.aspx.

FIGURE 3-4 PHI-4.1 Increase the proportion of 4-year colleges and universities that offer public health or related majors.

<u>PHI-4.1 Increase the proportion of 4-year colleges and universities that offer public health or related majors</u>

Four-year colleges and universities offering public health majors (percent)

2020 Baseline (year): 7 (2008)   **2020 Target:** 10.0   **Desired Direction:** ↑ Increase   [Display Years]

POPULATIONS	◁	2008	▷
TOTAL		7	

Courtesy of U.S. Department of Health and Human Services. *Healthy People 2020*. Available at http://www.healthypeople.gov/2020/data/Chart.aspx?pgid=1&topicid=35&objective=PHI-4.1&years=2008&showCI=False&showSE=False.

available for all *Healthy People 2020* objectives where appropriate data are available. These types of charts allow evaluators to compare their local data, goals, and objectives to the national data.

Evidence-Based Resources

As with DATA2020, the evidence-based resource tab allows the user to click on the topics and categories of interest and then click "Search" to view the data. See **Figure 3-7**.

FIGURE 3-5 Four year colleges and universities offering public health majors.

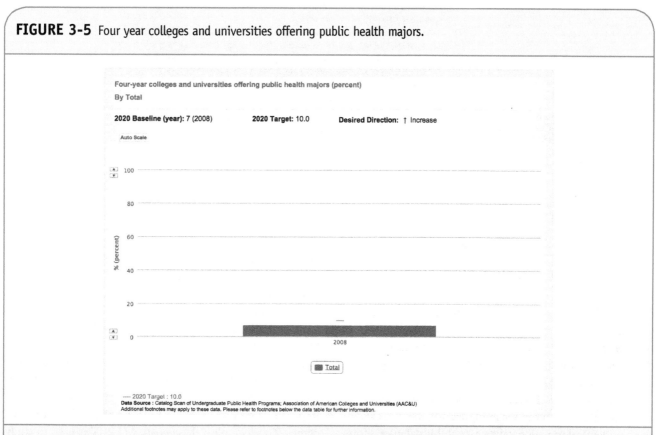

Four-year colleges and universities offering public health majors (percent)
By Total

2020 Baseline (year): 7 (2008)   **2020 Target:** 10.0   **Desired Direction:** ↑ Increase

Auto Scale

---- 2020 Target : 10.0
Data Source : Catalog Scan of Undergraduate Public Health Programs; Association of American Colleges and Universities (AAC&U)
Additional footnotes may apply to these data. Please refer to footnotes below the data table for further information.

Courtesy of U.S. Department of Health and Human Services. *Healthy People 2020*. Four Year Colleges and Universities Offering Public Health Majors. Available at: http://www.healthypeople.gov/2020/data/Chart.aspx?pgid=1&topicid=35&objective=PHI-4.1&years=2008&showCI=False&showSE=False.

FIGURE 3-6 Increase the proportion of 4-year colleges and universities that offer public health or related majors.

PHI-4.1 Increase the proportion of 4-year colleges and universities that offer public health or related majors

National Data Source	Catalog Scan of Undergraduate Public Health Programs; Association of American Colleges and Universities (AAC&U)
Changed Since the Healthy People 2020 Launch	Yes
Measure	percent
Baseline (Year)	7 (2008)
Target	10.0
Target-Setting Method	3 percentage point improvement
Numerator	Number of US four-year colleges and universities that offer majors in public health
Denominator	Number of US four-year colleges and universities which offer undergraduate degrees and are members of the (AAC&U)
Data Collection Frequency	Periodic
Comparable Healthy People 2010 Objective	Not applicable

Comments

Methodology Notes	The Catalog Scan used the content of course requirements to determine if specific programs fulfill Public Health criteria. Majors, minors, and concentrations in Community Health and other related fields were considered Public Health if they included the primary components of public health education for undergraduates (including courses in Epidemiology, Health Systems, and others).
	National efforts are currently underway to increase 4-year undergraduate public health programs, which will help achieve this objective. The following organizations have all created resources to help spur development of undergraduate offerings in public health: AAC&U's Educated Citizen and Public Health; ASPH's Undergraduate Public Health Learning Outcomes Development Project; APTR undergraduate public health effort; and APHA's policy statement on undergraduate public health education.
Description of Changes Since the Healthy People 2020 Launch	The target setting method was changed from projection/trend analysis to 3 percentage point improvement because the baseline was less than 10. The target itself remains unchanged.

Courtesy of U.S. Department of Health and Human Services. *Healthy People 2020*. Public Health Infrastructure Goal. Available at: http://www.healthypeople.gov/2020/topics objectives2020/TechSpecs.aspx?hp2020id=PHI-4.1.

Healthy People in Action

Healthy People in Action focuses on data from states and territories rather than national data. Again, this section allows evaluators to compare their local data to state data rather than only national data. When you click on each state, a document is provided with a plan for the state. **Figure 3-8** shows a sample of the link.

At this point, you select a specific state and review the available data. As you can see in **Figure 3-9**, the data categories are identical to national data except this database shows state-level statistics. For evaluators, state data are often more useful for making comparisons than using only the national data. Note that in this example, the high school graduation rate for Delaware is 78.0%, and the target goal is 82.4%.

Now that you have learned about two of the three tools of implementation for *Healthy People 2020*, it is time to explore how to use MAP-IT (*Mobilize, Assess, Plan, Implement, Track*). As previously stated in this chapter, *Healthy People 2020* reflects the nation's high-priority health issues and the need to decrease health disparities and improve determinants of health for enhanced health outcomes. To accomplish these goals, MAP-IT is used to study ways to achieve optimal health for individuals, communities

FIGURE 3-7 Evidenced-based resources.

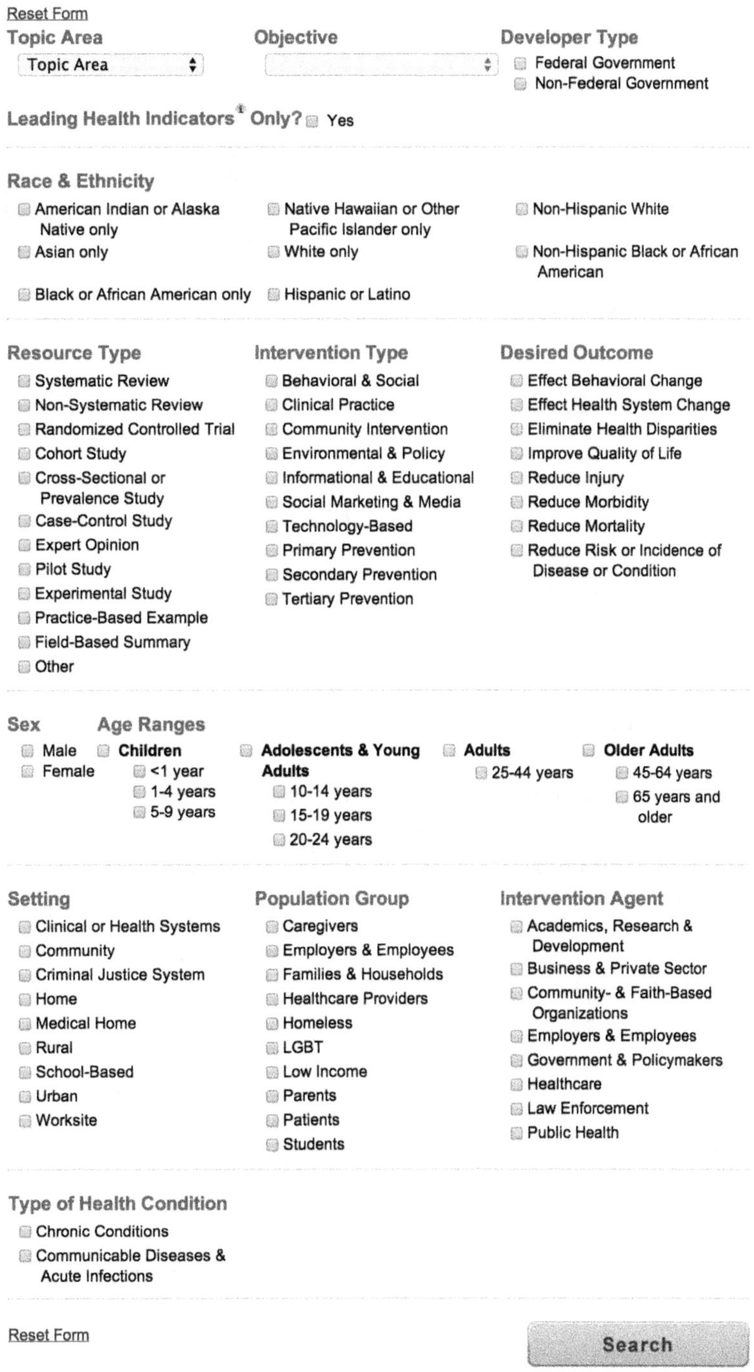

Reset Form

Topic Area

[Topic Area   ▼]

Objective

[▼]

Developer Type

☐ Federal Government
☐ Non-Federal Government

Leading Health Indicators[①] Only? ☐ Yes

Race & Ethnicity

☐ American Indian or Alaska Native only
☐ Asian only
☐ Black or African American only

☐ Native Hawaiian or Other Pacific Islander only
☐ White only
☐ Hispanic or Latino

☐ Non-Hispanic White

☐ Non-Hispanic Black or African American

Resource Type

☐ Systematic Review
☐ Non-Systematic Review
☐ Randomized Controlled Trial
☐ Cohort Study
☐ Cross-Sectional or Prevalence Study
☐ Case-Control Study
☐ Expert Opinion
☐ Pilot Study
☐ Experimental Study
☐ Practice-Based Example
☐ Field-Based Summary
☐ Other

Intervention Type

☐ Behavioral & Social
☐ Clinical Practice
☐ Community Intervention
☐ Environmental & Policy
☐ Informational & Educational
☐ Social Marketing & Media
☐ Technology-Based
☐ Primary Prevention
☐ Secondary Prevention
☐ Tertiary Prevention

Desired Outcome

☐ Effect Behavioral Change
☐ Effect Health System Change
☐ Eliminate Health Disparities
☐ Improve Quality of Life
☐ Reduce Injury
☐ Reduce Morbidity
☐ Reduce Mortality
☐ Reduce Risk or Incidence of Disease or Condition

Sex

☐ Male
☐ Female

Age Ranges

☐ **Children**
  ☐ <1 year
  ☐ 1-4 years
  ☐ 5-9 years

☐ **Adolescents & Young Adults**
  ☐ 10-14 years
  ☐ 15-19 years
  ☐ 20-24 years

☐ **Adults**
  ☐ 25-44 years

☐ **Older Adults**
  ☐ 45-64 years
  ☐ 65 years and older

Setting

☐ Clinical or Health Systems
☐ Community
☐ Criminal Justice System
☐ Home
☐ Medical Home
☐ Rural
☐ School-Based
☐ Urban
☐ Worksite

Population Group

☐ Caregivers
☐ Employers & Employees
☐ Families & Households
☐ Healthcare Providers
☐ Homeless
☐ LGBT
☐ Low Income
☐ Parents
☐ Patients
☐ Students

Intervention Agent

☐ Academics, Research & Development
☐ Business & Private Sector
☐ Community- & Faith-Based Organizations
☐ Employers & Employees
☐ Government & Policymakers
☐ Healthcare
☐ Law Enforcement
☐ Public Health

Type of Health Condition

☐ Chronic Conditions
☐ Communicable Diseases & Acute Infections

Reset Form

[Search]

Courtesy of U.S. Department of Health and Human Services. *Healthy People 2020*. Evidence Based Resources. Available at: http://www.healthypeople.gov/2020/implement/EBR.aspx.

FIGURE 3-8 Sample of state and territorial healthy people plans.

Alaska
- 2010 🗐
- 2020 🗐

Arizona
- 2020 🗐

Arkansas
- 2010 🗐
- 2020 [PDF - 1.75 MB] 🗐

California
- 2010 🗐
- 2020 🗐

Connecticut
- 2020 🗐

Delaware
- 2020 🗐

Nevada
- 2010 🗐
- 2020 🗐

New Hampshire
- 2010 🗐

New Jersey
- 2010 🗐

New Mexico
- 2010 [PDF - 340 KB] 🗐

New York
- 2010 🗐

North Carolina
- 2020 🗐

Courtesy of U.S. Department of Health and Human Services. *Healthy People 2020*. State and Territorial Healthy People Plans. Available at: http://www.healthypeople.gov/2020/implement/StateSpecificPlans.aspx.

FIGURE 3-9 Sample of data from Delaware.

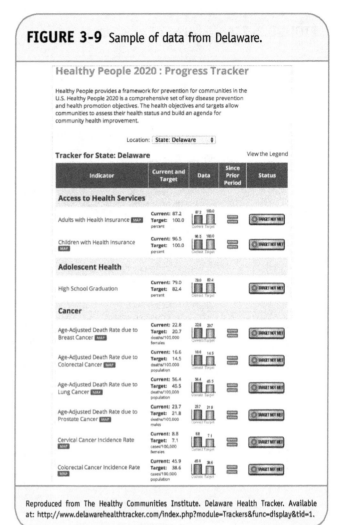

Reproduced from The Healthy Communities Institute. Delaware Health Tracker. Available at: http://www.delawarehealthtracker.com/index.php?module=Trackers&func=display&tid=1.

(e.g., organizations, institutions, corporations, universities), and the nation.[14] See **Figure 3-10** for the topic of interest for the MAP-IT example.

Table 3-5 presents how to use MAP-IT with an example aimed at increasing the number of state health departments that have at least one health promotion program aimed at improving the health and well-being of people with disabilities.

FIGURE 3-10 Topic for MAP-IT example.

DH-2.2   Increase the number of State and the District of Columbia health departments that conduct health surveillance of caregivers for people with disabilities

Baseline: 2 States and the District of Columbia conducted health surveillance of caregivers for people with disabilities in 2010

Target: 51 States and the District of Columbia

Target-Setting Method: Retention of Healthy People 2010 target

Data Source: Behavioral Risk Factor Surveillance System (BRFSS), CDC/PHSIPO

Data: HP2020 data for this objective

Details about the methodology and measurement of this HP2020 objective

HP2010 data for this objective

Close Details ▲

Courtesy of U.S. Department of Health and Human Services. *Healthy People 2020*. Disability and Health. Available at: http://www.healthypeople.gov/2020/topicsobjectives2020/objectiveslist.aspx?topicId=9.

INDIVIDUAL HEALTH RISKS AND BEHAVIORS

With a general understanding of health determinants, health disparities, and health equities at the population level, the discussion moves to individual health, including risk factors and behaviors. As public health evaluators, it is important for individuals to understand their personal health risks as well as the health risks they may have inherited from their families. The best way to become familiar with individual risk factors is by becoming familiar with your own personal risk factors.

TABLE 3-5 Using MAP-IT

MAP-IT	Objectives	Questions to Ask	Increase Health Promotion Programs for People with Disabilities
Mobilize	Gather a broad representation of key individuals and organize a partnership/coalition. Identify roles for partners and organizations. Assign responsibilities to move process forward.	What is the vision and mission of the coalition? Who should be represented?	The vision of the health department to improve health and wellness among people with disabilities Representative sample of individuals with disabilities, family members, caregivers, administration, and staff

Assess	Assess both needs and resources in the community.
	Set priorities: Feasibility, effectiveness, and measurability
	Collect state and local data to determine local needs.
	Explore social determinants of health related to the issue.
	   Is the health of the individuals with disabilities affected by the physical environment of the health department?
	   Does every individual with disabilities have access to multiple health program choices?
	   Does the health department accommodate individuals with disabilities through the social environment (e.g., location, hours of operation, adequate parking)?
	   Do individual lifestyle behaviors affect the health issue being addressed?
	   What will it take to improve the health programs of the health department?
		Who is affected and how?
		What resources do we have and what resources do we need?
			Retrieve health department medical chart data to determine percentage of individuals with disabilities.
			Review the syllabi from health courses to determine amount of time spent on issues related to individuals with disabilities.
			Determinants of health:
			   Does the health department offer health programs for individuals with disabilities?
			   Are there health programs offered with emphasis for individuals with disabilities?
			   Are individuals with disabilities able to register for health programs to increase their physical activity and well-being?
			   Do individuals with disabilities have access to one-on-one classes to address personal needs?
			   Are the hours of operation of the health department compatible with needs of individuals with disabilities?
			   Are individuals with disabilities in poor physical condition supported for starting to become physically active?
			   Do only individuals with disabilities in excellent physical condition go to the health department wellness classes?
			   After reviewing the data, what will it take to increase and improve the number of individuals with disabilities that participates in the health classes and wellness program at the health department?

(continues)

TABLE 3-5 Using MAP-IT (Continued)

MAP-IT	Objectives	Questions to Ask	Increase Health Promotion Programs for People with Disabilities
Plan	Use *Healthy People 2020* to determine the goals and objectives. Clear objectives are needed in a good plan. Write concrete steps for achieving each objective. Assign responsibilities and activities to each team member. Search for best practices and other tested interventions.	What is the goal? What is needed to reach the goal?	Goal: Increase the proportion of college and university students who receive information from their institution on inadequate physical activity. Write clear objectives and concrete steps for achieving each objective. Assign responsibilities and activities to each team member. Conduct a review of the literature for best practices of increasing physical activity for university students.
Implement	Create a detailed work plan. Share responsibility by assigning a specific person to each activity. Celebrate accomplishments.	Is the plan being followed? Is there a way to improve the plan?	Determine if the plan is being followed. Determine if improvements are needed in the plan.
Track	Evaluate each segment to track progress over time. Check data collection for standardization, reliability, and validity. Share progress with partners. If you see a positive trend in data, issue a press release or announcement.	Is the plan evaluated at each step? Is the plan being followed? Was the goal reached?	Evaluate the participation levels of individuals with disabilities at each step of the health and wellness programs. Are the individuals with disabilities at the health department increasing their participation in the health and wellness programs?

Courtesy of U.S. Department of Health and Human Services. *Healthy People 2020.* Available at http://www.healthypeople.gov/2020/implement/mapit.aspx.

Health Risks and Life Expectancy

Now that you have explored what is known about your family tree, it is time to investigate some of your other personal health risks. Check out the following links:

1. Check your life expectancy: http://www.ssa.gov/OACT/population/longevity.html or http://www.socialsecurity.gov/oact/STATS/table4c6.html
2. Assess your weight and health risk: http://www.nhlbi.nih.gov/health/public/heart/obesity/lose_wt/risk.htm
3. Life expectancy by country comparison—*The World Factbook*: https://www.cia.gov/library/publications/the-world-factbook/rankorder/2102rank.html

Although it is easy to blame health policy, social and physical barriers, and lack of health services, it is essential to remember that individuals' behavior also greatly impacts their health status. Some individuals assume that physicians can "cure" whatever ails them regardless of their poor choices in personal lifestyle health behaviors, such as eating a poor diet, failing to exercise, and engaging in high-risk substance abuse. A healthy lifestyle is a combination of all aspects of positive personal lifestyle behaviors rather than exploring only one behavior at a time. For example, suppose there are two 50-year-old females who have lived in the same neighborhood their entire lives, have similar job descriptions, and work in the same office building. One woman named Rachel is overweight and eats snacks and candy out of the vending machine when she is stressed at work. Rachel has a difficult time sleeping due to breathing problems caused by sleep apnea, a disorder that sometimes affects individuals who are overweight. The other woman, Cindy, maintains an average weight and also has a high-stress job. Cindy handles stress by running 3 miles every morning and packs a healthy sandwich and fruit for lunch each day in order to save money. Her exercise routine is exhausting, so she sleeps well at night. Both females have the same high-quality access to health care, but each woman has different personal health behaviors. Even though their determinants of health are similar, their overall health is influenced by their personal lifestyle choices.

Biology and Genetics

Up until now, the determinants of health have described external factors that may be changed to improve health, even though it may be very difficult to do so. This last category deals with the internal and nonchangeable factors of biology and genetics. First, let's begin with definitions. Biology is defined as the study of living organisms including their physical structure, function, growth, origin, evolution, and distribution, whereas genetics is a branch of biology related to the study of heredity, including the genetic constitution of an individual, group, or class. For this discussion, biology includes factors such as age and sex, and genetics involves inherited conditions (e.g., sickle cell anemia, hemophilia, and cystic fibrosis). The definitions can become blurred when thinking about health conditions, such as heart disease. Although heart disease is influenced by lifestyle choices, also important in whether or not a person will develop heart disease are biological factors (structure and function of the heart muscle) and genetic factors (family history). See **Figure 3-11**.

Now let's put the population and individual-level components of health determinants into one example of an evaluation case study. Recently, Dr. Jackie Williams, a clinic manager,

FIGURE 3-11 Your health risks and life expectancy.

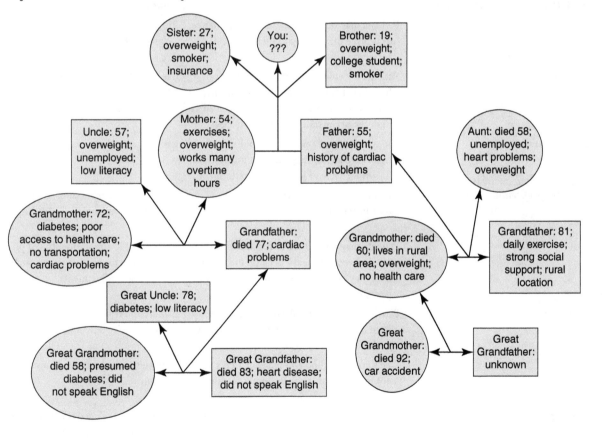

FAMILY tree: Draw what is known about your family tree to explore your health risks. Once you are aware of some patterns, you can make behavior and lifestyle choices based on your genetic health risks. Try to identify the health risks in this family tree.

reviewed his appointment database and noticed some trends in the appointment "no show" data. She knows that one of her clinic nurses, Sharee, is completing her master's in public health degree with a focus in evaluation studies. She asks Sharee to review the data and give her some ideas on why patients were not coming for their scheduled appointments. After studying the data, Sharee developed **Table 3-6** for Dr. Williams.

HEALTH LITERACY

As evaluators begin to plan programs, it is important that they assess the literacy level of the target population. Without proper planning and attention to health literacy, the evaluation of the program will not yield valid results. When written documents or verbal instructions are above the literacy level of the recipient, the result is a lack of comprehension.

It is up to the evaluators to verify that the written and verbal information provided by the health program is at the proper health literacy level. According to the U.S. Department of Health and Human Services, health literacy is defined as the extent that individuals have "the capacity to obtain, process, and understand basic health information and services needed to make appropriate health decisions."[15] It is estimated that 12% of adults lack the health literacy skills required to manage their health needs.[16] Adults with health disparities also have low health literacy and are more likely to report their health as poor and to lack health insurance.[17] As noted previously in this chapter, the same individuals dealing with health disparities are also the populations most likely to experience low health literacy (e.g., elderly, racial and ethnic minorities, people with less than a high school degree or GED

TABLE 3-6 Linking Missed Clinic Appointment Data to Disparities and Determinants of Health

Issue: Increasing number of patients who do not attend a scheduled medical appointment.		
Health Disparities and Determinants	**Issue**	**Solution**
Education	Patients may not understand the importance of routine monitoring of their medical condition.	Provide low literacy health education classes related to their chronic disease.
Employment	Patients are employed full-time but do not have benefits linked to vacation and sick time. Missing work for what is perceived as unnecessary means a reduced paycheck.	Use flexible scheduling of staff to extend the available clinic hours for evening appointments.
Language barrier	Some patients may not speak English as their first language, so they may not understand the importance of follow-up appointments.	Use translation services.
Lack of transportation	Patients may not have reliable transportation.	Have public transportation routes and schedules available in the waiting room.
Stress	Patients may not adhere to recommended medical appointments, because their daily lives may be too stressful, with other complex situations.	Allow flexible appointments and phone counseling for routine issues, such as medication adjustments.
Social support	Patients may lack social support and suffer from depression; no willingness to improve health.	Explore interest in social support groups and health education classes.
Safety	Due to neighborhood violence, patients do not feel safe leaving their homes for the medical appointments.	Explore telephone case management options.
Economic issues	Patients do not have money for a copayment or do not have clean clothes to feel presentable at a medical appointment.	Explore social service needs through telephone case management.
Patients have numerous reasons for missing appointments. As evaluators learn more about health disparities and determinants of health, they begin to understand why their patients are missing medical appointments.		

certificate, people with low income levels, nonnative speakers of English, and people with compromised health status). Low health literacy is also linked to poor health outcomes, less utilization of preventive services, and higher healthcare costs.[17]

When evaluators plan health programs, it is common to collect participant's demographic data for the final evaluation report. If the participants have low literacy skills, they may become overwhelmed with stress because of the unfamiliar situation. When health information is not written and explained for those with low literacy, individuals are unable to give truly informed consent to participate in the program or evaluation. Whether or not the health information is connected to a health program or a medical procedure, individuals with low literacy skills need basic health education to understand and retain the medical information needed for self-care, medication regimens, follow-up treatment, or the initial cause of their illness and prevention of a future reoccurrence.

Evaluators also need to realize that health literacy skills involve not only the written word but also numbers. For example, if a health educator is planning and evaluating a new diabetes education course for the county health departments, the health educator needs to explore the health literacy level for math and reading during the development of the course. Some basic math is needed when tracking blood glucose levels, measuring liquid medications, and reading prescription labels. For reading, the health educator needs to be aware of the reading literacy level for any written materials or hand-outs used in the diabetes course. All healthcare providers and evaluators benefit by communicating in plain language for maximum comprehension and understanding.[18] Documents written in plain language include:

- Placing the most important information first
- Grouping information together to increase understanding
- Writing in active voice
- Using simple, one- to two-syllable words rather than standard medical terminology
- Providing a phonetic pronunciation of medical terms

The readability score of plain language documents should not exceed a 5th-grade reading level.[18] Most word-processing software packages include readability-level tools.

From an evaluator's standpoint, it is important to create written materials prior to the implementation of a new program. It is too late to wait until the program is in place and ready for evaluation. The best way to determine if the written materials are appropriate for the intended audience is to pilot-test the materials several times using the target population during the development process. After achieving a 5th-grade readability score, the next step is to consider the spoken word. When explaining health information, it is essential to avoid using medical terminology, abbreviations, and medical jargon. Plain language applies to written and spoken health information.[19] See **Box 3-2** for an example of plain language.

BOX 3-2 Example of Plain Language

High Literacy: Employee Benefits	Low Literacy: Employee Benefits
Good morning, Mr. Smith. Welcome to the EOH Division of the XYZ Corporation. I am sure that you are excited to start your career since you just graduated with your MPH and passed the CIH exam. My name is Cathy and I am from HR and I will help you understand and enroll in your benefits package. We have a wide variety of PPO and HMO benefits including, of course, PTO and FMLA. You will also need to determine if you wish to enroll in a 401K plan or a defined benefit plan for retirement.	Good morning, Mr. Smith and Mr. Williams. My name is Cathy. I work for Human Resources. I am so glad that your partner was able to join us this morning, so both of you understand the employee benefits that we offer to domestic partners at XYZ Corporation. I do not know a lot about your recent master's in public health degree and your certification in industrial hygiene. I will try to avoid acronyms used in my field, and you can tell me about your job without acronyms when we are finished. For health insurance, we offer Preferred Provider Options, or PPO, and Health Maintenance Organization, or HMO, health insurance plans. PPO costs more per month, but you get to select your healthcare providers. HMO is less expensive, but you have less choice in healthcare providers. We also offer personal time off. We call this PTO. It means that since XYZ is open 24 hours and 7 days per week, your vacation, sick, and holiday paid days off are merged together. Another wonderful benefit is the Family Maedical Leave Act. Fortunately, in this state, we have the privilege of offering this benefit to domestic partners. Let me stop here and ask if you have any questions, then I will explain the retirement options.

TABLE 3-7 Example of English to Spanish Translation

English	Spanish
I speak only a bit of English.	Yo sólo hablo un poco de Inglés.
Where is the nearest clinic? I feel weak. Please help me. I have no money.	¿Dónde está la clínica más cercana? Me siento débil. Por favor, ayúdame. No tengo dinero.
I need to find inexpensive housing in this area.	Tengo que encontrar una vivienda barata de esta zona.
Where is the closest bus stop?	¿Dónde está la parada de autobús más cercana?

Lastly, evaluators should be aware that individuals attending public health programs may have excellent literary skills in one language, but limited language proficiency in another language. Many global citizens experience this situation during international travel, especially when faced with unfamiliar alphabets. Even with a limited working knowledge of another language, individuals struggle to explain their health history and immediate need for treatment. It is important for healthcare providers to determine an individual's level of literacy in their native language before assuming a lack of health knowledge. For example, if an English-speaking patient became ill while traveling to Mexico or if a patient from Mexico became ill while traveling to the United States, a translator would be required for understanding. See **Table 3-7**.

SUMMARY

This chapter presented information about health disparities and determinants of health. From this discussion, it is apparent that health is "a state of complete physical, mental, and social well-being and not merely the absence of disease or infirmity."[20] While some individuals reach optimal health, other individuals lack optimal health due to factors outside of their control. In other cases, individuals make poor personal health choices, such as use of tobacco products, lack of exercise, and improper weight management. In any case, evaluators planning, implementing, or evaluating health programs need to understand the impact of health disparities and social determinants of health on health outcomes.

CASE STUDY

After reading the following case study, make a list of the health disparities and social determinants of health that shape the health outcome of the individuals living in this federally subsidized housing complex.

This case is focused on three families that reside in an inner city, federally subsidized high-rise housing unit. There are 90 apartment units in this high-rise complex with a total of 450 residents with an average of five people per unit.

However, some units have two residents, while some have multigeneration families with a total of eight individuals in a single unit.

Family One

The Hawthornes—Jim, age 58, and Nancy, age 54—have been married for 35 years. Jim teaches elementary students in a small church school a few blocks from their apartment. Nancy, a former teacher, stays home to care for her parents. Jim and Nancy are both about 35 pounds overweight and have a family history of diabetes and hypertension. Due to their hectic schedules, they do not take time to exercise. Their net income is $47,000 annually, or $3916 per month. Because Nancy's parents live with them, they qualify for federally subsidized housing. With a tight budget for household expenses, they set aside a little money each month to pay a portion of living expenses for their two children in college. Nancy's parents live on the minimum fixed Social Security retirement income. Jim and Nancy's health insurance is available through the school district and costs $260 per month for themselves and their two children. Because the family does not have any chronic health conditions, they selected the lower monthly cost premium with the higher annual deductible cost of $1000 per person for an annual cost of $4000 for the Hawthorne family. For example, after Nancy pays $1000 of her medical bills, the insurance company begins to pay 80% of medical bills, and then Nancy pays 20% of her medical bills for the remainder of the calendar year. They admit that they probably do not know enough about health, nutrition, and exercise, but they feel fine. In May, Jim experienced moderate chest pain while playing basketball with friends at the local park. After some cardiac tests in the emergency department, he was admitted to the hospital. The next day, the cardiologist conducted a heart catheterization and placed three stents in Jim's blocked arteries with minor complications. The total $120,000 hospital bill included the emergency department tests, anesthesiologist, radiologist, nuclear medicine, operating room time, cardiologist, medications, and hospital room charges. Because Jim had not yet paid his

$1000 annual health insurance deductible, he was required to pay the first $1000 of the medical bill + 20% of the remaining $119,000 bill, which totaled $24,800. Jim and Nancy did not have enough money in savings, so they established a 36-month payment plan of $688 per month with the hospital. Fortunately, the hospital did not charge any interest. This additional monthly expense put further strain on all aspects of the family budget. Due to his declining heart condition, Jim was required to retire early from teaching, and they sold their second car. Living on Jim's small retirement check, they struggled to pay any portion of their children's college expenses. Their children moved home and got part-time jobs. Currently, there are six individuals in their two-bedroom apartment.

Family Two

Lynette, age 23, lives down the hall from Jim and Nancy. She has three children all under the age of 6 years. She works full-time at the Head Start preschool that her two youngest children attend. The oldest child is in first grade. Lynette earns $9 per hour, and her monthly take-home salary is about $1400 after taxes. Because the Head Start program is federally subsidized, whenever there is a federal budget cut, her hours are reduced or the preschool closes for a few days. Because Lynette is a kind person, she is willing to look in on Nancy's parents whenever Nancy needs to attend to personal appointments. Nancy takes care of Lynette's children occasionally in the evening, so Lynette can get some time to study. Currently, she is enrolled in two online courses that are required before she enters cosmetology school in the fall. She will need to quit her preschool job when her cosmetology courses begin full-time in August. At that time, two children will be in the nearby elementary school. She qualifies for a federal loan to help pay for living expenses. She hopes that no disaster happens and that none of her children get sick during the 3-month cosmetology course. She decided to get licensed as a nail technician and cosmetologist at the same time to expand her employment options upon graduation.

Family Three

Bob, age 77, and his wife, Charlotte, age 76, live downstairs from Lynette. They both worked full-time on an assembly line for a large steel manufacturing company. They retired at age 65 in hopes of receiving full-time company retirement benefits and Social Security for the rest of their lives. The manufacturing company went bankrupt and closed in 2009 during the economic downturn in the United States. As a result, their retirement benefits were cancelled and their Medicare supplement healthcare monthly premium doubled. They had to sell their home of 40 years and move into this one-bedroom federally subsidized unit. They do not have any adult children, and their siblings live in a different state. Their faith-based community of many years is located across town, so they feel displaced from friends and embarrassed about living in this low-income apartment. They do have one car in good condition, but no longer drive at night. Their health is good, but Bob has some issues with hypertension, and Charlotte is coping with arthritis in her knees. They feel depressed and isolated. Their limited monthly income prevents them from participating in enjoyable activities such as dining out or going to the movies. They visit the local library each week because it is within walking distance. They enjoy reading and discussing books with each other. They never expected their retirement years to be so miserable.

STUDENT ACTIVITY

Web of Social Determinants

Review the diagram of the five key areas of the social determinants of health according to *Healthy People 2020*. These five key areas are: economic stability, education, social and community context, health and health care, and neighborhood and built environment.

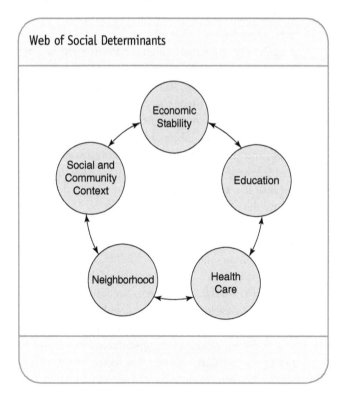

Web of Social Determinants

The following is a story about a woman named Angela. After you have read each portion of the story, think about which social determinant of health affects the story. For example, if you believe education and economics are factors in that part of the story, draw a line from the education circle to the economics circle. Continue drawing lines between social determinants of health for that section until you can think of no more. Then, continue to the next section of the story.

1. Angela lives in an urban city of approximately 2.5 million people. Angela's neighborhood is in an older section of town where not many jobs are available. When Angela was 16 years old, she got pregnant. She had not been on any birth control because Planned Parenthood was on the other side of town and she did not have a car of her own. She was not in a stable, good relationship with the baby's father and decided to break off her relationship with him because of her child.

2. The school asked that she leave school until after she had the baby. Angela's parents did not make a lot of money, but they helped her as much as possible with her pregnancy. Her mother tried to get her enrolled in Medicaid while she was pregnant, but the rules and regulations were very confusing, and there was a lot of paperwork that she had to fill out. Because of this, Angela did not go to her first doctor's appointment until she was almost 6 months' pregnant. Angela's son was born 6 weeks early and was a little bit smaller than most other babies.

3. Angela never returned to high school after she had her baby, because her mother worked during the day and was only able to help watch her son at night. Angela worked stocking shelves at a local store at night, so that she could earn some money to take care of her son. However, her job only let her work 30 hours a week, and she was ineligible for health insurance coverage. Angela couldn't afford to buy her own insurance because it was very expensive, and she needed every penny she could get.

4. When Angela was 23 she met a man who worked as a day laborer in construction and married him. Over the next 5 years they had two children. In order to save money, they moved into an aging two-bedroom, government-subsidized apartment. Not long after moving in, Angela developed a regular cough. She thought it had to do with some mold that she noticed growing in a bedroom closet. Because she could not afford to move, she regularly cleaned the mold, but it always seemed to come back.

5. When Angela was 29 years old, her husband was injured in an accident at work. Because he was a day laborer, he did not have any insurance, and they had to pay all of his hospital bills out of pocket. He was hurt for a long period of time and could not go back to work. He started drinking more than usual as a result of his accident. Angela was forced to pick up extra hours at work and an extra job in order to put food on the table. Thankfully, one of Angela's neighbors helped by watching her children while she was at work.

6. When Angela turned 32 she divorced her husband. She found out that after his accident he had been abusing prescription pain medication. After begging him to stop several times, the final straw came when he was arrested for driving while under the influence. Their youngest child was with him in the car at the time.

7. When Angela was 34 she applied for and received a promotion at her job. She was finally eligible for full-time benefits and health insurance.

8. When Angela was 42, she passed out while at work. When she went to the doctor, she learned that she has diabetes and that her blood sugar had gotten too low. Her doctor recommended that Angela start exercising and making better food choices, as she had gained a lot of weight over several years. Angela found it very hard to make better food choices, as there are a lot of fast food restaurants in her neighborhood, and getting food from them is often cheaper than buying it from the grocery store. Exercising is hard because she doesn't want to walk at night in her neighborhood because it is poorly lit.

9. Now Angela is 47, and she has gotten her diabetes under control and no longer needs to take medication. Her church started a walking club three times a week at a local high school track. Because all of her children have grown and are out of the house, she also has more money for healthier food options.

After you have finished, think about these questions:

1. What did this exercise show us?
2. What social determinants of health are often linked?
3. We often think about social determinants of health as things that are risks. What social determinants of health were benefits to Angela?

REFERENCES

1. Joint National Committee on Prevention, Detection, Evaluation, and Treatment of High Blood Pressure. *Arch Intern Med.* 1997;157:2413–46.

2. Burt BA, Eklund SA. *Dentistry, Dental Practice, and the Community.* Philadelphia: WB Saunders Company. 1999:204–20.

3. Bolen JR, Sleet DA, Chorba T, et al. Overview of efforts to prevent motor vehicle-related injury. In: *Prevention of Motor Vehicle-Related Injuries: a Compendium of Articles from the Morbidity and Mortality Weekly Report,*

1985-1996. Washington, DC: U.S. Department of Health and Human Services, Centers for Disease Control and Prevention; 1997.

4. Centers for Disease Control and Prevention. Fatal occupational injuries—United States, 1980-1994. *MMWR*. 1998;47:297–302. Available at: http://www.cdc.gov/mmwr/preview/mmwrhtml/mm5016a4.htm. Accessed January 12, 2012.

5. Bunker JP, Frazier HS, Mosteller F. Improving health: measuring effects of medical care. *Milbank Q*. 1994;72:225–58.

6. Mokdad AH, Marks JS, Stroup DF, Gerberding JL. Actual causes of death in the United States, 2000. *JAMA*. 2004;291(10):1238–1245.

7. *Healthy People 2020*. About Healthy People. Available at: http://www.healthypeople.gov/2020/about/default.aspx. Accessed May 3, 2012.

8. Kline R, Huang D. *Defining and measuring disparities, inequities, and inequalities in the Healthy People initiative*. National Center for Health Statistics. Centers for Disease Control and Prevention. Available at: http://www.cdc.gov/nchs/ppt/nchs2010/41_Klein.pdf. Accessed October 2, 2013.

9. *Healthy People 2020*. Disparities. Available at: http://www.healthypeople.gov/2020/about/disparitiesAbout.aspx. Accessed October 2, 2013.

10. Braveman PA. Monitoring equity in health and healthcare: a conceptual framework. *J Health Popul Nutr*. 2003;21(3):181.

11. Whitehead M. The concepts and principles of equity and health. *Health Prom Int*. 1991;6(3):217.

12. Kawachi I. A glossary for health inequalities. *J Epidemiol Comm Health*. 2002;56(9):647.

13. *Healthy People 2020*. Implement. Available at: http://www.healthypeople.gov/2020/Implement/default.aspx. Accessed October 2, 2013.

14. *Healthy People 2020*. Implementing Healthy People 2020. Available at: http://www.healthypeople.gov/2020/implementing/default.aspx. Accessed May 3, 2012.

15. Kirsch IS, Jungeblut A, Jenkins L, Kolstad A. *Adult Literacy in America: A First Look at the Results of the National Adult Literacy Survey (NALS)*. Washington, DC: National Center for Education Statistics, U.S. Department of Education; 1993.

16. Centers for Disease Control and Prevention. *Simply Put: A Guide for Creating Easy-To-Understand Materials*. Atlanta, GA: Centers for Disease Control and Prevention; 2010. Available at: http://www.cdc.gov/healthliteracy/pdf/Simply_Put.pdf. Accessed April 18, 2014.

17. National Center for Education Statistics. *The Health Literacy of America's Adults: Results from the 2003 National Assessment of Adult Literacy*. Washington, DC: U.S. Department of Education; 2006.

18. Plain Language Action and Information Network. What Is Plain Language? Available at: http://www.plainlanguage.gov/whatisPL/index.cfm. Accessed January 12, 2012.

19. U.S. Department of Health and Human Services. *National Standards for Culturally and Linguistically Appropriate Services in Health Care*. Washington, DC: Office of Minority Health; 2001.

20. World Health Organization. Definition of Health. Available at: http://www.who.int/about/definition/en/print.html. Accessed April 18, 2014.

CHAPTER 4

Theories and Models

CHAPTER OBJECTIVES

By the end of this chapter, students will be able to:

1. Explain the difference between inductive and deductive reasoning.
2. Evaluate theories and models to determine the most appropriate application for the proposed evaluation.
3. Produce action plans and time management charts for projects.
4. Assess each segment of a strengths, weaknesses, opportunities, and threats (SWOT) analysis for quality improvement.

KEY TERMS

action plans
models
SWOT analysis
theories

INTRODUCTION

This chapter begins with a discussion of theories and models, by exploring various theories and models related to building, planning, and evaluating frameworks. First, the chapter focuses on community theories and then moves on to individual behavior change theories. It is important to note that some references in this chapter are several decades old. These older references are linked to established theories and models that have been stable, valid, and reliable when used in research and evaluation over an extended period of time. This chapter also introduces some theories and models that are current, but have only been used in a few studies. Following

this discussion, the end of the chapter explores strategic planning techniques to achieve goals in the allotted time.

Let's begin with definitions. Depending on the discipline, theories and models are defined using approximately the same terms. In other disciplines, models are used to develop theories or are used independent of theories. A theory is a set of related concepts that present a systematic view of events, issues, and situations in order to explain them or make predictions, while models generally represent interactions between concepts in order to show patterns.[1] In science, theory is based on tested and observable facts. Once a scientific theory is developed, the facts may be interpreted or investigated by other scientists, but the facts remain the same. Theories are based on fact, laws, and principles, while leaving room for unanswered questions. Over time, theories are challenged and tested. Scientists confirm or refute theories based on reviews within the scientific community. Theories either stand the test of time or are deemed to be lacking credibility. Theories are used to increase and validate knowledge. Some theories are limited to one discipline, while other theories are used across disciplines. For example, behavioral change theories are used across disciplines to modify individual behavior to improve health outcomes. Theories are used to test a hypothesis, investigate a phenomenon, or validate an existing body of knowledge. In some disciplines, such as nursing, theories are used to establish and guide practice. The remainder of this chapter provides examples of universal scientific theories followed by theories and models related to systems, communities, and individual behaviors. The chapter ends with a presentation of theories used for strategic planning.

TYPES OF THEORIES AND MODELS

Communities and Organizations

This section describes various types of theories and models used in planning programs and evaluations. The theories and models described begin with the Ecological Model,[2,3] because it shows broad associations from individuals to organization to community policy development. The discussion introduces theories and models related to communities and organizations, including the PRECEDE-PROCEED Model, Social Networks and Social Support Theory,[4] Diffusion of Innovations Theory,[5] and the RE-AIM Model.[6] Last, numerous theories attempt to explain, predict, or change human behavior. As with any theory, these theories have been modified for improvement. The theories presented include the Health Belief Model,[7] Stages of Change Model or Transtheoretical Model,[8] and Social Learning Theory or Social Cognitive Theory.[9]

Ecological Model

In 1979, Bronfenbrenner developed the Ecological Model,[2,3] also sometimes called the socio-ecological model or ecological framework, with a focus on the interaction between behavioral patterns and social environmental factors. Five main constructs of this model include the following (see also **Figure 4-1**):

- *Intrapersonal factors*: Is an individual willing to change one or more characteristics, such as knowledge, attitudes, skills, or intention, to conform to social norms? For example, individuals with a desire to begin a weight-loss program seek information, because they are trying to conform to the social norm.
- *Interpersonal relationships*: Are social networks (family, friends, coworkers, and acquaintances) providing positive or negative influences on a person's health behavior? For example, an alcoholic individual enjoys a social network of alcoholic friends because negative health behavior is the social norm of the group. When individuals join Alcoholic Anonymous, they establish a

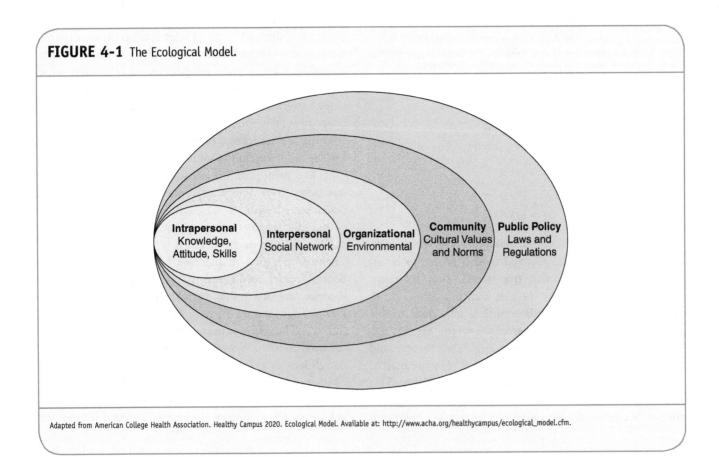

FIGURE 4-1 The Ecological Model.

Adapted from American College Health Association. Healthy Campus 2020. Ecological Model. Available at: http://www.acha.org/healthycampus/ecological_model.cfm.

new positive social norm with new friends who strive to remain free of drinking alcohol over time.

- *Organizational factors*: Is the organization providing positive or negative influences on the wellness of the employees? For example, the campus recreation center offers a substantial discount to all university employees. This incentive shows the university's commitment to the health and wellness of the employees as well as the students.
- *Community factors*: Are the individuals in power at the community level providing positive or negative influences on the overall health of others? Community can be defined as family, church, informal social networks, or geographic area. Because communities compete for scarce resources, there needs to be a coordinated effort to allocate resources equitably. Too often, individuals with the lowest literacy skills (e.g., poor, rural, disabled, homeless, minorities, and unemployed) receive the least amount of educational services. For example, the city council voted to build a new library with ample classroom space, free daycare services, and adult education programs on the campus of the elementary school in a low-income housing development. This library changed the environment and provided numerous positive educational, health, and social benefits. The educational programs, such as high school equivalency classes, computer skills training, English as a second language, adult reading, and book clubs, were offered at convenient times for working parents. The full service library became a focus for enhanced social support networking among neighbors, improved safety, and community pride.
- *Public policy*: Is the purpose of the proposed national, state, or local public policy aimed at improving and protecting the population's health? For example, the decision to make a law requiring that bike helmets be worn by all riders 16 years of age and younger was based on research on types of bike injuries that could have been avoided or minimized if the child had been wearing a bike helmet.

PRECEDE-PROCEED Model

The PRECEDE-PROCEED Model[10] is used for community-based program planning, implementation, and evaluation. For maximum effectiveness, it is recommended that the entire community should be involved from the beginning. The PRECEDE-PROCEED model serves as a guide for individual and long-term community projects. As with most models, it guides the process rather than being a step-by-step procedure. Now let's break the model into two parts. PRECEDE determines what needs to be done prior to the implementation and stands for *Predisposing, Reinforcing,* and *Enabling Constructs in Educational/environmental Diagnosis and Evaluation*.[10] PROCEED stands for *Policy, Regulatory,* and *Organizational Constructs in Educational and Environmental Development* and determines how to progress to the intervention.[10] Together, there are eight phases: four phases in PRECEDE and four phases in PROCEED. See **Figure 4-2**. Notice that Figure 4-2 is circular. The model begins in the upper right-hand corner with quality of life issues and goes counterclockwise through PRECEDE. Across the bottom, PROCEED begins with Phase 5 and ends with Phase 8 as the outcome evaluation.

PRECEDE (Phases 1–4) Phase 1: Social assessment— Determine the ultimate desired goal of the program or intervention.[10] The goal of most health programs is to improve quality of life. For this discussion, let's use the example of how quality of life improves when air pollution decreases. For social assessment, evaluators collect information from hospital records to determine if hospital admissions increase due to asthma during times when there are rates of high air pollution. Besides hospital records, this information is also obtained by conducting community surveys, focus groups, interviews, and public town hall meetings. It is important to involve the community at the first step of social assessment and throughout the entire process to achieve maximum participation and buy-in.

Phase 2: Epidemiological assessment—Investigate the data associated with the health and community issues (behavioral, environmental, lifestyle) that might help or hinder attaining the goal of the program.[10] Using the previous example, the environmental community issue of insufficient public transportation hinders the goal of decreasing air pollution levels. The health and community issues can be defined as follows:

- *Behavioral* issues relate to specific and measurable actions based on data. For example, counties collect information on public bus ridership per route to determine how to change bus routes to meet the needs of the community and increase ridership.
- *Environmental* issues relate to the natural and physical characteristics of the community. Issues such as garbage pickup, sewer repair, housing density, and general street maintenance affect the overall quality of the air. Social environment refers to community attitudes regarding certain actions such as increasing bike lanes, enforcing bike laws, and requiring bike helmet usage for all ages.

FIGURE 4-2 PRECEDE-PROCEED model.

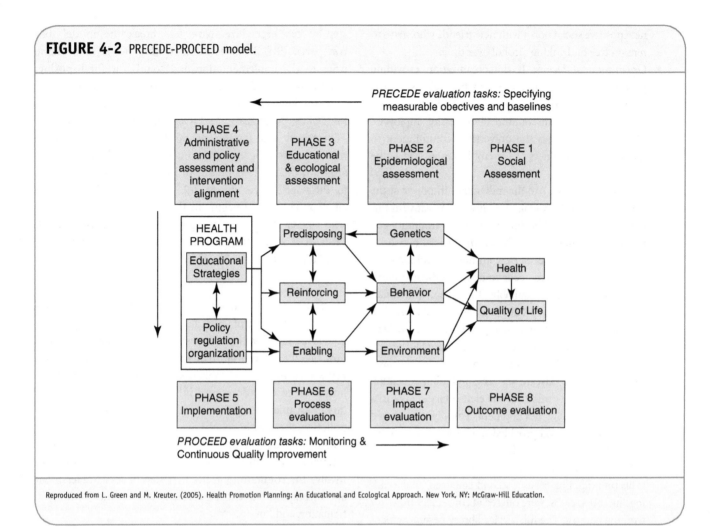

Reproduced from L. Green and M. Kreuter. (2005). Health Promotion Planning: An Educational and Ecological Approach. New York, NY: McGraw-Hill Education.

Economic environmental issues include low bus fares to increase ridership, incentives for carpooling, and convenient parking lots for individuals who choose to utilize public transportation.

- *Lifestyle behaviors* are a collection of behaviors that form a pattern of living that positively or negatively influence health outcomes. For example, if a family lives in an industrial and manufacturing neighborhood, the children have a greater likelihood of exposure to toxic air pollutants that may induce asthma at a younger age. This high level of air pollution. also decreases participation in outdoor activities for children and families.

Phase 3: Identify the predisposing, enabling, and reinforcing factors that influence the issues noted in Phase 2:[10]

- *Predisposing factors* influence whether or not an individual is likely to adopt healthy or risky behaviors. Predisposing factors include knowledge, attitude, beliefs, values, and confidence. For example, if an individual

has never learned the connection between air pollution and asthma, he or she may engage in outdoor activities during peak times of air pollution. A second example relates to confidence. If individuals with asthma are not confident in their skills regarding when to use their inhalers, they are less likely to use the inhaler daily to prevent asthma attacks and instead use their inhaler as a rescue inhaler as needed.

- *Enabling factors* are the internal and external factors that determine if an individual adopts and maintains positive or negative health behaviors; these include availability and accessibility of resources, laws, policies, and community commitment. For example, the community commits to incorporating adequate bike lanes into all existing main streets and new road construction. This type of road construction shows a community commitment to increasing safe bike ridership and increasing healthy weight management of the population.

- *Reinforcing factors* support the effort to encourage and support the planned health efforts. For example, there is support for clean industry and manufacturing corporations in communities that provide tax incentives for decreasing emissions of air pollutants, thus fostering healthy environments. In addition, city council members vote to impose tax penalties on those corporations that fail to reduce polluting emissions within a 3-year time frame.

Phase 4: Identify administrative and financial polices needed to influence what needs to be implemented.[10] For example, if the city council votes to add bike lanes, there needs to be adequate funding available in the city budget. Without funding, votes from city council members show commitment, but no ability to make the changes actually happen.

PROCEED (Phases 5–8) Monitoring the evaluation

Phase 5: Design and conduct the intervention. Based on the data from Phases 1–4, the program planner sets up and implements the planned intervention.

Phase 6: Evaluate the process. Process evaluation determines if the intervention is doing what was planned. This phase is about the procedures rather than the results. For example, if the intervention was to offer incentives for carpooling to reduce traffic congestion and pollution, the process evaluation investigates if there are more people carpooling to work on a daily basis as planned.

Phase 7: Evaluate the impact. Impact evaluation involves whether or not the intervention had the desired impact on the target population. For example, if the public transportation adds more routes and busses, how many people have started riding the bus to work?

Phase 8: Evaluate the outcomes. Outcome evaluation determines to what extent the intervention led to the planned outcome. For example, if the numerous interventions are initiated in a community (increased tax for industry with high air pollution emissions, incentives to attract clean industries, increased bike lanes for all new highway construction, enforced bike helmet laws, improved bus routes to enhance ridership, incentives for carpooling, etc.), is the air pollution decreasing and are the hospital admissions for asthma decreasing? Keep in mind that some interventions take years before the results are noted in community statistics. Each phase in PROCEED involves conducting a formal evaluation.[10]

RE-AIM Model

The purpose of RE-AIM is to evaluate program interventions to determine the impact of programs.[6] Programs are assessed at the individual, organization, and community levels using five dimensions—reach, efficacy, adoption, implementation, and maintenance:

- *Reach* pertains to the individual level and establishes the number or percentage of people who receive the program. To calculate the percentage, it is necessary to know the denominator (total population) and number of participants. Although it is ideal to collect demographic data on participants and nonparticipants, ethical issues arise because nonparticipants may not have consented to participate. In some cases, if a large community intervention is studied, evaluators use census data. At this level, similarities or differences between participants and nonparticipants are verified at the baseline.
- *Efficacy* relates to the individual's assessment of positive and negative program outcomes and the need to include physiologic, behavioral, quality of life, and participant satisfaction outcomes.
- *Adoption* refers to the organization or community and establishes the percentage of locations, such as worksites, health departments, and schools, that adopted the program. Direct observation, interviews, and surveys determine the level of adoption. At the same time, barriers to adoption are investigated.
- *Implementation* is the fidelity of the program, or the extent to which the program was provided as intended. At the individual level, participant adherence and follow through is measured as the outcome. At the organization or community level, implementation is measuring staff involvement and implementation fidelity.
- *Maintenance* is the most challenging at the individual, organization, and community levels. Individuals relapse into previous behaviors. Unless polices are changed and enforced at the organization and community levels, health behavior programs are not sustained. See **Box 4-1**.

Social Networks and Social Support Theory

In 1985, Gottlieb developed the Social Networks and Social Support Theory[4] to recognize how behavior change occurs when individuals have social networks and social support in their community. Social networks are groups of family members or friends and include the following characteristics:

- *Structure*: Is there a defined group size with common goals or activities?
- *Interaction*: Does the relationship among members include mutual sharing? Do the members contact each other frequently? Are the relationships long term?
- *Function*: Do the relationships offer social support, resource connections, and a sense of social identity?

BOX 4-1 RE-AIM Case Study

One year after the implementation phase, the furniture factory manager hired an external evaluator to determine the success of the worker safety policy. This factory is the main source of income for this rural county. The RE-AIM Model was used for the worker safety policy evaluation:

Reach: It was necessary to determine approximately how many individuals worked at the furniture factory. Once that number was estimated, the factory used personnel files to determine how many employees were injured and how many employees were not injured 1 year after the worker safety training. Surveys and interviews were conducted with representative groups to determine knowledge, attitudes, and beliefs about the current worker safety policy and how the policy was implemented.

Efficacy: The furniture factory initiated a number of worker safety classes and provided free hard hats, gloves, back support belts, and steel-toed shoes for all employees who worked in the factory excluding office staff. Over the year of implementation, data were collected on the positive and negative consequences and on the participants' satisfaction.

Adoption: To ease the implementation, the furniture factory hired a part-time health educator to answer questions, teach the safety classes, and direct individuals wishing to obtain the free safety equipment. Surveys were collected and interviews were conducted by the health educator to determine the success of the adoption phase with a special emphasis on the barriers to adopting the worker safety policy. Throughout the year, data were collected on the number of individuals injured after completing the worker safety classes and utilizing the safety equipment provided.

Implementation: After 1 year, the pre-policy data, first month of policy data, and end-of-year data were analyzed to determine the effectiveness of the implementation. Were fewer employees injured? Were the injuries less severe than before the worker safety policy? How many employees registered, attended, and completed the four-session worker safety classes? How many items of worker safety equipment were distributed?

Maintenance: One year after the worker safety policy was enacted, data were collected again to verify that the policy had been institutionalized and the number of employee injuries in the furniture factory decreased in number and severity.

Social supports include the following characteristics:

- *Emotional support*: Do the individuals listen and show concern toward each other?
- *Instrumental support*: Do the individuals offer actual tangible or physical support, such as financial support or time?
- *Informational support*: Do the individuals give genuine advice, directions, or resource referral information?
- *Appraisal support*: Do the individuals provide positive feedback to each other? Keep in mind that not all social networks offer genuine social support to the individuals involved.

When evaluating social support organizations, it is good to review the mission statement of the organization and to learn a little about the retention of individuals in the social support groups. For example, the American Cancer Society offers Reach To Recovery social support groups for women with breast cancer. The groups are free, open to the public, and provide advice and support to those women going through breast cancer treatment and recovery. Another well-known and positive social support group is Alcoholic Anonymous. It is open to all members worldwide with no fee attached for the support. On the other hand, some organizations claim to offer social support, but upon further investigation, social support ends when individuals fail to pay mandatory membership fees, question the organizational mission statement, or miss too many meetings. For example, a weight-loss organization requires weekly dues and offers support, advice, and positive feedback for reaching weight-loss goals. However, as soon as the individual stops paying weekly dues, the support, guidance, and praise stop immediately.

Diffusion of Innovations Theory

Diffusion of Innovations Theory[5] explains how individuals adopt new ideas, products, and social practices across a community or from one community to another. For the diffusion process to work, it is necessary to describe adopters and rate of adoption. Adopters are individuals that accept change at various rates:

- *Innovators*: Individuals that seek out the latest technology, product, or activity

- *Early adopters*: Individuals that like innovation, but are not the first in line at the store
- *Early majority*: Individuals that wait until they receive some external motivation before getting involved in the change
- *Late majority*: Individuals that are not willing to make any change until most people have made the change; they have a wait-and-see attitude toward change
- *Laggards*: Individuals that are last to buy into the change in spite of constant exposure or that have limited access to the typical communication networks

Engaging innovators is critical for success and involves studying the characteristics of innovation. These characteristics include:

- *Relative advantage*: Is this change or innovation perceived as better than the current product or service?
- *Compatibility*: Is the change or innovation perceived as consistent with the past experiences?
- *Complexity*: Is the change or innovation perceived as difficult to understand or use?
- *Flexibility*: Is it possible for the adopter to try out the change or product prior to adopting the change?
- *Observability*: Is it possible for the adopter to observe others using or adapting to the change or innovation?

For example, when "hybrid cars" were first available, manufactures emphasized the advantages over other new cars on the market. At the time, the price of gasoline was increasing rapidly, so car dealerships did not have to offer incentives for purchasing them. In fact, most dealerships had trouble keeping enough hybrid cars in stock to meet the demand. Soon the price of gasoline plateaued, so the hybrid car–buying surge flattened. Car dealerships had to start promoting their product to gain the market share of early adopters and early majority buyers. In the meantime, more car manufacturing brands started producing their own hybrid cars. Some car dealerships began offering discount pricing and rebates to first-time buyers. Last, as more and more consumers purchased hybrid cars, their social network observed the comfort and cost savings of driving a hybrid car.

Keep in mind that an individual may be an early adopter for one behavior or product and a late adopter for another innovation. For example, an individual may be an early adopter for driving a hybrid car, but may be the late majority when it comes to exchanging their green lawns for xeriscaping with draught-resistant plants and using less water and pesticides in drought-prone areas. Over time, individuals accept or reject the innovation or perhaps adopt a later

version of the same innovations after further modifications are made to increase consumer satisfaction. For example, the homeowners' association may vote to convert all green space to xeriscaping to decrease the overall cost of lawn and grounds maintenance.

Last, without successful communication, innovations are not successful. There are two basic communication channels: interpersonal and mass media. First, interpersonal or face-to-face communication is considered the most effective method of innovation adoption. Second, mass media channels are a rapid and effective way to create awareness and knowledge about the innovation. Mass media channels include radio, television, newspapers, billboards, magazines, brochures, direct-mail marketing, phone solicitation, and social media websites. Although mass media reaches a larger audience, it is less effective in changing individual behaviors. For example, when manufacturers developed a gum to help people stop smoking, they used communication to make the product successful. The company gave free nicotine gum samples to health educators teaching smoking-cessation classes. This technique allowed health educators to distribute the nicotine gum to patients face-to-face and talk about the health benefits related to smoking cessation. At the same time, the nicotine gum manufacturer focused on mass media by advertising in print media with discount coupons and mail-in rebates, along with radio and television advertising. Many smokers considered the nicotine gum as a way to stop smoking, even though limited research was conducted on the effectiveness of the gum in smoking cessation.

Individual Behavior Theories and Models

Health Belief Model

The Health Belief Model[7] was developed in the 1950s by psychologists who assumed that individuals fear disease and that the degree of fear determines their motivation to seek preventive health services. Simply, actions to reduce fear motivate individuals to act.[7] The Health Belief Model consists of four constructs related to perceived threats and net benefits. See **Table 4-1**.

The Health Belief Model incorporates cues to action, which are internal or external events that motivate individuals to act. An internal event is feeling a breast lump and scheduling a mammogram appointment. An external event is having a close relative be diagnosed with a specific disease or health condition, viewing a public service announcement, or reading a healthcare brochure. The external examples activate an individual's readiness to take action. For example, an overweight male who smokes two packs of cigarettes each day reads multiple brochures about weight loss and smoking

TABLE 4-1 The Health Belief Model Constructs

Construct	Question	Example
Perceived susceptibility	Does the individual think that he or she is at risk of getting the health condition or disease?	A 45-year-old Indian female living in a tribal area outside of Mumbai does not perceive a personal risk for cervical cancer because no one in her family has ever had cervical cancer.
Perceived severity	How serious does the individual think the health condition or disease is?	A 20-year-old female in Detroit, Michigan does not perceive the need to receive an HPV vaccine, because she is not aware of the potentially serious and long-term conditions that may result from an undiagnosed sexually transmitted disease.
Perceived benefits	Does the individual believe the suggested action would decrease the risk of impact of the health condition or disease?	An overweight, 48-year-old male attorney with a stressful job who has had diabetes for more than 10 years does not perceive any value or health benefits from exercising a few days per week to lose 10–15 pounds.
Perceived barriers	What is the individual's opinion on the real or psychological costs of the suggested action?	A 50-year-old African American woman is afraid to mention a changing mole on her ear, because she is very afraid that she might need surgery that requires removal of a portion of her ear.

cessation, but he does not begin to change his behavior until his health insurance premiums increase due to his risk status.

In 1977, Bandura[11] added self-efficacy to the Health Belief Model. Self-efficacy is the individual's confidence that he or she has the ability to perform the suggested action successfully. For example, if a woman does not believe that she has the ability to remember how to correctly use the exercise machines at her gym, she is less likely to use the machines for fear of sustaining an injury from misuse.

Stages of Change Model or Transtheoretical Model

In the early 1980s, Prochaska and DiClemente published the Stages of Change or Transtheoretical Model, which describes the stages of an individual's readiness to change a specific health behavior.[8] The six-stage model is used to predict either adding a positive behavior or dropping a negative behavior. See **Table 4-2**.

The Stages of Change or Transtheoretical Model is a circular rather than a linear model. Often, individuals revert to undesired behavior during the action or maintenance stage. It is common for individuals to go through the stages several times prior to achieving success of extinguishing a negative behavior or engaging in a positive behavior.

Theory of Reasoned Action

In 1975, the Theory of Reasoned Action was developed to predict and to understand human behavior; it has four constructs.[12] See **Table 4-3**.

Social Learning Theory or Social Cognitive Theory

Social Learning Theory combines interactive factors to understand human behavior.[9] See **Table 4-4**.

In addition, the theory involves three types of reinforcement to influence behavior change: 1) direct reinforcement—the individual receives a reward for performing the behavior; 2) vicarious reinforcement—the individual sees someone else receive a reward for performing the behavior; and 3) self-management, self-control reinforcement—the individual gains control by tracking personal behavior, and personal rewards reinforce the positive behavior. For example, when individuals join a weight-loss group, they learn how to eat healthy and exercise more (behavioral capacity). They see others in the group record their weight loss each week, so they have an expectation of losing weight. The weekly meetings offer the type of environment to assist individuals seeking a healthy weight-loss program. Their behavior is reinforced, because they lose weight each week (direct) and observe others (vicarious) receive applause and certificates each week for achieving weight-loss goals. After tracking their prescribed food and exercise plan, they gain control over food and exercise to achieve and maintain their ideal weight.

STRATEGIC PLANNING MODELS

Now that this chapter has covered several theories and models related to behavior change, the discussion moves to strategic planning skills that are required when planning a

TABLE 4-2 Stages of Change Model or Transtheoretical Model

Stage	Question	Example
Precontemplation	Is the individual aware that the behavior is a problem?	Patient experiencing tooth pain is not ready to schedule a dental appointment due to fear of dental procedures.
Contemplation	Has the individual seriously thought about changing the behavior in the near future?	Patient wants to have a dental exam in the next few months.
Preparation	Is the individual planning to take action? Is the individual making arrangements prior to changing behavior?	Patient is going to schedule a dental examination when he gets paid in a few weeks and is investigating the cost of dental procedures at several dental offices in his neighborhood.
Action	Is the individual implementing a specific action plan to modify behavior and surroundings?	Patient schedules the appointment and goes to the appointment. After the appointment, he schedules another appointment for 6 months later.
Maintenance	Is the individual continuing the desirable actions? Is the individual repeating the actions to prevent lapses and relapse?	Patient keeps the dental appointment that was scheduled 6 months earlier.
Termination	Does the individual have the ability to resist temptation and relapse?	Over the next 2 years, the patient scheduled and kept four dental appointments for routine cleaning.

TABLE 4-3 Constructs in Theory of Reasoned Action

Four Constructs in the Theory of Reasoned Action	Example
One: Individuals believe that if a behavior is performed a given outcome will occur.	If individuals quit smoking, they believe that their chances of staying healthy are increased.
Two: Behavior is influenced by motivation to comply with social norms.	If their workplace is sponsoring a smoking-cessation course, workers are likely to follow social norms and be motivated by coworkers to quit smoking.
Three: Attitude plays a role in behavior. If an individual has a positive attitude, the outcome is likely to be favorable, or if an individual has a negative attitude, the outcome is likely to be less favorable.	Individuals who tried to quit smoking with the nicotine patch and did *not* get sick while using it are more likely to remain nonsmokers by using the nicotine patch for a few weeks. Individuals who tried to stop smoking previously and felt sick while using the nicotine patch are less likely to keep using the patch. Also individuals who never tried to quit smoking and rarely get sick are less likely to quit smoking in the future.
Four: Subjective norms affect beliefs. If an individual believes that his or her social peer group is in favor or opposed to a certain behavior, this perception impacts the motivation to comply with peers.	If individuals believe (with or without evidence) that their coworkers quit smoking, then they are also more likely to quit smoking.

TABLE 4-4 Constructs of Social Learning Theory

Construct	Question	Example
Behavioral capability	Does the individual have the knowledge and skills necessary to perform a specific behavior that impacts future actions?	After attending five classes with a physical therapist, did individuals with work-related back injuries obtain the knowledge and skills necessary to prevent a reoccurrence of their back injury in the future?
Expectations	Does the individual expect a specific outcome for performing a behavior?	After attending five classes with a physical therapist, did individuals with work-related back injuries expect that the prescribed exercises would lower their chances of future back injuries?
Self-efficacy	Does the individual have an adequate sense of self to do what it takes to change a behavior?	After attending five classes with a physical therapist, did individuals with work-related back injuries have a personal desire to follow the prescribed exercise plan to lower their chances of future back injuries?
Environment	How is the individual changing his or her environment and at the same time being changed by the environment?	After attending five classes with a physical therapist, individuals with work-related back injuries learn how to lower their risk of future back injuries by changing their work habits and wearing a back brace during work hours. After this change, did the individuals report that it was easier to follow the prescribed exercise plan because not following the exercise plan caused their back to ache?
Reinforcement	What type of reinforcement is influencing an individual to change a behavior?	After attending five classes with a physical therapist, what type of reinforcement did individuals with work-related back injuries receive when attempting the required behavioral changes? Did the individuals receive praise from supervisors for wearing their back brace to prevent future back injuries?

new project, evaluating an existing project, or determining procedures to revamp an organization. The easiest way to define strategic planning is to answer the following questions:

- Where is the project currently?
- Where does the project hope to be in 1 year?
- How and what needs to be accomplished to meet the goal?

There are numerous benefits of strategic planning; it provides a roadmap for how the project is conducted from beginning to completion. A few examples of how a project benefits from strategic planning include: 1) establishing realistic and achievable objectives for each goal, 2) developing a sense of ownership among the team members, 3) prioritizing use of key resources, 4) allowing the opportunity to listen to team member opinions prior to initiating the first step of the project, 5) creating and reviewing the time management chart together to avoid time conflicts in the future, and 6) addressing potential internal conflicts among team members. To avoid complaints that strategic plans are developed but never used, it is important to update and refer to them

at regular intervals. Think of the strategic plan as a process rather than a final product. For example, it serves no purpose for a College of Public Health to spend several months revising the strategic plan, core values, and mission statement of the college if the changes and recommendations in the plan are never implemented or are not revisited by the administration, faculty, and students every few months to ensure implementation of the recommended changes.

There are two common types of strategic planning models. One is goal based and the other is issue based. Goal-based strategic planning involves starting with a goal or mission statement and then developing the action plan to meet the goals (e.g., improve air quality inside a sewing factory). Issue-based strategic planning begins with examining the issues or problems that need to be addressed, then prioritizing the issues and working toward an action plan to solve the problems (e.g., improving the types of air filters used in the sewing factory, lowering the cost of air filters to encourage more frequent changes, decreasing the number of hours worked per shift in the sewing factory to reduce exposure to fabric fibers, negotiating fair wages for sewing factory workers, negotiating union standards for sewing factory workers). For maximum collaboration and participation, engagement of diverse stakeholders is ideal in the development of either type of action plan. Once the action plan is developed and agreed upon, it is necessary to use a time management chart to ensure timely completion of the project.

This section describes several tools to assist with tracking the progress of the action plan over time. There are many ways to manage simple to complex projects, including elaborate computer software programs, Gantt charts, action plans, and SWOT analysis, all of which are described in the following paragraphs. Regardless of the tracking tool selected, it is important to utilize a management system tool for each project.

Gantt Charts

Gantt charts illustrate schedules, tasks, and activities over a specific time period of the project. See **Figure 4-3**. Because Gantt charts are viewed by the entire team, everyone is aware of start and finish dates of each aspect of a project. By using shading for percentage completed, the vertical line stays current to the present. Some Gantt charts provide details of relationships between activities and the team members responsible for completion of each task.

Action Plans

Action plans track each step related to goals, objectives, activities, and the person responsible. See **Table 4-5**. This type of action plan reduces confusion about who is responsible for assuring that each activity is completed on time. Action plans are developed with input and collaboration from team members to reduce conflict and misunderstanding of assigned tasks. It is also important to tie the name of the responsible person to job descriptions and personnel

FIGURE 4-3 Example of a Gantt chart.

Project Name: ABC Health

	Tasks	Task lead	Start	End	Duration weeks	% Done	Work Days	Days Complete	Days Left
1	1.1	Sue	1/2	1/20	3	100%	15	15	0
2	1.2	Jane	1/9	1/20	2	80%	10	10	0
3	1.3	Rob	1/9	1/20	2	90%	10	10	0
4	1.4	Sue	1/23	3/31	10	40%	50	15	35
5	2.0	Kelly	1/23	2/6	2	80%	10	10	0
6	2.2	Jane	2/13	3/19	5	2%	25	0	25
7	2.3	John	3/5	3/12	1	0%	5	0	5
8	3.0	Sue	3/5	3/12	1	100%	5	0	5
9	4.0	Rob	3/5	3/19	2	0%	10	0	10
10	4.1	Kelly	3/5	3/26	3	0%	15	0	15
11	4.2	Rob	3/5	3/26	3	0%	15	0	15
12	4.3	Sue	3/5	4/2	4	100%	20	0	20
13	4.4	Jane	3/5	4/2	4	0%	20	0	20
14	4.5	John	3/12	4/2	3	50%	15	15	0

Date columns: 1/2/12, 1/9/12, 1/16/12, 1/23/12, 1/30/12, 2/6/12, TODAY, 2/13/12, 2/20/12, 2/27/12, 3/5/12, 3/12/12, 3/19/12, 3/26/12, 4/2/12

TABLE 4-5 Example of a Detailed 2-Month Action Plan

Goal: Initiate a 3-year plan study to increase usage of public transportation in order to decrease traffic congestion and air pollution from car emissions in the county.

Month	Objective	Activity	Responsible Person(s)
March	By the end of the 2nd week of March, form a community task force with 4 members representing city administrators and 26 individuals representing a cross-section of individuals who ride public transportation and individuals who do not ride public transportation to initiate a 3-year plan to improve the satisfaction of public transportation services within the city limits.	Purchase print, radio, television, and social media advertisement to solicit citizens' participation in the community task force, inviting interested individuals to attend an organizational meeting on March 29 to form a task force to improve the city's public transportation.	Stephen Westin, City Administrative Assistant for Public Transportation Services
		Assign four city administrators from different city units to chair four subcommittees (secondary data, qualitative data, quantitative data, and feasibility) within the task force plus administrative support for each subcommittee.	Lilly Knowles, MBA, Human Resource Director Stephen Westin, Administrative Assistant for Public Transportation Services
	By the end of March, hire two graduate public health students to work on this initiative as part of their thesis related to air pollution from car emissions.	Contact the College of Public Health located on the university campus; place an advertisement; review applications; interview at least three graduate public health students; hire two students; complete paperwork for their salary and tuition payment.	Lilly Knowles, MBA, Human Resource Director Stephen Westin, Administrative Assistant for Public Transportation Services
	By the end of March, a minimum of 26 interested community members will attend the first task force meeting.	Make attendee name tags; have laptop and screen; make colored markers and large white paper tablets on easels available; order nutritious food for meeting; prepare PowerPoint slides for introductory remarks to describe the goals and objectives of task force.	Lilly Knowles, MBA, Human Resource Director Stephen Westin, Administrative Assistant for Public Transportation Services
		Have each participant sign up on the white tablets for their 1st and 2nd choice of the four subcommittees. If interested community members were not able to attend the meeting due to work conflicts, they are invited to email their subcommittee choices to Stephen within 3 days.	Stephen Westin, Administrative Assistant for Public Transportation Services
		Assign participants to subcommittees based on their desired choice so each subcommittee represents a variety of neighborhoods and public transportation ridership. Each subcommittee is overpopulated with members in anticipation of attrition and work schedule conflicts.	Lilly Knowles, MBA, Human Resource Director Stephen Westin, Administrative Assistant for Public Transportation Services
		Arrange date, time, and location for each of the four subcommittees; email or call participants with their subcommittee assignment and other pertinent information.	Stephen Westin, Administrative Assistant for Public Transportation Services

April	By the end of the 4th week in April, the Secondary Data task force subcommittee will meet with the chair and a minimum of four community members.	Agree upon goals and objectives and most convenient time, date, and location for future meetings. For example, a subcommittee goal may be gathering existing secondary data, such as current ridership on each route over the last year.	Janet Johnson, MBA, Public Service Manager Evelyn Schwenzer, Administrative Assistant for Public Service Manager
	By the end of the 4th week in April, the Qualitative Data task force subcommittee will meet with the chair and a minimum of four community members.	Agree upon goals and objectives of this subcommittee and most convenient time, date, and location for future meetings. For example, a subcommittee goal may be interviewing a select number of community members (qualitative data) about their public transportation opinions.	Mark Kendall, City Manager Margaret Riley, Administrative Assistant for City Manager
	By the end of the 4th week in April, the Quantitative Data task force subcommittee will meet with the chair and a minimum of four community members.	Agree upon goals and objectives of this subcommittee and most convenient time, date, and location for future meetings. For example, a subcommittee goal will be to develop a 10-question postcard public transportation satisfaction survey (quantitative data) with return postage for mailing to 1000 randomly selected households within the city limits. The same survey will be posted on the city website and social media sites.	Chris Mitchell, MS, Information Technology Director Bradley Hanson, Intern, Information Technology
	By the end of the 4th week in April, the Feasibility task force subcommittee will meet with the chair and a minimum of four community members.	Agree upon goals and objectives of this subcommittee and most convenient time, date, and location for future meetings. For example, a subcommittee goal may be investigating long-term contracts with current city bus contractor (feasibility data) to determine ability to change bus routes.	Davis March, MBA, Financial Services Coordinator Simon Patel, Administrative Assistant for Financial Services Coordinator

TABLE 4-6 Sample Strengths, Weaknesses, Opportunities, and Threats (SWOT) Analysis

Strengths What is working? Even if the internal team effort is strong, how can it be improved?	Weaknesses Are there problems that could be minimized? Where are the problems located? Are the community stakeholders involved?
Opportunities Are we missing something that would improve the project? Are there additional grants or funding opportunities that we are overlooking?	Threats Are we overlooking a problem? How can we eliminate a possible funding cut? Is any agency providing the same type of program or services?

performance reviews. It is unfair to assign extra or unfamiliar duties to individuals without proper training and support. The preferred method involves having individuals work in pairs within a collaborative work commitment.

Strengths, Weaknesses, Opportunities, and Threats (SWOT) Analysis

While Gantt charts or action plans are valuable tools for tracking progress, it is also important to step back, revisit the strategic plan, and assess the big picture. A SWOT analysis allows the team members to explore the project from various viewpoints that may be overlooked in the daily routine. The most appropriate time to conduct a SWOT analysis is during a team meeting. After starting the discussion with a broad question (e.g., What is this project trying to accomplish?), the discussion moves to the SWOT analysis. **Table 4-6** shows an example of some questions to begin a SWOT analysis. As more questions and responses are added to each box, the big picture emerges for further discussion. The discussion is not a time for finger pointing, complaints, or criticism, but it is a collective way to improve what is working and reduce any problems.

SUMMARY

This chapter covers a variety of theories and models. The theories and models can be applied and used as a framework for designing and evaluating programs in communities and organizations as well as in modifying individual behaviors. The chapter ends with a description of strategic planning models including Gantt charts, action plans, and SWOT analysis.

CASE STUDY

At the university student health clinic near Pune, India, the team members (administrators, clinic staff, health educators, and students) determined the need to promote the human papillomavirus (HPV) vaccine to university students. India ranks highest in number of deaths from cervical cancer (72,825 annually) and represents 26.4% of all women dying of cervical cancer globally.[13,14] Because Rajal, the health educator, has a master's in public health degree with a concentration in evaluation, she was given the task of designing a program plan and evaluation for the HPV vaccine campaign. First, Rajal conducted 10 student focus groups and two faculty focus groups to obtain a general opinion of the HPV vaccine. The focus group data revealed that the male and female students were not interested in receiving the HPV vaccine because they did not perceive any risk of acquiring HPV. Because this perception was the most common response, Rajal decided to utilize the Health Belief Model for the HPV vaccine campaign. After presenting the focus group data to the clinic team members, they made the decision to focus the HPV campaign on female students first, then expand the HPV campaign to include male students in the following semester. See **Table 4-7**.

Case Study Discussion Questions

1. What other theories could have been used?
2. Create the first few steps of the logic model for this case study.

STUDENT ACTIVITIES

1. Write two research questions related to improving community participation in an exercise initiative for diabetes prevention. Select a theory, and write a description about how this theory serves as the framework for designing the clinic intervention.
2. Describe a personal behavior that you would like to change. Select an individual behavior change theory, and write how you could apply the principles of the theory to your personal behavior change.
3. Using a Gantt chart, plot the calendar of assignments for a course that you are taking this semester. Be sure

TABLE 4-7 Health Belief Model Constructs for the HPV Vaccine Campaign

Construct	Question	Example
Perceived susceptibility	Do the female students think that they are at risk of acquiring HPV from a sexual partner?	Even though the female students admit to being sexually active, they did not perceive their susceptibility to HPV. They stated in the focus groups that they would not date anyone with HPV, even though they have no way of determining which males have HPV without a confirmed medical diagnosis.
Perceived severity	How serious do the female students think the HPV is?	Most female students have known an older female relative or friend that died of cervical cancer.
Perceived benefits	Do the female students believe that receiving the HPV vaccine would decrease their risk of acquiring cervical cancer?	Most female students do not believe that receiving the HPV vaccine would decrease their risk of acquiring cervical cancer.
Perceived barriers	What is the individual's opinion on the real or psychological costs of the suggested action?	Female students believe that if other students find out that they received the HPV vaccine, their reputation will be diminished. Other students might think that they are promiscuous. Also, if married females receive the HPV vaccine, the male spouse might question the fidelity of the marriage.

to include a vertical line indicating the current week of the course.

4. Describe a group or organization in which you are a member. Using a SWOT analysis, describe how the group or organization might be improved.

REFERENCES

1. Kerlinger FN. *Foundations of Behavioral Research.* (3rd ed.) New York: Holt, Rinehart and Winston; 1986.

2. McLeroy KR, Bibeau D, Steckler A, Glanz K. An ecological perspective on health promotion programs. *Health Educ Q.* 1988;15(4):351–77.

3. Bronfenbrenner U. *The Ecology of Human Development: Experiments by Nature and Design.* Cambridge, MA: Harvard University Press; 1979.

4. Gottlieb BH. Social networks and social support: an overview of research, practice, and policy implications. *Health Educ Behav.* 1985;12:5–22.

5. Rogers EM, Shoemaker FF. *Communication of Innovations: A Cross-Cultural Approach.* New York, NY: The Free Press; 1971.

6. Glasgow RE, Vogt TM, Boles SM. Evaluating the public health impact of health promotion interventions: the RE-AIM framework. *Am J Public Health.* 1999;89(9):1322–7.

7. Rosenstock IM. Historical origins of the health belief model. *Health Educ Quarts.* 1974;15(2):175–83.

8. Prochaska JO, DiClemente CC. Stages and processes of self-change of smoking: toward an integrative model of change. *J Consult Clin Psychol.* 1983;51(3).

9. Bandura A. *Social Learning Theory.* Englewood Cliffs, NJ: Prentice Hall; 1977.

10. Green L, Kreuter M. *Health Program Planning: An Educational and Ecological Approach.* New York, NY: McGraw-Hill Publishing; 2005.

11. Bandura A. Self-efficacy: toward a unifying theory of behavioral change. *Psychol Rev.* 1977;84(2):191–215.

12. Fishbein M, Ajzen I. *Belief, Attitude, Intention and Behavior: An Introduction to Theory and Research Reading.* Reading, MA: Addison-Wesley; 1975.

13. Chhabra S, Bhavani M, Mahajan N, Bawaskar R. Cervical cancer in Indian rural women: trends over two decades. *J Obstet Gynaecol.* 2010;30(7):725–8.

14. The World Health Organization. Human papillomavirus (HPV) and cervical cancer. Available at: http://www.who.int/mediacentre/factsheets/fs380/en/. Accessed October 2, 2013.

CHAPTER 5

Reliability and Validity

KEY TERMS

external validity
internal validity
pilot testing
random errors
reliability
systematic errors
validity

INTRODUCTION

This chapter introduces the concepts of reliability and validity. Briefly, in quantitative and qualitative evaluation, reliability refers to consistency. The two forms of reliability discussed include stability and internal consistency. Next, the chapter defines validity and discusses the types of validity as well as threats to internal and external validity. It is essential to remember that it is more important to be valid than reliable. Validity is defined as the extent to which a test measures what it purports to measure. Therefore, if the test does not measure the correct concept, it does not matter if it is reliable. Last, the chapter ends with a detailed description of how to conduct a pilot test.

RELIABILITY

If you are asked to describe the word *reliable*, you might think of dependability or trustworthiness (e.g., a dependable car or trustworthy friend). In evaluation, reliability is focused on consistency of the instrument or survey being used, not the respondents. Reliability is related to consistency or ability to repeat results.[1] For example, if you weigh a package on your bathroom scale several times in 2 hours, you are likely to get the same weight of 2.6 pounds each time. This exercise shows that your bathroom scale is reliable and consistent. Next, you take the same package to the post office. The package weighs 2.1 pounds on the official post office scale, which determines the cost of postage of mailing the package. Because the post office scale is frequently calibrated for accuracy, the scale at the post office is reliable (consistent in reporting the same weight each time) and valid (measures what it reports to measure).

Evaluators know that a test is reliable if the results are the same each time it is used with the same individuals. Let's explore why reliability is important. If the test results are not approximately the same each time an individual completes the test, evaluators have no way of determining which of the scores is correct. If the results are different each time the test is used, the test is deemed faulty or unreliable.[2] For example, when environmental scientists send water samples to test for the presence of contaminants, they expect that the machine used to test the water sample is reliable. If the machine is not reliable, environmental scientists may fail to provide the correct information to the county or corporation regarding the level of contaminants in the water supply. This inaccurate result could affect the lives of hundreds of people using this water supply. Environmental scientists count on the reliability of countless tests for clean air and water. These tests keep the population healthy and safe. In another example, if standardized exams are not reliable and an individual obtains a professional license because of those test scores, how may we be certain that they *really* have the knowledge necessary for performing their jobs accurately and safely? From an evaluation standpoint, unreliable tests lead to inaccurate conclusions. The developers of the program that is being evaluated may make important decisions based on these inaccurate conclusions. They may decide to continue a program that truly does not work well or cease one that actually does. Other evaluators may try to duplicate the study or build on the faulty results. Time and resources are unnecessarily wasted until the lack of reliability is discovered.

This section introduces two ways to establish reliability: stability and internal consistency. Because it is not possible to calculate reliability, evaluators can only estimate it. Reliability measurement is beyond the scope of this chapter, so definitions are provided for greater understanding, but without calculations.

Stability

Stability is when the results of a survey or instrument are consistent over time. You can check the stability of an instrument by giving it to an individual to take and then give it to him again to retake after a certain period of time has lapsed; this is called the test-retest technique. Test-retest involves two assumptions. First, the items or observations do not change over time. For example, survey questions are not changed between the first and second administration. Second, the time between the first and second administration is long enough (e.g., several days or weeks depending on the instrument) that participating individuals do not remember their responses. If the results remain stable, then the test is reliable. For example, if students take the Graduate Record Exam the first Saturday of each month for 3 consecutive months, their scores remain somewhat consistent. Another example is the Myers-Briggs Type Indicator of personality types. This instrument claims to remain stable over a person's adult life.[3] However, it should be noted that there are also instruments that are specifically designed to show change over time, such as the Hassles and Uplifts Scales (HSUP), which measures attitudes about daily situations instead of focusing on major life events.[4]

Internal Consistency

Internal consistency is defined as the extent to which each question in a survey is related to the same topic. Internal consistency is also called homogeneity. In quantitative research, evaluators use a split-half technique to measure homogeneity. This technique is done by dividing the entire test or survey into two equal halves (e.g., odd-numbered and even-numbered questions). The two forms are administered to the same individuals. If the odd-numbered questions yield the same results as the even-numbered questions, the entire test is deemed reliable. For example, instructors write 40 questions about information provided in Chapter 26 of an epidemiology textbook. The even-numbered questions are used for Test A and the odd-numbered questions are used for Test B. Both sets of questions for Tests A and B are printed on one form and distributed to the students. Evaluators grade Test A questions to obtain one score, and then grade Test B questions to obtain another separate score. If the whole exam has internal reliability, the Test A and Test B scores should be approximately equal, with all questions measuring concepts related to material covered in Chapter 26. If questions draw from topics in other chapters, the exam lacks internal reliability.[5]

Related to the discussion of internal consistency, readers may see the term *coefficient alpha* or *Cronbach's alpha* used in the literature.[6] Cronbach's alpha is defined as a measurement of internal consistency among a group of items (e.g., survey, test, or interview questions). This measurement allows evaluators to determine how well the items measure different aspects of the same topic.[7] Although the statistical formula to calculate coefficient alpha or Cronbach's alpha is beyond the scope of this chapter, readers should note the range of reliability scores. Cronbach's alpha values range from zero to one. Values closer to one indicate a higher internal consistency than values closer to zero (see **Table 5-1**).[8]

TABLE 5-1 Range of Reliability Scores

Reliability Score	Rating
Equal to or greater than 0.9	Excellent
Equal to or greater than 0.8	Good
Equal to or greater than 0.7	Acceptable
Equal to or greater than 0.6	Questionable
Equal to or greater than 0.5	Poor
Less than 0.5	Unacceptable

For qualitative data, internal consistency is called inter-rater reliability or inter-observational reliability. These terms mean that the scoring or observations remain consistent regardless of the person who is doing it. For example, instructors participate in training on how to score essay exams. Following training, instructors receive identical essay exams from 10 students. When instructors have reliable grading skills, each student grade is consistent among all instructors. If instructors have very different scores on identical students' essay exams, their skills are unreliable and more training is required. For inter-observations, evaluators use a checklist to standardize and increase reliability. For example, evaluators observing adolescents and parents use a checklist to record the number and duration of conversation interactions, the number of family members present, the language spoken, the individuals who initiate conversations, and distractions (television, cell phone, eating, etc.) used by adolescents and parents to pass time while waiting for their food to arrive at a restaurant. Checklists ensure that evaluators are collecting the same type of observational data. Evaluators use the following formula to calculate an inter-rater reliability score:

$$\frac{\text{Number of concurrences}}{\text{number of opportunities for concurrence}} \times 100$$

For example, two evaluators use a predetermined checklist to observe 80 patients in the clinic waiting room. According to their checklist, they agree on 68 out of the 80 ratings. The calculation is $68/80 = 0.85 \times 100 = 85\%$. Therefore, evaluators agree 85% of the time, or their observations have a reliability of 85%.[9] There is an acceptable range of reliability scores for qualitative research, with 90% being excellent and less than 50% being unacceptable. Of the two ways to estimate reliability, each one has advantages and disadvantages.[10] See **Table 5-2**, then practice your skills using **Box 5-1**.

As we move from reliability to validity, it is important to understand the relationship between the two concepts. If a scale is valid, the results should be the same over and over. However, the reverse is not always true. Reliability is about consistency and repeatability. Validity is defined as whether the scale measures what it was intended to measure and if results are generalizable to other populations.[11] **Figure 5-1** illustrates relationships between reliability and validity.[12] Keep in mind that the center of the target is the concept that you are trying to measure. Each dot represents one individual who is completing a survey or interview.

VALIDITY

Let's begin the discussion of validity by looking at how reliability and validity are related. As noted in Figure 5-1, it is possible for a test to have low reliability and low validity, high reliability and low validity, and high reliability and high validity. For example, a depression test appears to be consistent

TABLE 5-2 Estimating Reliability: Advantages and Disadvantages

Ways to Establish Reliability	Type	Advantage	Disadvantage
Stability	Test-retest	Single rater is adequate No need to train teams of raters Less expensive and time consuming	Often difficult to recruit same respondents to respond twice Individuals may not respond as seriously the second time
Internal consistency	Quantitative: Split-half forms	Respondents take both surveys at the same time No need to recruit respondents twice	Need to create a large pool of items
	Qualitative: Inter-rater or inter-observation reliability	Best for observational research, especially when video recording is used Possible option: One rater reviewing video at two different times	Expensive Time consuming Requires team of raters for best results

Data from Trochim MK. Types of Reliability. Research Methods Knowledge Base. Available at: http://www.socialresearchmethods.net/kb/reltypes.php. Updated October 20, 2006. Accessed September 2, 2013.

BOX 5-1 Evaluation Practice Case Study: Reliability

The College of Public Health at State University offers two sections each semester of an epidemiology class, which is required for all newly admitted public health students during their first year. Each semester, professors rotate this teaching assignment. In the fall semester, Dr. Nice taught one section and Dr. Stern taught the other section. Over the years, whenever Dr. Nice teaches, students earn higher final grades than when other professors teach the same course. The administrators are concerned that Dr. Nice is teaching students the test questions rather than teaching the broad application of concepts related to epidemiology. Administrators also note that professors are responsible for creating their own exams. Because the administrators do not have time to investigate their concern, they hired Acme Evaluation Team to investigate the situation. The Acme Evaluation Team began by investigating the internal consistency of the tests offered in the epidemiology classes. They obtain copies of the midterm exams from Dr. Nice, Dr. Stern, and several other professors from previous semesters. Using the split-half technique, the Acme Evaluation Team concluded that the midterm exams were not internally consistent. Some professors emphasized certain topics while other professors highlighted different subject areas on the midterm exams. Once this result was known, the Acme Evaluation Team developed a checklist for observing professors' lectures. The checklist was based on the general concepts from a few specific chapters from the textbook. During the second half of the fall semester, Dr. Nice's and Dr. Stern's lectures were observed by two Acme Evaluation Team members. Based on the checklist, it was apparent that Dr. Nice stressed some textbook materials in particular while Dr. Stern covered each area equally. The inter-rater reliability score of 96% showed consistency on the part of the Acme Evaluation Team. Based on the results of reliability research, the Acme Evaluation Team made the following recommendations to administrators:

1. Standardize the epidemiology course syllabus, so every semester the course remains the same for all professors teaching the course and all first-year public health students enrolled in the course.
2. Update courses as needed to stay current with knowledge.
3. Have professors develop a commonly shared test bank based on the major points from each chapter of the textbook.
4. Have all students take online exams in the computer lab during the regularly scheduled class period; exam questions would be randomly generated by the computer from the commonly developed test bank so that teaching to the test would be prohibited.
5. Students would learn the same material regardless of the professor teaching each section, and professors would save time by not having to develop and grade exams.

The administrators incorporated the recommendations and everyone agreed that the Acme Evaluation Team solved the problem for the College of Public Health.

and reliable. However, after analyzing the data, evaluators discover that it is actually measuring self-esteem rather than depression. In this case, the scale is reliable, but not valid, because it is consistently measuring the wrong construct. It is more important for a test to be valid than to be reliable.

Types of Validity

Validity is defined as the extent to which a test measures what it purports to measure, whereas reliability is focused on consistency.[13] There are several types of validity called internal validity, including face validity, criterion-related validity, construct validity, and content validity.

Face Validity

Face validity examines how the test appears. Does the test look reasonable? Does it appear to be well designed? Is the test appealing? Face validity is not based on theory, but merely the appearance of the test (e.g., potential ease of completion, comprehension, and readability). Evaluators strive for excellent face validity. Even though the test may not be reliable, it at least looks good. Think of face validity as "showing up in the correct outfit." The individual looks good at the job interview, but there may or may not be enough experience to back up the good looks to land the job. However, keep in mind that first impressions are important, and without the

FIGURE 5-1 Comparing reliability and validity.

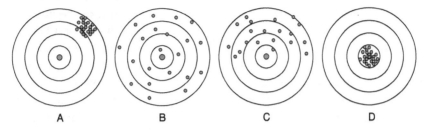

A   B   C   D

A: Reliable but not valid: Dots are consistently measuring the wrong concept.
B: Low reliability and low validity: Dots are spread across the target; low consistency and low measurement of concept.
C: Neither reliable nor valid: Dots are inconsistent, measuring the wrong concept and missing the target.
D: Both reliable and valid: Dots are packed closely in the center; consistently measures the correct concept.

Reproduced with permission of William M.K. Trochim. Available at http://www.socialresearchmethods.net/kb/relandval.php.

right outfit, the interview may begin poorly. The same is true with evaluation surveys; if the survey does not "show up in the right outfit" (i.e., look appealing) then individuals are less likely to complete it.[14] Face validity also refers to the logical sense of the survey. For example, if respondents are told that the survey they are about to complete is seeking their level of satisfaction with clinic services, but the survey questions are all related to utilization of clinic services, the survey would lack face validity.

Criterion-Related Validity

Criterion-related validity measures one topic in two different ways. In other words, just because students pass the written test does not mean that they can perform a specific skill. For example, suppose evaluators are establishing criterion-related validity for intravenous (IV) placement technique among military disaster management students. First, the military disaster management students complete a written test related to proper procedures for IV placement techniques. Following this written test, evaluators use a checklist when observing military disaster management students during the step-by-step procedure as they insert IV catheters into the patient's forearm. The written test is validated by using the criterion-related strategy of the observation checklist. It is essential that the military disaster management students know the didactic information, but they must also know how to perform the required skill.

Construct Validity

Construct validity is used to measure a concept that is not actually observable. For example, while heart rate during exercise on a treadmill may actually be observed and felt, something like memory or intelligence cannot.[15] Evaluators establish construct validity by exploring relationships with similar measures, experimental measures, and comparison scores among defined groups.

Relationship with Similar Measures Evaluators are interested in using a newly developed shorter depression scale for adolescents. Adolescents are asked to complete both the older, longer depression scale with established validity and the newly developed shorter depression scale. If the measurements of the established depression scale are similar to the measurements on the new scale, then evaluators conclude evidence of construct validity.

Relationship with Experimental Measures Evaluators create a controlled environment that increases anxiety among assembly workers by turning off the air conditioning in the factory. After 1 hour the workers are uncomfortable, and workers are asked to complete two anxiety scales: one with established validity and a newly developed scale. In the midst of potential anxiety, workers should score higher on both scales. If both scales show similar levels of anxiety, evaluators conclude evidence of construct validity. Note that this scenario serves as an example only, and the reader should recognize the ethical issues in such an evaluation.

Comparison Scores among Defined Groups Evaluators use a newly developed dexterity aptitude test with the hypothesis that adults have varying degrees of dexterity. More than 1000 adults complete the new dexterity aptitude test. If results show that adults in specific fields (e.g., lab technicians, dentists, musicians, chefs, hairstylists) score higher on the new dexterity aptitude test than adults in nondexterity occupations (e.g., lawyers, truck drivers, writers, accountants), then there is evidence of construct validity.[16]

Content Validity

Content validity is defined as how well a test measures the specific content it is intended to measure.[11,17] For example, if evaluators wish to study how global health students learn commonly used prophylactic malaria medications, they design a test. If the test includes questions about tuberculosis pharmacological agents, their test fails content validity.

Threats to Internal Validity

Threats to internal validity are defined as those things that confuse or confound test and survey results and overall findings. Evaluators need to consider threats to internal validity as an alternative explanation for some results. The following discussion explains the nine threats to internal validity. These threats include history, maturation, testing, instrumentation, regression, ceiling and floor effects, attrition, selection, and the Hawthorne effect:

- *History*: History is defined as when an event happens during research that influences the behavior of participating individuals. For example, evaluators are conducting an evaluation on the effectiveness of reducing gun violence on campus by increasing knowledge about personal safety and reporting all suspicious activity. They conduct pretest surveys among undergraduates and offer 3 weeks' worth of seminars on reducing gun violence in all resident halls on campus. Prior to collecting posttest surveys, a campus shooting that receives wide media attention happens at another university. This campus shooting completely changes posttest results.

- *Maturation*: Maturation is defined as the natural changes that occur over time with individuals. For example, evaluators design an evaluation to determine reading comprehension changes from August to May among third-grade students. Results show improvement in reading comprehension skills. Evaluators need to ask if scores improved due to the natural maturation of students and their improved ability to sit still and focus on test questions as they age or if their reading comprehension improved over the school year.

- *Testing*: Testing refers to differences noted from pretest to posttest that can be attributed to students becoming familiar with the test. Changes may not occur due to the intervention, but rather because respondents are familiar with the test. For example, evaluators conduct a food choice seminar for newly diagnosed type 2 diabetic patients and their families. A pretest is conducted at the beginning of the seminar and again at the end. Because the time frame between pretest and posttest collection is less than 3 hours, posttest responses are influenced by familiarity with the survey, perhaps even more so than retention of presented information.

- *Instrumentation*: Instrumentation measures changes in respondent performance that cannot be credited to the treatment or intervention. For example, observers get bored and record data less accurately after 2 hours than they did at the beginning of the observation. Respondents experience fatigue when completing long surveys, so questions at the end are less accurate than questions near the beginning.

- *Regression*: Regression may be defined as some respondents performing well on pretests and poorly on posttests or vice versa merely by chance. This widespread performance for some respondents may have no explanation other than chance. Data from these high pretest/low posttest performances cancel each other, and the overall score is similar to the average mean scores for all participants. This effect is called "regression to the mean." For example, an individual may have an upper respiratory infection and is taking medication during the posttest, but did not have an infection when the pretest was collected. Generally, it is impossible to know what factors influenced the very high or very low test scores.

- *Ceiling effect and floor effect*: These are two subsets of this threat to internal validity. Ceiling effect is when all participating individuals perform extremely well on a pretest and posttest, therefore making it difficult to determine any changes the intervention may have had. Evaluators need to consider if scores are artificially inflated by the observer and not related to treatment. The floor effect occurs when individual performance starts out low and remains low. This effect leads evaluators to think that individuals are unresponsive to treatment, when in fact the low performance may be due to a factor outside of the intervention or treatment altogether. For example, the floor effect could occur if individuals are so ill with the flu that neither standard-of-care flu medication nor new flu treatment medication will achieve therapeutic improvements.

- *Attrition*: Attrition refers to individuals lost from the study. Evaluators match demographics of participating individuals and then randomly assign individuals to treatment or control groups. If a large portion of individuals leaves the study for a variety of reasons, results may reflect more about the individuals that stayed in the study than the treatment conditions of the study. For example, evaluators conduct a 10-year longitudinal study to document benefits of communal living among senior citizens over 70 years of age. Evaluators match individuals living in the community with individuals living in a retirement community. Many participants are lost to follow-up due to natural changes (e.g., illness, disabilities, and death). Results are inconclusive due to characteristics of the remaining participants rather than the living conditions.

- *Selection*: Selection is defined as when participating individuals are different at the onset of the study. Therefore, results are inconclusive based on differences rather than treatment. For example, evaluators are exploring the effectiveness of two different malaria treatments. In India, they recruit individuals to participate in the malaria evaluation for 6 months. When results are inconclusive, evaluators realize that most individuals in Group A treatment were exposed to one type of malaria and most individuals in Group B were exposed to another type of malaria due to geographical locations. Therefore, it is not possible to know if the malaria treatment or type of exposure influenced the results.

- *Hawthorne effect*: The Hawthorne effect gets its name from the workers at the Western Electric Company in Hawthorne, Illinois, who improved their performance when they knew that they were being watched. For example, individuals working on an assembly line perform better when they know that their annual salary increase is based on the number of widgets they make during a given time period. The Hawthorne effect does not only take place in research settings.[18]

Before moving onto the next section, it is important to remember that threats to internal validity should be considered prior to finalizing any evaluation results, and plans should be made about how they will be avoided during survey creation, data collection, and data analysis.[19–21]

Threats to External Validity

External validity is defined as the generalizability of results. In other words, if the evaluation is repeated with different populations, situations, time, or environments, the results are expected to be the same. A threat to external validity might explain how generalizations are incorrect.[22] Repeating the evaluation in different populations is the best way to access generalizability. This section explores factors that influence generalizability including population, environment, temporal/sequential factors, participants, testing and treatment interaction, reactive arrangements, and multiple treatment conditions.

Generalizability is linked to independent variables. Just as a quick review, there are independent and dependent variables. Independent variables are the variables that researchers manipulate and control. Dependent variables are fixed and not manipulated. For example, if evaluators are interested in how the amount of sleep affects athletic performance, the independent variable is sleep, and the dependent variable is athletic performance; the amount of sleep can be manipulated (e.g., 4 hours, 6, hours, 8 hours, and 10 hours). Evaluators control the number of hours of sleep by having participants stay in a sleep lab at night and waking them up after 4, 6, 8, and 10 hours of sleep. They have each participant walk on a treadmill at a comfortable speed for 30 minutes and do bicep curls with 5-pound weights at 8:00 a.m., noon, and 8:00 p.m. The evaluators would determine if the participants with less sleep were more likely to walk a shorter distance and do fewer bicep curls. Now let's apply this example to factors that influence generalizability, or threats of external validity:

- *Population (also known as selection and treatment)*: When population selection is too specific, treatment is matched to a specific sample and not applicable to a wider population. For example, the sleep study was conducted with a specific age group, so the evaluators need to repeat the evaluation with another group. If the sleep study was conducted with young adults and found that lack of sleep had minimal effect on athletic performance, evaluators need to repeat the study with older adults to determine if results are statistically similar or different. If athletic performance was more affected for older adults, then results would reflect lack of external validity. Given these results, evaluators would design another evaluation.

- *Environmental*: The sleep study was conducted in a controlled university sleep lab. If it was repeated by having participants stay at home and set their alarm clocks so that their sleep was still limited to 4, 6, 8, and 10 hours, how would changing the environment affect the athletic performance results for young and older adults? It is possible that (1) both age groups sleep better in their own beds than in a university sleep lab, (2) one group sleeps better in their own beds, or (3) both groups sleep better in the university sleep lab. Regardless, these results would always reflect the possible lack of external validity.

- *Temporal/sequential factors*: The sleep study was conducted during the winter months in a northern geographical area. If the study was conducted during summer months in a southern geographical location, would results be any different? Is it possible that the increase or decrease in sun exposure during daytime hours might affect sleep patterns?
- *Participants*: The following factors regarding participating individuals are linked to threats of external validity:
  - Animal-to-human links: When evaluators use rats or other animals to test specific drugs, it is questionable whether humans will react to the new drug in the same way as rats.
  - Human-to-human links: Evaluators use college students for many studies because the students are a convenient sample. However, results are questioned because data gathered from college students may not be generalizable to other groups of young adults not attending college.
  - Gender bias: Evaluators who include only men or only women in an evaluation find it is not generalizable to the nonrepresented gender group. The same is true for studies that include only heterosexual individuals and fail to recognize lesbian, gay, bisexual, and transgender (LGBT) individuals.
  - Racial bias: Evaluations conducted on only African Americans do not yield generalizable results to other racial groups. In today's world of linking genetics to health conditions, issues of racial inclusion are more important than ever.
  - Cultural and ethnocentric bias: Evaluation conducted on one specific cultural group is not generalizable to other cultures. For example, evaluators studying the Mexican Hispanic population in Texas may not generalize the results to other Hispanic groups in the United States. Spanish-speaking individuals do not share the same cultural background (e.g., the cultures of Puerto Rico, Mexico, Nicaragua, Honduras, Venezuela, and Spain are different). Also keep in mind that some religions contribute to cultural differences among various populations.
- *Testing and treatment interaction*: If participants learn from the pretest, then they may be less likely to learn as much from treatment. For example, a pretest is given at the beginning of a "new to diabetes" cooking class. If participants are sure that they received a perfect score on the pretest, they are less likely to listen intently during

the class, because they already know the information. When evaluators split the sample into two groups—one receiving pretest, treatment (cooking class), and posttest, the other receiving treatment (cooking class) and posttest—evaluators can calculate the differences.

- *Reactive arrangements (also called Hawthorne effect)*: The Hawthorne effect was described under threats to internal validity, yet it also applies to external validity. If individuals change their behavior when observed (threat to internal validity), results are not generalizable to real-world conditions (threat to external validity).
- *Multiple treatment conditions*: In some evaluations, the same individuals are exposed to multiple treatments. Because multiple treatments may create an artificial setting that does not exist in the real world, results may not be generalizable. For example, if the sleep study is conducted in the university sleep lab, individuals sleep alone (space) in a cool (temperature), quiet (sound) room with soft pillows and luxurious sheets (environment). The setting is artificial, exposing individuals to multiple treatments not linked to real-world bedrooms. At home, they may have a hot bedroom, an uncomfortable bed with old sheets, lumpy pillows, a snoring spouse, and loud neighbors. Results from multiple treatments in the sleep lab are not generalizable to populations trying to sleep in less than ideal conditions.

Last, evaluators need to be aware of all possible threats to external validity that affect independent variables. Results reporting threats to external validity are not regarded as a weakness in the evaluation, but rather an opportunity to design further studies. For example, if season and geographical location affect sleep study results, evaluators have the opportunity to explore this newly identified issue. It is possible that lack of generalizability from threats to external validity could lead to exciting and groundbreaking lines of new studies.

RELATIONSHIP BETWEEN INTERNAL AND EXTERNAL VALIDITY

Evaluators remain aware of threats to internal and external validity, but they know that internal validity is more critical than external. Without internal validity, the evaluation is not testing what it reports to measure. However, it is important to keep in mind that as the inclusion criteria becomes more selective, the results become less generalizable. For example, evaluators wish to study a new indoor air quality air filter. Their selection criteria are limited to office buildings constructed more than 20 years ago. These older buildings are more likely to have poor indoor air quality, thus limiting the sample criteria, which in turn limits the generalizability of results.[20]

MEASUREMENT ERROR

There are two types of errors that influence the results, surveys, tests, and instruments: random errors and systematic errors.

Random Errors

Random errors occur by chance and are inconsistent across the respondents. Random errors increase or decrease results in an unpredictable manner; therefore, evaluators have no control over the occurrence of random errors. Keep in mind that reliability is influenced by random errors because reliability is concerned with the degree of consistency of the measurement.

Random errors influence consistency in various ways. First, participating individuals may change from day 1 to day 2. For example, they get more or less sleep, take or stop taking cough medicine, or forget or remember to bring their reading glasses. Second, tasks change between day 1 and day 2. For example, the day 1 observer may not be available to observe on day 2, or on day 1 the participants mark their responses on the survey and on day 2 participants are asked to mark their responses on a separate answer sheet. Third, if there is a small sample of participating individuals, outside forces have a greater impact on the outcome. For example, if there are only 10 individuals completing a survey and 3 did not get enough sleep, then 30% of the scores might be affected. However, if

25 individuals complete the survey and 3 did not get enough sleep, only 12% of the responses will be affected. Let's put these three sources of random errors into an example for greater comprehension. See **Box 5-2**.

From the example in Box 5-2, it is easy to see how one, two, or three random errors occur by chance during evaluations. Each random error alters the reliability of knowing if a 10-week course was reliable in teaching adolescents how to provide safe self-care for their newly diagnosed medical condition.

Fourth, random errors occur within written tests. There are three examples under this source of random errors:

1. If the test is too short, individual scores are based more on chance and luck than on knowledge. If the exam covers all human bones, but there are only 10 questions, there is a chance that some students know only the bones asked about on the test and some students know all of the bones *except* for the ones asked about on the test. Either way, random error occurs due to the inconsistency of the exam.
2. If the test is not graded precisely the same way for each student, random errors cause inconsistent reliability. For example, if a professor does not follow an objective grading rubric, student scores are compromised due to subjective and indefensible grading procedures.
3. If the test is not administered consistently, random errors occur. For example, when students take a makeup exam, professors should provide an environment similar to the

BOX 5-2 Random Errors Case Study

Evaluators want to evaluate the current community-based education program to determine whether newly diagnosed type 1 diabetic adolescents know the correct procedure for testing their blood glucose levels, determining the correct amount of insulin needed, and injecting the insulin. The adolescents are enrolled in a 10-week health education program sponsored by the local health department. The evaluators observe the adolescents during the week 7 class and again during the week 8 class.

- First, adolescents may change between week 7 and week 8. If they performed the task poorly in week 7, they may have received extra practice at home while their parents watched and critiqued their insulin technique.
- Second, the task may change slightly from week 7 to week 8 because the instructor brought different glucose monitors during week 8, so the adolescents are not as familiar with the equipment. Also, the evaluator observing on week 7 is not available week 8, so the observer's own technique is slightly different for week 8.
- Third, there are five adolescents attending during week 7 and only three adolescents attending during week 8.

All three of the random errors occurred by chance, and all three random errors influenced the reliability of the diabetic class outcome data.

classroom (e.g., lighting, sound level, environment, vibration, time allotment) provided to the other students.

Random errors are often the result of the evaluator's ability to repeat the items (e.g., measurements, tests, surveys, and observations) the same way to obtain the same results. One way to minimize random errors is to collect data from a larger sample size. The random errors in either direction are less influential on the overall data with a large sample size. Last, random errors are reduced through statistical methods by averaging scores over a larger sample size.

Systematic Errors

Systematic errors are consistent in the same direction, so that no matter how many times the experiment is repeated the same error occurs. Validity is influenced by systematic errors. Systematic errors introduce inaccuracy into the measurement, cause a bias in data, and diminish the extent to which the test is measuring what it purports to measure.[23] Systematic errors are problematic to detect and eliminate. Unlike random errors, it is not possible to reduce the effect of systematic errors through statistical methods.[24] If evaluators suspect bias in their data, they investigate possible systematic errors.[25]

There are three areas to investigate when searching for systematic errors: environment, observation, and drift. Environment refers to how the setting changes over the course of the research. For example, if the evaluation was conducted outside, the temperature, humidity, wind speed, or heat index may cause variations in data and results that are difficult to pinpoint. Observation may change due to observer fatigue, time of day, room temperature, training of different observers, attitude of participants, and various other human behavior variables. Lastly, drift is defined as when evidence suggests that the data are slowly moving in one direction.[26] For example, drift may occur if the machine used for lab results is not calibrated each day prior to running water samples. The problem with each type of error is that even when the error is recognized, it is difficult to determine when it began in the data-collection process and how much the systematic error influenced the actual results.

Let's explore one example to illustrate how validity is affected by systematic errors. Public health students in occupational health are studying for a practicum exam on how to use various types of emergency clothing and equipment in situations where liquid and gas biohazard materials have contaminated an indoor workplace environment. Because knowing how to handle and remove biohazard materials is essential to occupational health, a perfect score is required on this practicum exam to move to the next phase of training. On the day of the exam, two professors decide to set up a biohazard materials spill in a simulated factory in one lab classroom, so students can demonstrate their biohazard materials practice skills. The students arrive at their usual classroom and are told to complete a worksheet while they wait. One at a time, the two professors call each student's name alphabetically to come to the simulated factory. They use a checklist to observe the students' skill in dressing in the protective clothing and using exact techniques for handling and cleaning up the simulated biohazard materials. After each student completes the skill test, they are told to return to the classroom without being told their exam score. As the exam continues for 3 hours, the students at the end of the alphabet become more anxious, because they see the stress of the returning students. The increased anxiety is likely to affect their test performance. This testing technique diminishes the validity of the practicum exam. As an evaluator of this exam, how would you suggest changing the format so that the practicum exam remains valid? There are numerous possible answers, but one solution is presented here. The professors could arrange several simulated biohazard material spills in five laboratory classrooms. Each classroom is equipped with a doctoral student observing the same biohazard materials clothing and clean-up activities with a prescribed checklist. All students would begin the practicum exam at the same time and rotate to the five laboratories for various types of biohazard material exercises. The standardized process would be complete in 1 hour with high validity.

With the awareness of measurement errors, how do evaluators reduce the chance of creating them? The following are ways to reduce measurement errors:

- *Pilot test*: Whether evaluation involves collecting quantitative or qualitative data, pilot testing is essential. Pilot testing is a complete dress rehearsal before data collection. Spending money on pilot testing is always a good investment and worth every cent. Near the end of this chapter, pilot testing is presented in detail.

- *Data-collection training*: Evaluators train data collectors for consistency (e.g., detailed checklists, machine measurement calibration checks, inter-rater comparisons to avoid creating errors). For example, data collectors read from a script for consistency with instructions prior to having an individual complete a survey.

- *Double data entry*: Evaluators enter a portion of the data twice and then compare the two entries. If there are multiple errors, evaluators go back to the original data and determine why the errors are occurring.

- *Statistical consultation*: Evaluators consult with statisticians to seek assistance with entering data and to determine ways to reduce and/or measure data errors.

- *Triangulate data collection*: To increase reliability and validity, evaluators choose to collect similar data using more than one method. For example, during the first week of the month, evaluators conduct interviews with adolescents about healthy food choices. With the same adolescents, evaluators conduct survey data on the same topic. Interview and survey responses are compared for consistency.[27]

RELIABLE AND VALID RESEARCH

Before leaving the discussion on reliability and validity, it is beneficial to step back and examine a broad view of research. Frequently, evening news programs reveal U.S. Food and Drug Administration (FDA) reports recalling specific medications for numerous reasons. Even though drug testing is intensely scrutinized during the research and development phase, FDA recalls are usually linked to research.[28] Researchers need to know how to distinguish between dependable and undependable research. Researchers build their study protocols on the previous research of colleagues in similar fields of study, because it is more efficient and economical. However, if previous original research is proven to be faulty, the entire line of research is built on flawed assumptions and results. Reliable research is based on several basic assumptions, including randomized controlled trial designs and adequate sample sizes, and is free of known bias.

Randomized Controlled Trial Designs

The gold standard of research design is the randomized controlled trial (RCT). Let's define the terms. When a study is *randomized*, it means that the research participants are randomly assigned to either a treatment group or a nontreatment group (placebo group). Some clinical trials can study more than one treatment group (e.g., Drug A, Drug B, or Drug C). Participants in each group have similar characteristics, such as age, gender, or length of diagnosis at the beginning of study. Random assignment technique allows researchers to draw conclusions with confidence if one group is significantly different at the end of the study.[29] A *controlled* study is defined as one group receiving treatment while another similar group receives no treatment. Control groups may be randomized from original groups of participants or control groups may be similar groups at a different location. For example, colon cancer patients over 50 years of age at University Cancer Center are randomized into two groups: Drug A and no treatment. In another study, colon cancer patients over 50 years of age at University Cancer Center are randomized into two groups: Drug A and Drug B. The control groups are similar colon cancer patients over 50 years of age

receiving the standard of care (nonexperimental treatment) at St. Mary's Cancer Hospital located in the adjacent county. Researchers compare similar patients receiving treatment to patients receiving either no treatment (placebo) or non-research-related standard-of-care treatment. Data explore variables such as reduction in tumor size, patient reaction to treatment, length of hospital stay, or time in remission. Even though randomized controlled trials offer the ideal design, such studies are not exempt from data-collection, measurement, and analysis errors that influence the reliability and validity of overall study results.

Adequate Sample Size

Evaluators seek an appropriate sample size for their studies. When a sample is too small, results are inconclusive and significant differences among groups are statistically harder to determine. On the other hand, when a sample is too large, cost, feasibility, and time become problematic. Evaluators strive for an ideal sample size to adequately represent the target population. However, a large sample is preferred over a small sample because of the increased precision and accuracy of the study.

Free of Bias

Bias occurs from numerous causes including selection, measurement, and intervention. Selection bias occurs if specific individuals or groups are purposely omitted from the evaluation. Measurement bias happens during data collection by evaluators or subjects because of systematic errors in measurement. Evaluators may influence individual responses by their body language during an interview, or a subject may provide socially desirable responses, such as telling interviewers they smoke a smaller number of cigarettes a day than they actually do or overstating the time and amount of physical activity achieved per week. Last, intervention bias involves how intervention groups are treated differently from control groups if the evaluators involved know which group is which.[30]

PILOT TESTING

Pilot testing is similar to a dress rehearsal for a theatrical performance. Pilot tests involve every aspect including environment, data collection, content, and outcomes of the evaluation. Pilot tests involve conducting a preliminary test of data-collection tools and procedures to identify and eliminate problems. When evaluators execute pilot tests correctly, they save time and resources during the actual data-collection process. When evaluators fail to conduct a rigorous pilot test, they risk collecting unusable data for a high price. Let's explore how to conduct a pilot study by category.

BOX 5-3 Participant Recruitment for Pilot Test

Use the same method of participant recruitment:

Phone Interviews

Are home phones, office phones, or cell phones going to be called?

How are phone numbers going to be obtained?

Will random digit dialing be used?

What is the cost incurred to obtain the phone numbers?

What time of the day is ideal for reaching participants?

Are the participants anonymous or are the names known to researchers?

Mailed or Online Surveys

How are postal or email addresses going to be obtained?

What is the cost incurred to obtain the postal or email addresses?

If email, are LISTSERV-type lists available?

In-Person Interviews or Surveys

How will participants be recruited?

Will incentives be used?

Are participants anonymous or known to researchers?

Sample of Respondents

Recruit a small number (< 10) of individuals with characteristics similar to the actual sample to test the method of recruitment, such as email, telephone, postal mail, or waiting room recruitment. If it is difficult to recruit individuals for the pilot test, then the recruitment methods for the actual study need revision (see **Box 5-3**).

Data Collection for Pilot Tests

Pilot tests allow evaluators the opportunity to determine if revisions are needed in the actual instrument or in the data-collection procedures (see **Box 5-4**).

Data Analysis

After the pilot test data are collected, evaluators enter the data and conduct a pilot test of the data analysis procedures (see **Box 5-5**).

Outcome

Following the pilot testing and modification phase, evaluators move forward with conducting the actual evaluation. Some evaluators may think that pilot testing is too labor intensive or too expensive to justify the results. These individuals are mistaken. Taking the time to conduct a thorough pilot test is always worth the time and money, because once data are collected, it is too late to fix mistakes that could prove to be fatal flaws for the entire study. Lastly, when reporting results, evaluators document the pilot study and revisions made based on results. This notation adds to the authenticity of the study.[31,32]

SUMMARY

This chapter introduced the concepts of reliability and validity. To briefly review, reliability refers to consistency, and validity is the extent to which a test measures what it purports to measure. The two different forms of reliability discussed include stability and internal consistency. The validity discussion included the types of validity, internal threats to validity, and external threats to validity. It is essential to remember that it is more important to be valid than reliable. Finally, the chapter concluded with a detailed description of how to conduct a pilot test.

CASE STUDY

The healthcare providers at the Glenville County Health Department pregnancy clinic have been using the same survey to screen patients for risk of family violence for several years. Only a small percentage of the women who take the survey obtain a score that would indicate that they are at risk for family violence. However, during the course of prenatal visits, when healthcare providers inquire if the women feel safe at home, it is not uncommon for women to disclose living with fear of violence. Because the survey results do not appear to be accurate, the clinic administrators decided it was time for a change. With a limited budget, the administrators decided to conduct an evaluation. A team of four staff members was formed and led by Michael Williams, PhD, MPH, Director of Quality Management for Glenville County Health Department. Fortunately, Dr. Williams has a background in public health and evaluation methods. Let's review the steps used by the team.

BOX 5-4 Data Collection for Pilot Test

Use the same method of data collection:

1. Create the exact environment that will be used for the actual data collection (e.g., location and time of day).
   a. If a certain meeting room is the intended site for participants to complete surveys, conduct the pilot test in the exact meeting room. Will the meeting room always be available during the actual data collection? Is the room quiet?
   b. If phone interviews will be conducted, verify that the digital sound recording devices work properly during the pilot test.
   c. If an online survey will be conducted, verify that the links are working and the survey responses are sent to a secure data-collection site.
2. When possible, observe participants while they complete surveys during the pilot test.
   a. How long did it take most participants to complete the survey or interview?
   b. Are they distracted by the environment or digital voice-recording device?
   c. Are there enough tables and chairs in the intended location?
   d. Are clipboards needed to provide a writing surface?
   e. Are sharpened pencils or pens available to complete the survey?
   f. Do respondents appear to be annoyed, fatigued, or bored near the end of the survey or interview?
   g. Do participants ask for an eraser to change their responses?
   h. Did respondents skip questions or look forward by skipping pages?
3. After the survey or interviews are complete, ask the participants a few questions.
   a. What was the purpose of the survey or interview?
   b. Were the directions clear?
   c. Were the questions easy to understand? Do any questions need clarification?
   d. Did any of the questions make them uncomfortable?
   e. Did the response choices allow the participants to enter their intended response?
   f. Was the survey or interview too long?
   g. Were there any questions that they did not understand?
   h. Were there any questions that they would change or reword?
   i. Did they skip any questions? Why?
   j. Would they tell their friends to participate in this study and complete the survey or interview?

BOX 5-5 Data Analysis Pilot Test

Begin the data analysis:

1. Prior to entering the data, read through the responses or interviews. Did participants interpret the question as evaluators intended?
2. Enter survey data as intended for actual evaluation. Although the sample size is limited in a pilot test, evaluators calculate mean, median, and mode for each question to determine the range of each question. For interviews, evaluators read responses for each question to obtain a general sense of answers from participants.
3. If paper surveys are going to be scanned, verify that the scanning machine is operating properly for scanning the completed surveys from the pilot test.
4. After viewing data, evaluators verify if results provided information needed to adequately address evaluation objectives.
5. Modify survey or interview questions as needed to clarify questions, response choices, or data results.

Step 1: Review Existing Survey Data

Before making any changes, the team reviewed the current survey. Immediately, they realized that the collected data had never been entered into a spreadsheet for analysis. The anonymous paper surveys were merely reviewed by a clinic nurse and placed in a large box for storage. There was no connection between the survey results and the discussion in the exam room nor was there evidence to confirm or refute the presumed percentage of women whose score indicated that they were at risk on the survey. One member of the team, Melissa Robinson, was a newly hired health educator with a graduate degree in public health. Instead of taking the time to analyze the existing anonymous surveys, Ms. Robinson suggested taking a random sample of 100 surveys and entering those responses to get an estimation of the survey results. Dr. Williamson agreed with her suggestion. In the meantime, after each new pregnant woman completed the survey, the clinic nurses scored the survey. This process eliminated the need to store boxes of surveys. The midwives continued to ask the women about their perceived level of safety at home and to enter the women's comments under the assessment tab. After the patient's appointment with the midwife, the clinic nurse entered the survey score in the woman's electronic medical records (EMR) under the assessment tab. This process continued for 3 months. Using the EMR database, Dr. Williams was able to provide evidence that survey results were not linked to what the women reported to the midwives.

Step 2: Reliability of Existing Survey

The team needed to determine the reliability of the existing survey before developing a completely new survey. Ms. Robinson suggested using the test-retest technique to see if the survey is stable. Because pregnant women have weekly clinic appointments near the end of their pregnancy, the team decided to ask 20 women to complete the survey for 2 consecutive weeks. The results showed that the survey was stable, because the responses remained the same from one week to the next week. Next the team decided to test the internal consistency of the survey. Using the existing 40-question survey responses, they analyzed the entire survey using the split-half technique. The even-numbered questions became Survey A, and the odd-numbered questions became Survey B. Ms. Robinson had a background in biostatistics, so she used the statistical measurement called Cronbach's alpha to determine how well the survey questions measured different aspects of the same topic. The Cronbach's alpha score was 0.62, which is low but acceptable.

Step 3: Validity of Existing Survey

Dr. Williams reminded the team that the survey may be reliable, but that does not mean that it is valid. She stated that the problem with the existing survey may be in that it is not valid; in other words, it does not measure what it was intended to measure. The team decided to focus on content validity and determine if the survey questions are closely related to domestic violence. Because none of the team members were involved in the development of the current survey, they did not have to be concerned about stepping on the toes of their colleagues. After a meeting in which each question was critiqued, it became evident that they had solved the problem. The majority of the survey questions were not related to family violence, but rather focused on topics such as neighborhood safety and satisfaction with community resources related to safety.

Step 4: Creating a New Survey

Dr. Williams suggested the team begin the process of creating a new survey by searching the literature. After a simple web search, one team member located a valuable website hosted by the Centers for Disease Control and Prevention (CDC). The website provides a free download book entitled "Measuring Intimate Partner Violence, Victimization and Perpetration: A Compendium of Assessment Tools." The book includes eight chapters: (1) Physical Victimization Scales, (2) Sexual Victimization Scales, (3) Psychological/Emotional Victimization Scales, (4) Stalking Victimization Scales, (5) Physical Perpetration Scales, (6) Sexual Perpetration Scales, (7) Psychological/Emotional Perpetration Scales, and (8) Stalking Perpetration Scales. Each chapter includes several scales with an explanation of how the scale has been used, published research using the scale, reliability and validity, and how to score and analyze each scale.[33]

The team was thrilled with the free and valuable information. Immediately, they began to compile the scales of interest to form their new patient survey.

Step 5: Pilot Testing

The team did not assume that they could skip the pilot-testing phase and begin to use the new survey. They carefully followed each step of the pilot-testing phase: participant recruitment, data collection, and data analysis. Ten pregnant women participated in the pilot test and were eager to provide feedback on the new survey. Some of the suggestions included lowering the literacy level of some questions, rearranging two subscales to improve the flow of the questions, and recommending the addition of some questions related to their children's safety. The edits were then made based upon the pilot test feedback. Because the clinic uses EMR check-in kiosks in the waiting room, it was possible to make the survey a required portion of the clinic visit at the first prenatal appointment and at the 25th weeks' and 37th weeks' gestation appointments. When the patients completed the electronic survey and hit submit, their score appeared on the assessment page with an explanation of patient's risk for the clinic staff to review at that day's appointment. After 6 months, the team met again to verify that the survey was working. Dr. Williams presented some data confirming that the pregnant women and midwives found the survey information to be valuable and that it facilitated open communication regarding risk of family violence.

Step 6: One Year Later

The prenatal clinic staff presented the family violence survey and results at the annual Glenville County Health Department board of directors meeting. Because the survey questions were not specific to pregnant women, or gender and age for that matter, the decision was made to have all new clinic patients over the age of 18 years complete the survey at their intake appointment and annually after that time.

Case Study Discussion Questions

1. How would you begin to modify the survey questions now that the survey has been used for a while in the clinic?
2. What are some of the possible threats to internal and external validity that might need to be considered?
3. If the clinic decided to conduct a second pilot test, what would you suggest that they modify in the procedure?

STUDENT ACTIVITY

This section asks several questions related to measurement reliability and validity. This student activity will require you to search the Internet for answers regarding reliability and validity of several of the questions.

The National Public Health Performance Standards Program (NPHPSP) is an effort by the Centers for Disease Control and Prevention (CDC) to create performance standards for state and local public healthcare systems. You can visit the NPHPSP website at http://www.cdc.gov/nphpsp/.

Questions

1. How many instruments are used by the NPHPSP? What do they measure?

2. To ensure that the standards of the NPHPSP measurement fully covered the gamut of public health action needed at state and local levels, the instruments were designed around what?

Complete an Internet search for the article entitled "Recommendations from Testing of the National Public Health Performance Standards Instruments" by Beaulieu, Scutchfield, and Kelly published in the *Journal of Public Health Management Practice* in 2003. Read the article and answer the following questions regarding their study on the validity of the NPHPSP instruments:

3. What three types of validity did the authors of this article test the NPHPSP instruments on?
4. What two ways did the authors test the criterion validity?
5. Why did the authors say it was difficult to assess criterion validity for public health systems?

The Student Life Department of North East University has decided that in order to better support new students they will give all incoming freshman a survey about what kind of support they have in their lives to help them with the transition from being a high school student living at home with their parents to a college student living on campus. The university hopes that scores from the test will help reveal students who may need extra support. Brad Johnson, the director of Student Life, does some searching at the library and finds four different measures of social support: the Miller Support and Affection Scale, the Latino Community Social Support Inventory, the Young Adult Social Support Scale, and the Cancer Social Support Scale.

6. Of the four measures that Brad found, which is the most likely to be one that he should research further?
7. Brad decides to research one of the scales further, and finds that it has a Cronbach's alpha of 0.78. Is this score acceptable?
8. Brad reads more about the Young Adult Social Support Scale and finds out that it has been tested against other social support scales for adults. When the Young Adult Scale is compared to a social support scale for adults, what kind of validity does this represent?
9. After his research, Brad decides that he will use the Young Adult Social Support Scale for his survey of new freshmen students. After the initial survey, the Student Life Department identifies 20 students who they feel have low social support. The Student Life Department decides to pair them up with students who have high levels of social support in a "buddy system." At the end

of the year they decide to give the Young Adult Social Support Scale survey back to the 20 students to see if the buddy system worked. All of the students showed improved levels of social support. The improvement in social support levels is an example of what threat to internal validity? Why?

Answers

1. There are three instruments used by the NPHPSP. They measure the state public health system, the local public health system, and the local public health governance.

2. The NPHPSP instruments were designed around the CDC's 10 Essential Public Health Services.

3. Beaulieu, Scutchfield, and Kelly tested the NPHPSP on face, content, and criterion validity.

4. The authors tested the criterion validity first by using documentary evidence through site visits and conference calls. Second, they used external judges to test criterion validity.

5. Beaulieu, Scutchfield, and Kelly state that there is no "gold standard" external criterion measure for public health systems that has been used on the national level before.

6. Brad should research the Young Adult Social Support Scale further. Because we are searching only about social support among college students, we probably do not want to look at the Miller Support and Affection Scale because we do not want to measure affection among the new freshman students. Further, we would not want to look at the Latino Community Social Support Inventory or the Cancer Social Support Scale because those measures have been made for very specific populations. While there are surely freshmen students of Hispanic ethnicity, not all the students are. Further, while there may be some freshmen who are dealing with or have dealt with cancer in the past, again, most have not.

7. Cronbach's alpha measures are a measure of internal consistency. A 0.78 score of Cronbach's alpha is considered to be between "acceptable" and "good." Therefore, Brad would continue to consider this test for use among freshmen students.

8. This represents criterion-related validity. When we test a new scale using another scale that has recognized reliability and validity properties, this is called criterion-related validity.

9. The most likely source of the threat to internal validity is maturation. We do not know that the buddy system was the reason that the students had higher levels of social support or because it was due to simply becoming older, becoming more relaxed with being away from home, and making friends in college. We don't know if this would have happened with or without the buddy system, particularly because there is no control group to measure them against.

REFERENCES

1. Trochim MK. Theory of Reliability. Research Methods Knowledge Base. Available at: http://www.socialresearchmethods.net/kb/reliablt.php. Last updated October 20, 2006. Accessed June 3, 2012.

2. Shuttleworth M. Definition of Reliability. Explorable. Available at: http://www.experiment-resources.com/definition-of-reliability.html. Last updated 2009. Accessed June 3, 2012.

3. MBTI Basics. The Myers and Briggs Foundation. Available at: http://www.myersbriggs.org/my-mbti-personality-type/mbti-basics. Accessed June 3, 2012.

4. Lazarus RS, Folkman S. The Hassles and Uplifts Scales. Mind Garden, Inc. Available at: http://www.mindgarden.com/products/hsups.htm. Accessed June 3, 2012.

5. Types of Reliability. Statsam Blog. Available at: http://statssam.wordpress.com/2012/02/05/types-of-reliability/. Last updated February 5, 2012. Accessed June 3, 2012.

6. Cronbach LJ. Coefficient alpha and the internal structure of tests. *Psychometrika*. 1951;16(3):297–334.

7. Litwin MS. *How to Assess and Interpret Survey Psychometrics*, 2nd ed. Thousand Oaks, CA: Sage Publications; 2003.

8. George D, Mallery P. *SPSS for Windows Step by Step: A Simple Guide and Reference*, 4th ed. Boston, MA: Allyn & Bacon; 2003.

9. Miller MJ. Reliability and Validity. Lecture Notes from Western International University. Available at: www.michaeljmillerphd.com/res500_lecturenotes/Reliability_and_validity.pdf. Accessed June 3, 2012.

10. Trochim MK. Types of Reliability. Research Methods Knowledge Base. Available at: http://www.socialresearchmethods.net/kb/reltypes.php. Last updated October 20, 2006. Accessed June 3, 2012.

11. Howell J, Miller P, Park HH, Sattler D, Schack T, Spery E, Widhalm S, Palmquist M. Reliability and Validity. Writing@CSU. Colorado State University. Available at: http://writing.colostate.edu/guides/research/relval/pop2b.cfm. Last updated 2012. Accessed June 3, 2012.

12. Shuttleworth M. Validity and Reliability. Explorable. Available at: http://www.experiment-resources.com/validity-and-reliability.html. Last updated 2008. Accessed September 4, 2013.

13. Kramer GP, Bernstein DA, Phares V. *Introduction to Clinical Psychology*, 7th ed. Upper Saddle River, NJ: Pearson Prentice Hall; 2009.

14. Fink A, ed. *How to Measure Survey Reliability and Validity*. Thousand Oaks, CA: Sage Publications; 1995.

15. Westen D, Rosenthal R. Quantifying construct validity: two simple measures. *J Pers Soc Psychol*. 2003;83(3):608–618.

16. Carmines EG, Zeller RA. *Reliability and Validity Assessment*. Newbury Park, CA: Sage Publications; 1991.

17. Trochim MK. Reliability and Validity. Research Methods Knowledge Base. Available at: http://www.socialresearchmethods.net/kb/relandval.php. Last updated October 20, 2006. Accessed June 3, 2012.

18. Hawthorne Effect. *The Free Dictionary*. Available at: http://medical-dictionary.thefreedictionary.com/Hawthorne+effect. Accessed June 3, 2012.

19. Threats to Internal Validity. Psychometrics. Available at: http://www.psychmet.com/id12.html. Accessed June 3, 2012.

20. Ferguson L. External validity, generalizability, and knowledge utilization. *J Nurs Scholarship*. 2004;36(1): 16–22.

21. Yu C, Ohlund B. Threats to Validity of Research Design. Creative Wisdom. Available at: http://www.creative-wisdom.com/teaching/WBI/threat.shtml. Accessed June 3, 2012.

22. Mitchell M, Jolley J. *Research Designed Explained*, 4th ed. New York, NY: Harcourt; 2001.

23. Inspection Training—Linear Instrument Characteristics. ToolingU. Available at: http://www.toolingu.com/definition-350115-5902-systematic-error.html. Accessed June 3, 2012.

24. Allain R. Random Error and Systematic Error. Southeastern Louisiana University. Available at: https://www2.southeastern.edu/Academics/Faculty/rallain/plab193/labinfo/Error_Analysis/05_Random_vs_Systematic.html. Accessed June 3, 2012.

25. Loktik O. Systematic Errors. Physics Laboratory Tutorial. Columbia University. Available at: http://phys.columbia.edu/~tutorial/rand_v_sys/tut_e_5_2.html. Last updated September 1, 2005. Accessed June 3, 2012.

26. False System Errors. European Centre for Medium-Range Weather Forecasts. Available at: http://old.ecmwf.int/products/forecasts/guide/False_systematic_errors.html. Accessed June 3, 2012.

27. Trochim MK. Measurement Error. Research Methods Knowledge Base. Available at: http://www.socialresearchmethods.net/kb/measerr.php. Last updated October 20, 2006. Accessed June 3, 2012.

28. MedWatch. U.S. Food and Drug Administration. Available at: http://www.fda.gov/Safety/MedWatch/ucm287881.htm. Accessed June 3, 2012.

29. Seuc A. Randomization to protect against selection bias in health-care trials: RHL commentary. The WHO Reproductive Health Library; Geneva: World Health Organization. Available at: http://apps.who.int/rhl/education/MR000012_seuca_com/en/. Accessed May 14, 2014.

30. Gerhard T. Bias: considerations for research practice. *Am J Health-Syst Pharm.* 2008;65: 2159–2168.

31. Leon AC, Davis LL, Kraemer HC. The role and interpretation of pilot studies in clinical research. *J Psychiatr Res.* 2005;45(5): 626–629.

32. Taylor-Powell E. Pilot Test Your Questionairre. University of Wisconsin-Extension, Cooperative Extension. https://www.team-psa.com/brfss/2012/pres/K_Trepanier_questionnaire.pdf. Accessed September 4, 2013.

33. Thompson MP, Basile KC, Hertz MF, Sitterle D. *Measuring Intimate Partner Violence Victimization and Perpetration: A Compendium of Assessment Tools*. Atlanta, GA: Centers for Disease Control and Prevention, National Center for Injury Prevention and Control; 2006. Available at: http://www.cdc.gov/ncipc/pub-res/IPV_Compendium.pdf. Accessed September 4, 2013.

CHAPTER **6**

Qualitative Data

CHAPTER OBJECTIVES

At the end of this chapter, students will be able to:

1. Discuss the advantages and disadvantages of qualitative research.
2. Evaluate the reliability and validity of qualitative data.
3. Analyze the differences between the types of qualitative design.
4. Discuss some examples of ethical issues related to qualitative research.
5. Conduct a simple analysis of qualitative data including data organization, coding, and data display.

KEY TERMS

coding
data display
qualitative data
validity and reliability of qualitative data

INTRODUCTION

Qualitative research explores the insight into human behavior and seeks information by gaining more experience with a particular topic through unstructured evidence and data. Qualitative research explores the *process* of the topic rather than the results. For example, qualitative research asks hospitalized patients about the reasons why they were unable to take their medications rather than simply noting in the chart the numbers of times the patient refused to ingest the medication. The data include transcripts from interviews, focus groups, media clips or videos, emails, customer service feedback, field notes, open-ended survey questions, and print media. Data analysis does not rely on numbers and statistics as in quantitative research, but qualitative research is an interpretation of the collected words. Quantitative research involves large samples and standardized measures, while qualitative research explores smaller samples and unstructured methods. With qualitative data, the researcher gains detail but loses generalizability. Qualitative research does not assume preconceived notions but rather seeks trends and patterns in the data. The techniques are flexible and allow researchers to change the interview script and add probing questions during an interview as needed to gain more in-depth information. Field notes allow the researchers to describe the environment and document changes in the interviewee's facial and body expression, mood, and tone during the interview.[1] Researchers are also noting if the body language matches the response. For example, patient states approval of the new hospital policies during an interview, but he does not look up and nervously taps his leg with his fingers. Qualitative data results are used to formulate research questions, build knowledge, design policies, generate hypotheses, and guide the foundation for further research.[2] This chapter introduces types of qualitative data, data-collection methods, ethical issues, and data analyses. **Table 6-1** describes the advantages and disadvantages of qualitative research.

THE QUALITATIVE-QUANTITATIVE DEBATE

There are advantages and disadvantages to qualitative and quantitative research methods. The easiest way to remember the difference between qualitative and quantitative research is qualitative research focuses on mostly words and quantitative

TABLE 6-1 Advantages and Disadvantages of Qualitative Research Design

Advantages	Disadvantages
Useful for complex subjects	Not needed for simple hypothesis
In-depth and comprehensive information	Subjective; difficulty establishing reliability and validity
Greater understanding of entire situation	Limited scope due to data-collection approaches
Interactions between variables	Possible researcher bias
Generates useful data	Requires detailed planning
Not dependent on large sample sizes	No precise results with mathematical calculations
Unique results	Not able to be replicated; lacks generalizability

research contains mostly numbers. Instead of trying to have either side win the debate, it is useful to compare the two methods. It is important to keep in mind that there is a fair amount of overlap between the two columns in **Table 6-2**. For example, it is possible for quantitative data to contain some open-ended survey questions, while researchers may count the various types of responses from interviews.

From Tables 6-1 and 6-2, it is easy to see the reason why some researchers use a combination of qualitative and quantitative data, called a mixed-method approach. The term *mixed methods* is also called triangulation. There is value in conducting mixed-method research that uses qualitative data

to tell the story and quantitative data to provide generalizable data. For example, triangulation is used when researchers conduct interviews with 30 physical therapists representing various work environments, such as outpatient clinics, hospitals, and in-patient rehabilitation centers. The interviews focused on work satisfaction, salary, and benefits. From the interview results, the researchers created survey questions for distribution to all licensed physical therapists in Ohio. This mixed-methods approach provides details from the interviews and generalizability from the large sample size of the survey. Other types of triangulation are: 1) methods triangulation, which involves combining data from multiple data

TABLE 6-2 Comparison of Qualitative and Quantitative Research

Qualitative Research	Quantitative Research
Quality	Quantity
Subjective, exploratory, and observational	Objective, confirming, and experimental
Description, discovery, hypothesis generating; evolve as data are collected	Prediction, confirmation, hypothesis testing
Flexible, evolving, emergent	Predetermined, structured
Search for patterns and meaning	Generalizable and structured
Natural setting, familiar conditions	Unfamiliar, artificial
Small and nonrandom	Large and random
Researcher as primary instrument, interviews, observations	Inanimate instruments (scales, tests, surveys, questionnaires, computers)
Inductive	Deductive
Comprehensive, holistic, expansive	Precise, narrow, reductionist

Data from Sharan Merriam's *Case Study in Research Education: A Qualitative Approach.* 1988. Published by Jossey-Bass.

sources on the same topic; and 2) researcher triangulation, which involves combining data from multiple researchers on the same topic.[3] Within triangulation, researchers corroborate the various types of data. Corroboration does not verify the accuracy of the participants' responses but rather confirms that the findings reflect what the participants were stating during the interview or focus group.[4]

QUALITATIVE RESEARCH: VALIDITY AND RELIABILITY

Before jumping in to the specifics, let's review the basic definitions. Validity is the degree to which the research tool measures what it was intended to measure. In qualitative research, validity is obtaining impressions, patterns, or trends of the experience or topic under investigation.[5] It is important to use skilled facilitators and moderators for qualitative research such as interviews, focus groups, or observations. Researchers try to eliminate as much personal bias as possible so that they do not hear or see what they want to see due to their bias. Researchers verify that the interview questions ask about the specific research topic to ensure validity. For example, if the research questions focus on patient satisfaction, the interview questions need to relate to the satisfaction of the patient's current clinic visit. Also, qualitative researchers address validity throughout the data-collection process. As more and more cases are reviewed, patterns, themes, and emerging hypotheses confirm the validity.[6] Another way to increase validity is to seek alternative explanations for the emerging patterns. For example, are the respondents providing honest responses or are they giving the type of answers that they think the interviewer wants to hear? This type of response is called social desirability. Or perhaps the respondents are trying to please the interviewer to ensure access to the incentive. Last, validity is increased when researchers reach a point of saturation, which is defined as when each additional interview, focus group, or observation does not yield any new information. For example, respondents keep stating approximately the same issues related to dissatisfaction with the clinic check-in process. The types of validity in qualitative research include:

- *Construct validity*: To what degree do the interview questions match the concepts and operational definitions in the research questions? For example, do the interview questions about workplace stress match the definition of workplace stress as defined in the research questions?
- *Content validity*: Does the research method match what is expected to be measured? For example, are

the researchers observing behavior when interviewing would be a more appropriate research design to answer the research questions?

- *Face validity*: Does the research method selected show that common sense was used? For example, if the researchers want to know about quality of hospital cafeteria food, did they conduct a taste test with employees, patients, and visitors?[7]

The validity of qualitative research is criticized for several reasons. First, because researchers are present during interviews or observations, the participant's behavior may change. This is called reactivity. For example, children act differently during playtime if they know that they are being observed by an adult. Second, researchers may use selection bias when recruiting participants. Third, researchers may inadvertently influence or bias the participants' responses during the interview. Fourth, researchers may not observe all factors in the situation or event under investigation. Fifth, researchers' bias may influence the data analysis.[8,9] For example, if researchers have strong positive or negative opinions about an interview topic, such as abortion, their body language and facial expressions may influence how the respondent is answering the interview questions.

Reliability is defined as the ability to yield the same results in repeated studies.[10] Qualitative research is criticized because it is difficult to replicate observations, patterns, and trends with the same phenomenon time after time.[5] Because it is not possible to use the same participants over and over, qualitative researchers address this criticism by using purposive participant sampling based on previous knowledge of the topic from literature reviews. To address researcher bias, researchers work in teams and read from scripted basic interview guides. During observations, research teams construct basic checklists and add field notes for additional details. Because interviews and focus groups are digitally recorded, research teams verify the reliability of the basic content of each interview. While it is possible to conduct test-retest procedures to verify reliability of quantitative data, it is also possible for qualitative researchers to do the same by repeating observations under varying conditions to verify emergence of similar findings.[11]

Lastly, the use of triangulation methods improves reliability and validity. By using different strategies to study the same topic, researchers gain different perspectives, for example by making observations under a variety of conditions, interviewing comparison groups (e.g., obtaining staff and patient perspectives), and having several researchers analyze the same data independently.[12] See **Box 6-1**.

BOX 6-1 Tips for Maintaining Validity in Qualitative Research

1. Listen carefully to each participant's response for proper interpretation.
2. Use two digital-recording devices to ensure accuracy of recording.
3. Write the report at each phase of the research.
4. Add sufficient details and primary data to final report so reader learns how conclusions were derived.
5. Provide researchers' reactions to data; reveal known bias.
6. Ask research team members to critique reports to ensure accuracy and completeness.
7. Establish balance between anticipated and actual significance of study.
8. Improve validity by checking grammar, consistency, and spelling.

Data from Wolcott, H.R. *Qualitative Inquiry in Education: The Continuing Debate.* Published by Teachers College Press; 1990.

TYPES OF QUALITATIVE DESIGN

For this chapter, the types of qualitative design include interviews, observational research, case studies, phenomenology, content analysis, ethnography, historical document analysis, and grounded theory.

Interviews

Structured interviews involve asking an agreed-upon set of questions. After conducting a review of the professional literature related to the research topic, researchers create a list of structured, open-ended interview questions. For example, an open-ended question is, "Describe what you did at work today," while a closed question is "On a scale of 1 to 10 with 10 being, 'I feel great,' how would you rate your health today?" All types of interviews are audio-recorded for transcription purposes, and the interviewer also takes notes during the session. Following each interview, researchers write field notes about observations made during the interview.

Unstructured interviews are different from structured interviews, because the researcher has guidelines rather than a set of questions, and the interview is more like a conversation. The interviewer moves the conversation in different directions to fully explore the topic of interest.[13] For example, if the research topic is physician-assisted suicide, the interviewer may move the conversation from religious beliefs to legal aspects to personal desires about end-of-life decisions, depending on what the participant says.

Focus groups are best defined as a group interview. Like interviews, focus groups have a predetermined set of questions, but also have the leeway to explore comments as desired to gain a deeper understanding of the topic. There

are advantages and disadvantages to using interviews versus focus groups. Interviews allow researchers to explore questions in-depth with each respondent, while focus groups allow a "group thinking" process with several individuals sharing their opinions at the same time. Interviews are more time-consuming and focus groups are faster. The cost is approximately the same, because respondents are paid for their time to participate in either an interview or a focus group.

When recruiting focus group participants, it is important that each focus group is composed of six to eight similar individuals. For example, it is not appropriate to host a focus group from a specific department in the clinic, because this configuration would have supervisors and staff in the same focus group. Instead, it would be appropriate to have a focus group with only administrative assistants from across the clinic. When hosting focus groups, it is useful to invite individuals with similar characteristics related to the topic of interest. For example, researchers studying the issues related to workplace injuries with an emphasis on back pain would recruit individuals receiving physical therapy from a work-related injury.

When conducting focus groups, there are at least two researchers in the room. One person is asking the predetermined questions followed by additional questions or probes to gain more details. For example, if the predetermined question is, "How would you describe your level of satisfaction with your last visit to this clinic?," the additional question or probe is, "Tell me more about your frustration with the patient check-in process." The probe questions are the researchers' opportunity to listen to the participants' answer to the predetermined question and gain more details by asking about one area of concern. A second researcher attends the focus group to take field notes and make sure that the audio-recording devices are working and the participants are comfortable. It is advisable to have one recording device at each end of the table. Each participant's name is written on a table tent, so the researcher may address individuals by their first name. It is important that the researcher receives a response from each participant for each question to ensure the broadest range of responses. As with individual interviews, extensive training is required prior to conducting a focus group. See **Box 6-2** for interviewing tips.

Observations

There are various types of observations. Let's look at **Figure 6-1** to see the broad view followed by a description of each type. In the descriptions of the observation types, it becomes evident that there is overlap. For example, researchers may combine participant and contrived observation for data collection. Keep in mind that observation research is filled with potential ethical issues and deceptive practices.

Participant and Nonparticipant Observation

Researchers participate in the activity or observe without involvement as a nonparticipant observer. There are two types of participant observations. First, participant observation involves a quick turnaround experience, while immersed in the situation for a brief period of time. For example, a secret shopper has a brief interaction at a fast food restaurant. The entire interaction could be less than 5 minutes. Second, other participant observations are more demanding and time consuming, because the researcher becomes a member of the

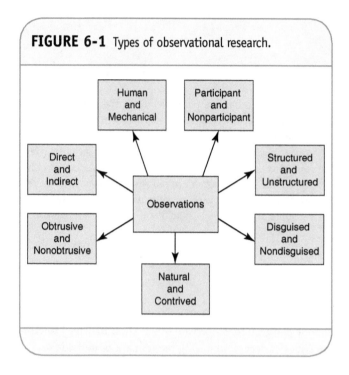

FIGURE 6-1 Types of observational research.

group, setting, or community. This research requires months or years of immersion into the culture, so the observation is the natural environment. The researcher writes volumes of field notes and collects documents, photos, and other pertinent data. Some researchers believe that participant observation with total immersion is the only way to gain insights into the setting.[14] See **Box 6-3**.

For example, the study involves watching family members in the emergency department (nonparticipant) or acting like a family member in the emergency department (participant).

Obtrusive and Unobtrusive Observation

Researchers trace or create physical evidence. For example, researchers use hidden cameras to collect data from individuals or collect data observing what types of food is left on the hospital cafeteria trays.

Natural or Contrived Observation

When researchers observe behavior in normal and ordinary settings, it may take a long time for the event to occur. In contrived observations, the setting is staged. Researchers collect the data faster because they do not have to wait for the event to occur. For example, researchers wish to observe how fathers alone interact with their children at an indoor shopping mall playground. They must wait until father-child dyads enter the playground without the mother or another adult. However, in contrived observation, father-child dyads

---

BOX 6-2 Tips for Interviewing

1. Practice interviewing how to ask unbiased questions without reacting to the response.
2. Select a comfortable location so participants feel at ease.
3. Avoid interview questions with possible "yes" or "no" responses.
4. Maintain a flexible approach by asking questions to receive broad responses and perceptions.
5. Ask repetitive, but reworded questions to validate responses.

BOX 6-3 Observation

Researchers are interested in improving the waiting room environment and efficiency within the hospital's emergency room, so a direct observation study is an appropriate qualitative research design. As with all research, approval from the hospital's institutional review board (IRB) is required prior to initiating research. Direct observation includes sitting in the waiting room and taking copious field notes on patients, family members, cleanliness, availability of restrooms, walking patterns, food brought in and food purchased from vending machines, placement of furniture and television screens, samples of nonidentifiable conversations, and other pertinent information and events. Observations would also include patient flow from parking options, signage to main entrance, check-in procedures and forms, total wait time and wait time between each phase, involvement of family, attitude of staff, and availability of WiFi and cell phone usage.

are invited to come and "try out" new outdoor toys at a staged indoor playground. Contrived observation may lead to ethical issues of deception during recruitment of individuals.

Disguised and Nondisguised Observation

Researchers observe behavior by posing as one of the group members. Nondisguised researchers inform individuals that they are conducting research. Both observations create ethical dilemmas. Disguised observations are deceitful, while nondisguised observations yield inaccurate data because individuals act differently when watched.

Structured and Unstructured Observation

To standardize data collection, researchers use checklists when conducting structured observations. With unstructured observations, researchers record field notes for data collection. For example, researchers utilize a checklist when observing the first 3 minutes of the patient–nurse interaction in the emergency department.

Direct and Indirect Observation

Researchers collect direct observations in real time, while indirect observations are collected after the event (e.g., secondary data). For example, direct observation would involve recording the time and procedures used by nurses to administer patient medications, while indirect would involve reviewing the digital medical administration record (MAR) to record only when medications were administered.[15]

Human and Mechanical Observation

Human observation involves researchers collecting data, such as field notes and checklists, while mechanical observation

uses audio and/or video cameras to collect data. For example, researchers are in the room with the physician when a cancer diagnosis is presented to a patient versus using digital cameras to record the physician–patient interaction. Digital recordings are more accurate for this type of data collection.[16]

Case Studies

A case study is defined as thorough exploration on a specific topic. A case study is an analysis of narrow and detailed variables describing individuals, groups, social units, or situations.[17] Case studies focus on the individual unit rather than the population. Case studies are not generalizable but concentrate on greater understanding of specific topics.[18] For example, if healthcare providers see a patient with extremely unusual symptoms, they could publish a case study describing the presenting symptoms, disease course, treatment, and outcome. Once the manuscript is published, other healthcare providers have the opportunity to share similar experiences in their patient populations.[13] See **Box 6-4**.

Phenomenology

Phenomenology is the study of human experiences and interpretations of an occurrence within a population. Unlike a case study, phenomenology explores an event or situation within a study population. Researchers wish to understand how the event is viewed or constructed by others. For example, a phenomenological study of the September 11, 2001 terrorist attacks would yield a wide variety of perceptions of the events. Individual perceptions may not be accurate, but researchers are not searching for accuracy, but rather perceptions of events.

BOX 6-4 Case Study of AIDS: June 5, 1981

On June 5, 1981, *Morbidity and Mortality Weekly Report* (*MMWR*) published a report of five cases of *Pneumocystis carinii* pneumonia (PCP) among previously healthy young men in Los Angeles. The men were described as "homosexuals"; two died. The Los Angeles County Department of Public Health prepared a case study that suggested an immune deficiency disease with possible sexual contact. The report prompted additional case studies from health departments in New York City, San Francisco, and other cities. In June 1981, the Centers for Disease Control and Prevention (CDC) in Atlanta created an investigative team to identify risk factors and to develop a case definition for national surveillance. Within 18 months, epidemiologists conducted studies to identify the major risks factors for acquired immunodeficiency syndrome (AIDS). In 1983, the CDC reported recommendations for prevention of sexual, drug-related, and occupational transmission.

Courtesy of Centers for Disease Control and Prevention. *Morbidity and Mortality Weekly Report*. First Report of Aids. MMWR 2001; 50(21);429. Available at: http://www.cdc.gov/mmwr/preview/mmwrhtml/mm5021a1.htm.

Historical Documents

Relying on inductive reasoning, researchers conduct historical research to study the details of past events. Possible source materials to study include newspapers, magazines, legal and medical documents, textbooks, periodicals, training manuals, photographs, and so forth. This information is useful in planning future events. As with any research, the first step is formulating the research question. For example, how was the polio vaccine distributed to the U.S. population in a short period during the 1950s? Is this historical model useful in planning the dissemination of vaccines for a newly emerging virus, such as H1N1 influenza? Prior to starting historical research, researchers establish the historical data to include in the study collection. Keep in mind that there are specific procedures to follow when seeking the authenticity of historical documents, but this discussion is beyond the scope of this chapter.[19]

Content Analysis

A content analysis is a collection of existing documents on a specific topic. Examples include:

- One type of document over time, such as all Seaside Hospital annual reports for the past 10 years
- Different types of documents on a specific topic during a specific time period, such as 1 year of identified health magazine articles and medical websites related to cervical cancer information for the layperson audience; media transcripts on a specific topic, such as whether television health news coverage about cardiovascular disease emphasizes lifestyle changes (e.g., maintaining healthy

weight, adequate daily exercise, and smoking cessation) or if the emphasis is on the latest research about cardiovascular drug therapies and surgical procedures
- Various personal documents on a specific topic, such as diaries, transcripts of videos, journals, social media entries from patients receiving cancer treatment

Each document collection is analyzed to get an in-depth view of the media reporting, public reaction, personal insight, and trends related to the topic of interest. For example, if hospital administrators are seeking a certificate of need from the county in order to build a new hospital, they would hire health researchers to conduct a content analysis related to the press coverage, newspaper editorials, emergency room overcrowding reports, and documentation of public opinion. The analysis of whole collections of documents would highlight a positive or negative need to build an additional hospital in the county.

Ethnography

Ethnography is a combination of interviews, observations, and case studies with emphasis on the relationship between behavior and culture.[19] A researcher team studies a particular location or population to gain greater understanding to address researcher questions. As with other types of qualitative data, researcher teams observe a setting, collect field notes, conduct interviews, and collects artifacts (e.g., unofficial and official documents). If case studies are used, researchers conduct life stories with specific individuals. Ethnographic research is labor intensive and involves extensive time on location.

Grounded Theory

Grounded theory is qualitative research used to generate a new theory based on a process of comparison. The first step is to develop a hypothesis and then begin to collect data about the topic from a variety of sources, such as literature reviews, public records, interviews, observations, and surveys.[20,21] By using the technique of grounded theory, researchers select published research or other documentation and make constant comparisons. Researchers compare the first two documents to each other. If the documents yield similar results, researchers continue the process with the third document and so on. With each additional document, researchers are searching for a bit of novel information that is new but similar to their existing information. If the comparative document yields conflicting or dissimilar results, that document is put aside for further review. As each document is compared to the others, it is either accepted or rejected. Through the process, the purposed hypothesis gains strength or it is determined that it needs further modification. The process is repeated over and over until all known documents are compared and either accepted or rejected. There is no clear endpoint. Researchers stop when it appears that no new information is available. This endpoint is called saturation.[22,23] The "rejected" documents are revisited to determine if there are any unexplored patterns or situations that need further consideration.

ETHICAL ISSUES IN QUALITATIVE RESEARCH

Some types of qualitative data collection require the consideration of possible ethical issues. In all situations, researchers guarantee participants assurances of confidentiality as stated on the informed consent document that was approved by the appropriate IRB. Regardless of what participants reveal in an interview or on a survey, the researcher's obligation is to maintain confidentiality of the information. To protect participant identity, researchers use pseudonyms and codebooks. For example, even if a participant shares with the researchers that he is involved in international drug trafficking, researchers are legally obligated to maintain the confidentiality of the information.[24]

In addition to protecting the confidentiality of the content, researchers are obligated to protect the actual storage of the data. This legal obligation involves protecting files within a locked cabinet or office, establishing computer password protection for digital files, determining the credentials of other researchers with access to the protected files, storage of paper copies of field notes, and various other data-storage issues. Last, there are issues related to who owns the data. This issue gets problematic when the agency funding the research wants access to confidential data held by the researchers.[25]

Some argue that researchers conducting participant observation must assume a deceptive role for full immersion into a community. For example, if the study involves documenting the quality of health care in a jail, the researcher would work with the legal system to become an inmate for a year to actually experience the quality of health care. Some researchers argue that this method is deceptive and unethical. Other researchers argue that it is the only way to gain reliable information, because they believe that individuals change their behavior if they know that they are being watched.[26] Some researchers believe that unethical studies yield poor quality results.[27] Generally, all agree that research is only as ethical as the researchers conducting the study, whether it is qualitative or quantitative research.

ANALYSES OF QUALITATIVE DATA

The qualitative researcher analyzes data continually—from the initial research phase to the final report. This constant process was labeled analysis and interpretation by Goetz and LeCompte.[20] There are several approaches to overall analysis, starting with the research questions and choice of data collection involving: 1) broad holistic or big picture view of the data, 2) collaborative partnerships from various and opposing viewpoints, and 3) detailed descriptions of the studied topic across multiple data sources to seek regular patterns or trends. All approaches involve sifting through data, coding data, and sorting data over and over again as each observation or interview is added to the data collection. Each round of data analyses refines patterns and trends, while attempting to interpret ongoing observations and interviews to refine conclusions. This section describes each level of qualitative data analysis.

Data Organization

Because qualitative data analysis requires a constant process of examining, sorting, and reexamining data, researchers need to precisely organize the data. There are two basic ways to organize the large qualities of data: manually and by computer.

Manual

Although computers are more commonly used to store data, researchers continue to find notebooks and boxes a useful way to organize the data. First, researchers copy the original documents and then store the original documents in a safe. Second, the copied documents are coded, cut apart, recoded, stored with notes in the margins, and continually resorted throughout the analysis process. In each reiteration, researchers add more extensive notes in the margins. In the beginning the notes are general, but later the notes focus on specific concepts.

Computers

Computers are increasingly the tool of choice for gathering, entering, retrieving, managing, and analyzing qualitative data. There are numerous qualitative software programs available. Despite the advantages of using a qualitative software program, qualitative researchers still are required to explore the data for patterns and trends leading to theory construction, because computers cannot analyze all of the complex meanings and perceptions explored in qualitative research.[28] See **Box 6-5**.

Coding Data

Data reduction is an essential step in coding data. Interview questions and responses are typically audio-recorded and then transcribed verbatim before analysis is begun. Transcription is extremely time consuming.[33] Due to the large amount of data that can be generated in qualitative research, a data-reduction process must be used to aid analysis. This procedure includes organizing the data; identifying emerging themes, categories, and patterns; and testing hypotheses against the data.

There are two types of codes: preassigned, or a priori, codes and exploratory codes. A priori codes are described by researchers prior to starting data analyses. For example, if research focuses on the efficiency of the hospital outpatient admissions process, a priori codes include courtesy of staff, wait time, cleanliness, paper documents versus paperless electronic medical records, and scheduling. Exploratory codes are added to the a priori codes as data are collected

and analyzed once new themes emerge. For example, using the previous example, researchers may discover that the temperature of the waiting room and long wait times for valet parking are frequently mentioned patient complaints yet were not on the a priori code list.

As the data are collected, researchers store two electronic copies of the original document in case one document is damaged or lost. These stored files are not analyzed. Before starting to code any data, researchers read a third copy of documents several times to improve familiarity. Researchers begin coding into the a priori code files. For any portion of the document that does not fit into one of the a priori codes, researchers start a file for these "leftover" files. These files are revisited later, and new exploratory codes are created. In addition to the a priori codes, researchers may slice the data codes into general categories, such as activities, personnel, methods, events, and location; or into taxonomic codes, such as who, what, when, and how. Researchers code and recode data several times and into several different categories until the data begin to take shape as patterns and trends emerge. In all coding situations, each segment is labeled with an appropriate code related to the research objectives. When complete data files contain multiple collections, such as interviews, focus groups, and observations, coding categories become more and more complex.[33] It is then necessary to create subfiles and segmented subfiles, so that every data fragment is analyzed and considered in the results.

There are three coding strategies.[34] First, open coding is the simplest form and used first to sort the data into a priori

---

BOX 6-5 Examples of Qualitative Software Programs

There are open source (free) and proprietary (for pay) computer-assisted qualitative data analysis programs. Both have their advantages and disadvantages. The following are examples of both kinds.

Open Source
Coding Analysis Toolkit (CAT)[29] is a web-based program developed by the Qualitative Data Analysis Program of the University of Pittsburgh. Able to import data from other programs, CAT uses keystrokes and automation as opposed to the use of a mouse to speed up activities.

Compendium is a computer program that facilitates the mapping and management of ideas and arguments, allowing people to record and structure collaboration.[30]

Proprietary
ATLAS.ti is a computer program that assists researchers to uncover and systematically analyze data hidden in text and multimedia, allowing users to code and annotate.[31]

NVivo helps people to manage, shape, and make sense of unstructured information in text and multimedia formats.[32]

or exploratory code categories. Second, axial coding is the intermediate step. This coding allows the researcher to begin to link the data into logical connections between categories. Third, selective coding is the last step and involves establishing the patterns and trends within the data. At this point, the categories are further refined for theory development and validation. All three steps are repeated over and over as the data are revisited in the process of data collection and analysis.

During the coding process, researchers work individually and also in teams to determine if the coding strategies are appropriate. Sometimes the a priori codes are merged together to form new, broader code categories, and other times the codes are split apart into subcategories. Coding is time consuming and only ends when researcher teams agree that patterns and trends are identified to address the research questions. At this point, researchers have the option to quantify the responses in each code category. For example, researchers found that 18 (62%) respondents stated that the staff was friendly and efficient in completing the necessary paperwork for admission. This process is not an attempt to transform qualitative data into quantitative data or to remove the individual richness, but rather it is used to add description to code lists. Lastly, qualitative researchers provide direct quotes to illustrate examples and emphasize noteworthy findings.

TABLE 6-3 Frequency Table for Demographic Data

Demographic Variable (*n* = 150)		
Gender		
	Female	47 (31%)
	Male	103 (69%)
Geographic Place of Residence		
	Urban	81 (54%)
	Rural	69 (46%)
Employment Status		
	Unemployed	17 (11%)
	Part-time employment	55 (37%)
	Full-time employment	54 (36%)
	Retired	24 (16%)

Data Display

When displaying qualitative results, it is useful to use graphics. Qualitative research data are displayed using tables, diagrams, charts, and graphs. Frequency tables are used to describe categorical data, such as demographics. See **Table 6-3**.

Unlike paragraphs of description, diagrams provide a visual depiction of volumes of data. Data used for **Figure 6-2**

FIGURE 6-2 Word cloud.

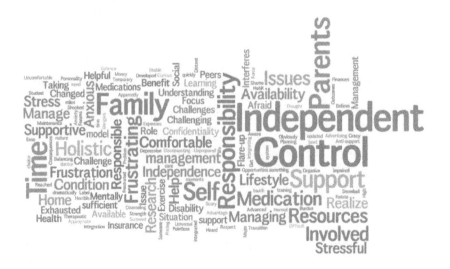

Diagram was made by using Wordle. Available at: www.wordle.net.

FIGURE 6-3 Number of patients admitted per month.

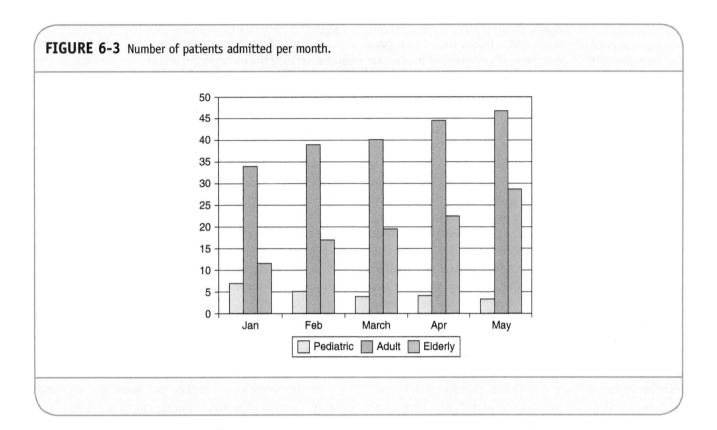

were the keywords taken from interview data of university students with chronic health challenges. The font size illustrates the number of times the word appeared in the interview transcripts. Obviously, the words "independent," "control," "family," "parents," and "support" comprise the key themes. Further analyses of the interviews showed the struggles between the students' desire to be independent and in control of their chronic health challenges, and their need for support from parents and family.

Charts and graphs show chronological order or categories. The two examples show the advantage of using charts and graphs over writing a descriptive paragraph. In **Figure 6-3**, it is easy to see that admissions of adults and elderly patients increased, while pediatric admissions decreased and then stayed about the same. This chart displays trend data used for making forecast projections for funding. The pie chart in **Figure 6-4** shows the patient satisfaction data requested by hospital administrators.

SUMMARY

This chapter focuses on all aspects of qualitative research design. The chapter begins with a discussion of the differences between qualitative and quantitative research designs,

FIGURE 6-4 Pie chart.

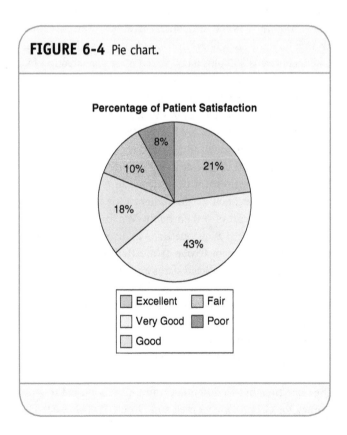

including the advantages and disadvantages of each design. The topic of reliability and validity of qualitative data is presented, followed by a description of each type of qualitative research design. After a discussion of possible ethical issues in qualitative research, the chapter concludes with a description of how to conduct a simple analysis of qualitative data including data organization, coding, and data display.

CASE STUDY

Research Question: Among Medicaid recipients, why do some women receive mammograms in a timely manner while other women never receive mammograms?

The results of this study will be used to design a brochure to encourage women receiving Medicaid to receive mammograms. Drs. Jackson and Graham design a qualitative study to answer the research question. After receiving approval from the institutional review board, they begin the recruitment process.

They decide to conduct a series of focus groups with two types of women: Group One includes women receiving Medicaid between ages 50 and 65 who have received at least two mammograms, and Group Two includes women receiving Medicaid between ages 50 and 65 who have never received a mammogram. Researchers wish to recruit a diverse group of women, so they post recruitment advertisements on social media sites and in local newspapers. They place brightly colored brochures in clinic waiting rooms, church bulletins, neighborhood laundromats, and local cafes. The incentive is $50 plus a taxi voucher for participating in a 90-minute focus group. The focus groups are scheduled for 90 minutes to give women a chance to arrive, locate the room, and get comfortable. However, the actual focus group takes only 1 hour. Focus groups are held at 10:00 a.m. and 6:30 p.m. on Tuesday, Thursday, and Saturday in the community rooms at two centrally located neighborhood libraries. From the flyer or advertisement, women are instructed to call an 800-number to schedule a convenient time to participate in a focus group nearest to their home. When women call, the scheduler asks them a few questions to determine their eligibility for Group One or Group Two. After the scheduler confirms their current Medicaid status and asks the women their age, ethnicity, and home address, the taxi voucher is mailed to each woman. The scheduler reminds each woman that she may not bring children or other family members to the focus group. Focus groups consist of six to eight women of similar demographics who arrive at the most convenient focus group location. In some cases, two focus groups are conducted at the same time in two different community rooms at the same library for Group One women and Group Two women. The

day before each focus group, the scheduler calls to remind each woman of the time, date, and location of the focus group and to verify if her taxi voucher was received.

To avoid researcher personal bias, Drs. Jackson and Graham hire six experienced qualitative researchers to conduct the focus groups. Within each focus group, one researcher serves as facilitator and the second researcher serves as moderator. After each focus group, researchers swapped roles to avoid exhaustion. By using paper name table tents for each participant, the researchers are able to state each woman's name. As women enter the community room, they are served a beverage and snack, given a pre-printed name table tent, and are asked to take a seat at the table. After the digital recording devices are checked at both ends of the table, the focus group begins with an explanation of the informed consent document, followed by the opportunity to ask questions. Each woman signs the informed consent document and gives the researchers one copy, keeping the other copy for future reference. Any woman not comfortable with the procedure is invited to leave at this time and still receive the $50 incentive.

As the focus group begins, the researcher asks each woman to respond to the following question: "When I say mammogram, what is the first thing that comes to mind?" After receiving a response from each participant, the researcher asks the next question on the predetermined interview guide. For the Group One women, the next question is, "How would you describe a mammogram to a woman who had never had a mammogram?" For the Group Two women, the next question is, "Because you have not had a mammogram, what would you like to ask a woman who has had a mammogram about the procedure?" Researchers have the flexibility of asking additional probing questions to gain further detail on any specific question. Each interview question requires a response from each participant, but the probing questions are directed at one or a few women. The process continues until each interview question is answered by each participant. The digital recording device remains on until the women are paid their $50 incentive and leave the room.

After each focus group, digital recordings are transcribed. Drs. Jackson and Graham review the transcriptions in a timely manner. If one question is consistently misunderstood by participants, they change the wording to improve clarity for future focus groups. Major revisions are allowed but require submitting an amendment to the IRB. Drs. Jackson and Graham, along with their graduate students, continue to review the transcripts and discuss possible emerging patterns and themes. Once some themes begin to emerge, the research team decides approximately how many

TABLE 6-4 Budget for One Focus Group

			Total
Facilitator and moderator	2 researchers for 2 hours	$150 per hour	$600
Beverages and snacks			$30
Room rental fee			$100
Incentives	8 women	$50	$400
Taxi vouchers	8 women	$30	$240
Supplies			$20
Transcriptionist	3 hours of typing for every hour of recording	$60 per hour	$180
Total			$1570

more focus groups to convene. Ideally, they want to reach a point of saturation where no new data are noted in the transcripts; however, each focus group is expensive and their funding is limited. See **Table 6-4**.

Fortunately, Drs. Jackson and Graham budgeted $35,000 for conducting the focus groups. After 16 focus groups are conducted and analyzed, the research team agrees that saturation is achieved and key themes have emerged. The challenging aspect of qualitative data analyses is that the actual words of the themes may or may not ever be stated by the focus group participants. For example, after reading and rereading the Group One responses to the first question, the emerging theme was labeled as "peace of mind." The women never stated that getting a mammogram gave them peace of mind, but the collective responses implied this theme, such as "I like to know that I'm ok"; "I get a mammogram, because breast cancer runs in my family. I need to get checked each year"; "I do it as an example for my daughters"; "It is just good to get checked out once in a while"; "I never know if I'm doing the breast self-exam correctly; I like the pros to tell me I'm ok for another year." Researchers agree that all of these quotes plus many more illustrate a "peace of mind" theme as to why women receive periodic mammograms. For the Group Two responses to the first question, the emerging theme is labeled "fear of the unknown." The quotes include: "You never know what they might find. I'd rather not know"; "I don't want to be exposed to that much radiation. I heard that it might cause breast cancer. I don't know about that"; "There is no cancer in my family and besides it is a scary and dangerous procedure anyway"; "I'm not sure that I need to know"; "I do not know what I would do if they found something."

Summary

By looking at only a few quotes from the first question, it is possible to see how researchers are challenged to juggle the data by looking at the big picture while not missing the tiny details. They want to make sure that the comments are unique and not the result of a "group thinking" process where everyone agrees with whatever the first respondent said. Researchers do not want to over- or under-analyze data, but they also do not wish to miss a central theme. Qualitative research data are not only challenging but also intriguing as researchers dig deeper and deeper to discover meaning and answers to their research question.

Case Study Discussion Questions

1. Besides focus groups, what other type of qualitative data could have been used to answer the research questions?
2. Describe the process of developing the codebook for retrieving the themes from the focus groups.

STUDENT ACTIVITY

For the following case studies, design a qualitative study that addresses the pertinent issues.

Case Study 1

Baxter Hospital plans to open a larger Pediatric Unit within 2 years. This unit houses a large waiting room with an indoor play area; two cafes; eight operating room suites; outpatient recovery rooms for 1-day stay procedures; 60 private inpatient pediatric rooms with a single bed for adults wishing to spend the night; three specialty rooms for art, music, and physical therapy; 12 pediatric intensive care beds; and one helicopter rooftop landing site. The hospital administrators wish to market the new pediatric unit as the leading facility in the state. The pediatric design architects know how to utilize the space for efficiency and utility, but they need help with creating a positive, healing atmosphere within the overall space as well as in the specific units. The space needs to work for children of all ages, parents, family members, nurses, therapists, and healthcare providers. What type of qualitative study would answer the concerns of the design architects?

Case Study 2

Sandersburg is located about 90 miles from a large city and has a population of about 30,000 people. For the past 5 years, the local community hospital has lost money. Because it is a small, 80-bed hospital, it is not able to offer the extensive services of the two larger regional hospitals. However, the people living in Sandersburg do come to the hospital for minor emergencies and outpatient surgeries. Because Sandersburg is near a popular ski resort, the tourists utilize the hospital during the winter months. Emergency medical transport teams work out of Sandersburg's emergency department for triage to the regional hospitals. Although the need for the hospital is well documented, financial experts are unable to determine how to make enough profit to justify keeping the hospital open. What type of qualitative study would address how to increase the hospital's profits enough to stay open?

Case Study 3

Greenleaf, a national health insurance company, decided to open a clinic in a busy downtown area near a metro station. Its marketing research team conducted a needs assessment prior to selecting this location. Using geographic information system (GIS) mapping, they learned that a large percentage of their policyholders worked in the tall buildings within a 1-mile radius of the clinic. Over the past year and after an extensive billboard, direct-mail, television, and radio advertising campaign, the clinic continues to be underutilized by the nearby workers. What type of qualitative study would address why policyholders are not utilizing the medical services of the nearby clinic?

Case Study 4

After 20 years in service, Serenity Hospice is a well established facility offering in-home palliative and end-of-life care to the people in Hills County. For the past year, Ms. Hudson, director of nursing, tracked the number of nurses who have left the facility after working there less than 6 months.

Because Serenity Hospice knows that this type of nursing is not for everyone, they offer nurses: 1) 2 weeks of paid hospice training prior to their first in-home assignment, 2) a buddy nurse with more experience, 3) 48 hours of paid time off after each patient death, and 4) 6 weeks of paid personal time off in the first year of employment. Even with these benefits, nurses are leaving after a few months. Ms. Hudson conducts exit interviews with each nurse, but she does not feel like she is getting enough information to solve the nursing staff problem. What type of qualitative study would address why Serenity Hospice is losing nursing staff after a few months of employment?

REFERENCES

1. Marshall C, Rossman GB. *Designing Qualitative Research.* Thousand Oaks, CA: Sage Publications; 1998.

2. Lindlof TR, Taylor BC. *Qualitative Communication Research Methods.* 2nd ed. Thousand Oaks, CA: Sage Publications; 2002.

3. Denzin NK, Lincoln YS. *The SAGE Handbook of Qualitative Research.* 4th ed. Los Angeles: Sage Publications; 2011.

4. Stainback S, Stainback W. Understanding and conducting qualitative research. In: *Conducting a Qualitative Research Study.* Reston, VA: Council for Exceptional Children; 1988.

5. Rubin A, Babbie E. *Research Methods for Social Work.* Pacific Grove, CA: Brooks/Cole; 1993.

6. The Association for Educational Communications and Technology. Ethical Issues in Conducting Qualitative Research. Available at: http://www.aect.org/edtech/ed1/40/40-05.html. Accessed May 3, 2012.

7. Kirk J, Miller M. *Reliability and Validity in Qualitative Research.* London: Sage Publications; 1986.

8. Maxwell JA. Understanding and validity in qualitative research. *Harvard Educat Rev.* 1992;62(3):279–300.

9. Whittemore R, Chase SK, Mandle CL. Validity in qualitative research. *Qual Health Res.* 2001;11(4):522–537.

10. McCall G, Simmons JL. *Issues in Participant Observation.* Reading, MA: Addison-Wesley; 1969.

11. Schaffir WB, Stebbins R. *Experiencing Fieldwork.* Newbury Park, CA: Sage Publications; 1991.

12. Golafshani N. Understanding reliability and validity in qualitative research. *Qual Rep.* 2003;8(4):597–607. Trochim M. Qualitative Methods. Research Methods Knowledge Base. Available at: http://www.socialresearch-methods.net/kb/qualmeth.php. Accessed May 3, 2012.

13. Adler PA, Adler P. Observational techniques. In: Denzin NX, Lincoln YS, eds. *The Sage Handbook of Qualitative Research.* Thousand Oaks, CA: Sage Publications; 1994:377–392.

14. Joppe M. The Research Process—Observation. University of Guelph School of Hospitality and Tourism Management. Available at: http://www.htm.uoguelph.ca/MJResearch/ResearchProcess/Observation.htm. Accessed June 3, 2012.

15. Parasuraman A. *Marketing Research.* 2nd ed. Boston: Addison-Wesley; 1991.

16. Polit D, Hungler BP. *Nursing Research: Principles and Methods.* 2nd ed. Philadelphia, PA: Lippincott; 1983.

17. Stake R. Case study methods in educational research: seeking sweet water. In: Jaeger RM, ed. *Complementary Methods for Research in Education.* Washington, DC: American Educational Research Association; 1988:251–279.

18. Key JP. Research Design in Occupational Education. Available at: http://www.okstate.edu/ag/agedcm4h/academic/aged5980a/5980/newpage19.htm. Accessed May 3, 2012.

19. Goetz JP, LeCompte MD. *Ethnology and Qualitative Design in Educational Research.* Lexington, MA: D. C. Heath; 1984.

20. Glaser B, Strauss A. *The Discovery of Grounded Theory.* Chicago: Aldine; 1967.

21. Kirk J, Miller M. (1986). *Reliability and Validity in Qualitative Research.* London: Sage Publications.

22. Strauss A, Corbin J. *Basics of Qualitative Research.* Newbury Park, CA: Sage Publications; 1990.

23. Taylor J. Toward alternative forms of social work research: the case for naturalistic methods. *Journal of Social Welfare.* 1977;4(2):119–126.

24. Gilgun JF. Steps in the development of theory using a grounded theory approach. *Qualitative Family Research Newsletter.* 1990;4(2):11–12.

25. Gilgun JF. Definitions, methodologies, and methods in qualitative family research. In: Gilgun JF, Daly K, Handel G, eds. *Qualitative Methods in Family Research.* Newbury Park, CA: Sage Publications; 1992:22–40.

26. McRoy RG. Qualitative Research. Available at: http://www.uncp.edu/home/marson/qualitative_research.html. Accessed May 3, 2012.

27. Fielding NG, Lee RM. *Using Computers in Qualitative Research.* London: Sage Publications; 1992.

28. Miles M, Huberman M. *Qualitative Data Analysis: A Sourcebook of New Methods.* Beverly Hills, CA: Sage Publications; 1984.

29. University of Pittsburgh. Coding Analysis Toolkit. Available at: http://cat.ucsur.pitt.edu/. Accessed May 3, 2012.

30. Compendium Institute. Available at: http://compendium.open.ac.uk/institute/. Accessed May 3, 2012.

31. Atlasti. Available at: http://www.atlasti.com/index.html. Accessed May 3, 2012.

32. QSR International/ NVivo. Available at: http://www.qsrinternational.com/products_nvivo.aspx. Accessed May 3, 2012.

33. QSR International. What is Qualitative Research? Available at: http://www.qsrinternational.com/what-Is-qualitative-research.aspx. Accessed May 3, 2012.

34. Marlow C. (1993). *Research Methods.* Pacific Grove, CA: Brooks/Cole Publishing Company; 1993.

CHAPTER 7

Evaluation Design

KEY TERMS

constructs
operational definition
quantitative design
variable

INTRODUCTION

This chapter introduces quantitative designs used in evaluation. Quantitative data are composed of numerical files used to answer specific goals and objectives and are analyzed using statistics. The focus of this chapter, evaluation, is built on determining the significance, accomplishment, and value of the program or project that is being evaluated.[1]

As social service budgets decrease, the need for quality evaluations increases in order to show effectiveness and efficacy of new and existing programs, procedures, and interventions. Evaluation results and recommendations focus on the strengths and weaknesses of various aspects of innovations and interventions and on the overall outcome.

ELEMENTS OF DESIGN

As evaluators plan, design, and implement evaluation programs, it is useful to think about the following questions:[1]

- What is the need for this program?
- Is this program based in theory?
- Is the program implemented correctly and according to the design plan?
- Is the program having the impact that was intended?
- Is the program within budget and cost effective?

Once the evaluator has the big picture in mind, it is important to think about the purpose of the evaluation. The purpose directs the design. For example, if the purpose of the evaluation is to determine the cost effectiveness, the design will be different than if the evaluation is to determine implementation fidelity. In all situations, the goals and objectives guide the evaluation design. Without specific goals and objectives, it is not possible to design the correct evaluation. Furthermore, without the correct design, incorrect data collection results in inadequate interpretation of the findings. Even with specific goals, objectives, and correct design, evaluators consider a range of plausible and alternative explanations when reviewing the results.

After the design is selected, the evaluator needs to consider several more issues. The next section introduces the concepts of operational definitions, variables, observations, and measurement.

Operational Definitions

Operational definitions are based on constructs and the goals and objectives of the program. It is up to the evaluator to provide clear and concise definitions for each construct. Evaluators may select a dictionary definition or provide a more specific definition suited to the evaluation. For example, if the evaluation involves interviewing senior citizens, it is necessary to provide an operational age definition for "senior citizens." The inclusion criteria may be individuals age 60 and older based on the population that the program serves, but others may define seniors as age 65 and older because that is how the federal government defines the concept. In cases like this, there is no absolute correct definition for the term *senior*, so the evaluator chooses that for this study the definition of "senior" is individuals 65 years of age or older on the day of the interview. For each construct, it is necessary to provide an operational definition in order to diminish bias in data analysis and interpretation.

Variables

Variables are defined as the items that can be changed or manipulated during the program or intervention. A variable may also represent an unknown quality or characteristic. There are different types of variables. The following list describes the purpose of each type of variable:

- *Independent variables* (IV) are what evaluators change or manipulate to understand their effect on the dependent or controlled variables. It is the variable believed to cause the change. For example, the independent variable may be the teaching simulation method used in the driver's education class. Any change in the independent variable is expected to have a change on the dependent variable.
- *Dependent variable* (DV) is affected by or reacts to the independent variable. For example, the quiz grades were higher (dependent variable) in the driver's education class after implementing the new teaching simulation method (independent variable).
- *Mediating variable* is defined as an intervening variable as it acts between the IV and DV. For example, a driver's education student taking the course for the second time may already have greater benefit from the simulation method than a student who obtained his learner's permit last week and has never actually driven a car.
- *Moderating variable* is used to show how relationships change with different variables. Using the same example, age is a possible moderating variable. Students with a driver's permit who are under the age of 17 may respond to the driver simulation differently from adult students who are enrolled in the course to get insurance points removed from their license due to a traffic ticket.
- *Confounding or extraneous variables* interfere with the independent and dependent variables. Sometimes evaluators are not aware of confounding variables until late into the study. For example, some of the drivers may share information in the parking lot during a break about how to "trick" the simulation equipment. Unbeknownst to the evaluators, the drivers try this simulation trick to make the evaluator think that the teaching method is improving their scores when, in fact, it is because of the information shared in the parking lot. These types of events are difficult and sometimes impossible to discover for evaluators.
- *Controlled variable* is held statistically constant so relationships between other variables may be analyzed without interference. For example, age may serve as the control variable, while the evaluators wish to know the relationship between gender and the effectiveness of the driver simulation method. When holding age constant, the evaluators can study if the driver simulation teaching method works better for one gender over the other.

Without intentionally causing confusion, it is important to note that previously defined variables are also viewed as either categorical or continuous for data analysis.

Categorical variables are defined as variables that name groups or categories, such as gender, ethnicity, ZIP code, employment status, or marital status. Within each group, the choices are independent or mutually exclusive from the other choices. For example, a survey question asks, "What is your current marital status?" The choices include: single, married, divorced, or widowed. Even if a person has experienced several of the listed choices, the question is asking for the respondent's current marital status. He or she selects one response choice for his or her current status and cannot choose any other. Second, continuous variables are measured over an incremental range, such as age, weight, height, resting heart rate, or cholesterol level. On a survey, respondents may be asked for the ZIP code of their primary place of residence (a categorical variable) and approximately how many miles the respondent drives on a typical day (a continuous variable). Evaluators could use these survey results to determine the level of public transportation usage.

Variables also have attributes. Once evaluators determine each variable, the next step is to assign attributes to the variables. First, the choices are mutually exclusive, which means that each choice is clearly different from the other choices. When a survey asks "If you drive to work most days each week, what type of motorized vehicle is driven to work daily?" the choices are: 1 = car, 2 = truck, 3 = sports utility vehicle (SUV), 4 = van or minivan, 5 = large motor coach vehicle, 6 = motorcycle, 7 = other, 8 = I take public transportation, 9 = I carpool, 10 = I walk to work, 11 = I work from my home, 12 = I do not work. It is important that each variable provides an exhaustive list of choices.

Second, a survey question asks respondents for their level of agreement. For example:

1. I feel happy most days. (*Circle the choice that best describes you.*)

> Strongly agree
> Agree
> Neutral
> Disagree
> Strongly disagree

Third, the attribute allows respondents to "check all that apply." In the example, it is possible that a respondent is working full-time and seeking a new job or a respondent is working one steady, part-time job as well as working a seasonal job on the weekends.

2. Describe your employment status today. (*Check all that apply.*)

> ☐ Full-time employment
> ☑ Part-time employment with steady, regular hours
> ☐ Part-time with unreliable hours
> ☑ Seasonal employment
> ☐ Temporary or day labor
> ☐ Contract employment, set hours for specific time period
> ☐ Seeking employment

Each type of variable attribute refines the information collected from respondents. The evaluator determines the attribute to use in each of the survey questions that best suits the objectives of the evaluation project.

Observations or Measurements

There are single and multiple observations. Observations are defined as watching an individual or group of individuals for the purpose of data collection. A single observation or measurement includes individual items such as observing workers for one hour at a factory assembly line to determine how often they make the same repetitive motion, watching children on a playground to determine favorite equipment, noting how many bikers are wearing bike helmets at a specific location and time of day, and so forth. The variable is observed and recorded only once per designated time and location. Multiple measurements involve measuring one variable several times over a defined period of time, such as watching bikers at the same intersection for 20 consecutive mornings from 7:00 a.m. until 9:00 a.m. Another multiple measurement involves collecting pretest survey data prior to an intervention and then again after the intervention. For example, public health students complete an online campus safety survey prior to attending the campus safety seminar; 3 weeks later the same students are asked to complete the same online survey again. The data analysis reveals the potential effectiveness of a campus safety seminar.

Treatments or Programs

Treatments or programs are defined as a single intervention, regardless of the time involvement or the number of sessions. A treatment can be one breastfeeding health education class, one epidemiology course offered during a 15-week semester, a 4-week safe driving course for elderly citizens, or a community-wide exercise program to promote walking in four specific neighborhoods. In evaluation, it is common to have one group of individuals participating in the treatment and one control group or nonparticipation group. It is also possible to have individuals or groups of individuals enter into the treatment or program in waves. For example, the 4-week free safe driving course for senior citizens is offered starting with the residents in one retirement complex, and then offered in a second retirement complex, and then a third and last retirement complex in the same county. Over 6 months, the driving residents in each of the retirement complexes have the opportunity to attend the driver safety course. Once the retirement complex drivers have completed the free safe driving course, the course is opened to all elderly drivers in the county. At the end of the free driver safety courses, the evaluators determine if the number of traffic tickets and auto crashes involving the senior drivers decreases or remains the same in the county.

Group Assignment

Depending on the evaluation design, evaluators assign individuals to a specific group prior to initiating the evaluation. There are several ways to make such group assignments, including random group assignment, quota group assignment, and every *n*th group assignment.

Random Group Assignment

Groups rather than individuals are assigned to random groups. For example, the evaluation team is evaluating a positive youth development program that is intended to increase certain positive aspects (e.g., leadership, teen pregnancy prevention, community service, and mentoring) among high school students. The random groups are assigned by schools rather than individual students. For the random group assignment, if there are 48 counties in the state, the first step is to match the county demographics depending on the goals and objectives of the evaluation. For example, there are many ways to match county demographics, including population size, number of square miles, social factors (income, education level, housing costs, age, etc.), geographic factors (urban, suburban, or rural), high school graduation rates, type and usage of public transportation, and unemployment rates. Once the county demographics are determined, the evaluators match similarly sized high schools in one county with similarly sized high schools in another county with comparable demographics. This process continues until all high schools are matched. Of the paired schools, one school is randomly assigned to the treatment group and the other paired school is randomly assigned to the control group. This random assignment can be done by writing the names of the first two matched schools on slips of paper. Fold the paper slips. Place the two slips in a hat and let someone draw out one slip of paper. The first name drawn is the treatment group, and the remaining slip becomes the control group. Repeat this process with the next two matched schools and so on until all matched schools are assigned to treatment or control.

Quota Group Assignment

For quota group assignment, evaluators use census data to determine what percentage of individuals are in each group of interest. For example, evaluators may wish to represent the population diversity in the United States according to the 2010 U.S. Census. Using **Table 7-1**, evaluators recruit specific groups of individuals based on their ethnicity and other inclusion research criteria. See Table 7.1.

Every nth Group Assignment

In the nth group assignment, evaluators select groups of individuals in a preset and specific pattern, such as every 10th or 20th individual on a list. For example, if evaluators wished to mail a satisfaction survey to a random sample of county employees who were hired in the last 12 months, the evaluation team might decide to use the nth group assignment. After receiving institutional review board (IRB) approval for the study, evaluators obtain a list of 250 new employees' names and mailing addresses. They select every 5th person to receive the satisfaction survey for a total of 50 mailed surveys. There is a limitation of concern when using this method. If the employee list of names was in alphabetical order, evaluators run the risk of selecting too many individuals from one common name group, such as Smith, Johnson, Rodriguez, or Patel, depending on the common ethnicity of the geographic area. To resolve this limitation, evaluators arrange the employees by date of hire rather than in alphabetical order prior to selecting every 5th individual to receive the mailed satisfaction survey.

Constructs

In evaluation, a construct is a concept, thought, or notion that is more challenging to measure, such as self-esteem, spirituality, motivation, or achievement, rather than a concrete concept, such as body mass index (BMI), height, weight, girth, or blood glucose level. Frequently, evaluators arrange several specific measures together to form a construct. For example, the construct of positive youth development may be a collection of leadership and public speaking skills, community service endeavors, and mentoring. By forming a positive youth development construct, evaluators determine if the youth are increasing and decreasing valuable skills or characteristics more or less than is typically expected. When defining a construct, it is important to seek agreement from experts on how to describe the terms and determine if the

TABLE 7-1 Sample of Quota Group Assignment

	Percentage from 2010 U.S. Census	Study Population (1500 Individuals)
White	72.4	1086
Black or African American	12.6	189
American Indian and Alaskan Native	.9	13.5
Asian	4.8	72
Native Hawaiian and Other Pacific Islander	.2	3
Some Other Race	6.2	93
Two or More Races	2.9	43.5

Data from Humes KR, Jones NA, Ramirez RR. Overview of Race and Hispanic Origin: 2010. The United States Census Bureau. Available at: http://www.census.gov/prod/cen2010/briefs/c2010br-02.pdf.

chosen items truly measure the construct. The term used is *construct validity* and is defined as the degree to which the construct measures the concept being studied. If the construct has low validity, then the study results yield low generalizability to other study populations. If the construct has high validity, when the construct is used with a different study population, similar results yield high generalizability.[2]

TYPES OF DESIGN

Evaluation design is the framework or scaffolding. In this section, three types of design are described, including true experimental, quasi-experimental, and non-experimental design. True experimental design is when random assignment is used to determine how participants are assigned to groups and the independent variable is manipulated. Quasi-experimental design does not use random assignment. Non-experimental design is used when there is no need for group assignment. For example, if the evaluators wish to know more about what customers think of having calorie counts listed on the menu for each item, they would place a postcard survey and pencil on each table and ask customers to complete a survey after each meal. If they took the survey to the check-out register, the customer would receive a 10% discount on their bill as an incentive for completing the survey. In this case, there is no need for a random assignment. Now, let's explore each type of design in greater detail. See **Figure 7.1**.

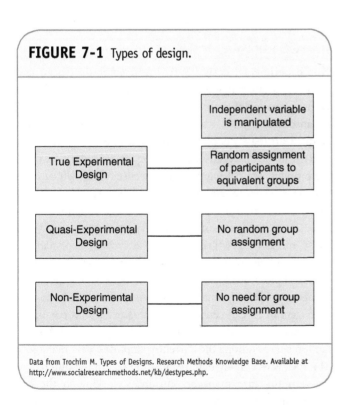

FIGURE 7-1 Types of design.

Data from Trochim M. Types of Designs. Research Methods Knowledge Base. Available at http://www.socialresearchmethods.net/kb/destypes.php.

True Experimental Design

True experimental design includes 1) manipulating the independent variable, 2) exploring cause-and-effect relationships, and 3) random assignment of participants to equivalent groups. Let's discuss each of these points in detail:

1. True experimental design allows evaluators to determine cause-and-effect relationships. As independent variables (IV) are changed, evaluators understand the effect on the dependent variable (DV). In addition, evaluators must control the other types of variables as much as possible to strengthen the cause-and-effect relationship. Because it is not possible to prove an absolute cause-and-effect relationship, evaluators use statistical calculation to determine whether the results are due to findings rather than probability due to random chance.[3]

2. With a causal relationship in the objectives, the manipulation of the treatment variable, also called the IV, produces different outcomes in the DV. Any differences in the DV are due to the applied treatment conditions or manipulation of the treatment. For example, suppose evaluators wanted to verify which prophylactic malaria treatment produces the least amount of adverse side effects. In the current prophylactic malaria treatment, the two most common adverse side effects are gastrointestinal symptoms and sleep disturbances. The IV is the type of prophylactic malaria treatment, and the DV is the reduction of adverse side effects. One hundred Fulbright scholars traveling to Southeast Asia agreed to participate in this evaluation: 50 individuals agreed to take Malaria Treatment A, and 50 individuals agreed to take Malaria Treatment B.

3. Random assignment determines how participants are assigned to a minimum of two equal groups: Malaria Treatment A and Malaria Treatment B. Keep in mind that random selection and random assignment are not the same. Random selection is a sample chosen from a population, while random assignment is used in true experimental design.

Another aspect of random assignment is called blinding. When individuals are not told which treatment they are receiving, it is called a blinded study. For example, after an individual agrees to participate in an evaluation, he is asked to select one of two envelopes. Each envelope contains either a blue (treatment) or yellow (control) card. Evaluators open the envelope and write down the individual's name and the color of the card selected. In this case, evaluators know if the individual is in the treatment or control group. When the random assignment is not conducted by the evaluator, it is called a double-blinded study, because the participant and the evaluators are not aware of which individuals are in the treatment and which are in the control group. In this situation, the individual still selects an envelope, but the evaluators are not aware what each colored card represents. This option is the strongest research design, because neither the individual nor the evaluator is aware of the treatment or control selected for each participant. This method reduces bias.

For example, 90 women are recruited to participate in three 60-minute sessions per week for a 10-week exercise program evaluation conducted by the College of Physical Therapy. Prior to the initiation of the program, the women are evaluated by a physical therapist to document their pre-exercise leg strength level, BMI, and lung capacity. After the physical therapy assessment, the 90 women are invited to participate in a true experimental randomized evaluation. After signing the informed consent documents, each woman selects an envelope with an enclosed colored card corresponding to Group A (cardio machines, strength exercises, and fitness information class), Group B (aerobics class and weight machines), or Group C (control = running outside only). Thirty women are assigned to each group. All recruited women work 40 hours per week and are between 50 and 60 years old. After 10 weeks of participating in the three different exercise programs, evaluators receive data from the physical therapy records to determine if there are statistically significant differences between the overall fitness improvement and post-BMI of Groups A, B, and C. In this example, the IV is the exercise program and the DV is the BMI. Because other variables were held constant (such as age), the cause-and-effect relationship is strong. See **Box 7-1**.

While randomized, controlled trials are considered the "gold standard," before moving to the next type of design, it is worth noting some limitations of true experimental designs. One limitation is that individuals in the control group may inadvertently be exposed to the treatment, for example, individuals sharing experiences in a common waiting room. When the evaluation setting is a school or a residential facility, it is not feasible to randomly assign each student or resident to various different treatment options, especially when the differences are noticeable. In this situation, evaluators would use a quasi-experimental design.

Quasi-Experimental Design

Unlike true experimental design, quasi-experimental design has no random assignment or matched groups, no control group, and evaluators do not manipulate the independent variable. Evaluation results yield limited generalizable conclusions. In quasi-experimental design, the assignment is based on factors such as cost, convenience, feasibility, or some other criteria. Evaluators may or may not have control over which individuals or groups are assigned to each treatment group. Also, if the design involves using multiple waves of enrollment, it is a quasi-experimental design. See **Box 7-2**.

The limitation of quasi-experimental design is that it cannot determine cause-and-effect relationships and cannot exclude *all* the reasons why a relationship does exist, including the lack of definitive causal inference and possible confounding bias cause by the dissimilarity among groups.[4]

Non-Experimental Design

Non-experimental design is the most common design and involves variables that are not manipulated by the evaluator. Non-experimental evaluation variables are not manipulated, because they involve attributes (e.g., gender, socioeconomic status, learning style, or any other personal characteristic or trait), a single observation, and survey or secondary data that were previously collected, such as census data. Unlike true and quasi-experimental research, non-experimental evaluation involves: 1) no manipulation of the independent variable, 2) no random assignment of participants, and 3) no cause-and-effect conclusions due to alternative explanations. This type of design uses mostly descriptive statistical analysis. For example, if evaluators were hired by a health insurance company to determine the job satisfaction of telephone case managers in its call centers, the evaluators would conduct a non-experimental design including: 1) a one-time job satisfaction survey among the currently employed case managers; 2) a review of employment records to explore the differences between the case managers currently working in the call centers and the case managers who left the call center critical

---

BOX 7-1 Example of a True Experimental Research Design

Pre-BMI	Treatment	Post-BMI
A_1	$X_{E\ Group\ A}$	B_2
A_1	$X_{E\ Group\ B}$	B_2
A_1	$X_{C\ Group\ C}$	B_2

E = Experimental group
C = Control group

Data from Gribbons B, Herman J. True and quasi-experimental designs. *Practical Assessment, Research & Evaluation*. 1997; 5(14). http://PAREonline.net/getvn.asp?v=5&n=14.

BOX 7-2 Example of a Quasi-Experimental Design

An evaluation team was hired by the State Department of Health to evaluate the level of satisfaction of consumers with their new federally sponsored health insurance plans sold through the State Department of Health website. Because the consumers had already purchased one of the three federally sponsored health insurance plans, the evaluators selected a quasi-experimental design. Also, there was no need to manipulate the independent variable. The evaluators developed a health insurance plan satisfaction survey. After pilot testing the survey, the State Department of Health supplied the evaluators with an email address list for the consumers who purchased one of the three new federally sponsored health insurance plans. The evaluators emailed the satisfaction survey to the first 1000 consumers who purchased each of the three new federally sponsored health insurance plans. Because there is no need for random assignment in quasi-experimental design, the evaluation team decided that the first 1000 consumers on each list would be adequate, because these consumers had the new federally sponsored health insurance longer and would have more experience using the new health insurance than consumers who purchased the insurance more recently. The online survey format entered the survey results into a database for easy data analysis and without the cost of data entry. A few of the limitations of this evaluation include that consumers who purchased the health insurance early may be different from those consumers who purchased the health insurance later. Also, the consumers who have access to email and the computer skills to complete an online survey may be different from consumers with limited computer access or skills to complete an online survey. The results showed that consumers reported different levels of satisfaction with the three health plans. Some consumers reported difficulty in finding healthcare providers who accept their type of health plan, other consumers reported satisfaction with healthcare providers but dissatisfaction with prescription medication coverage and high copayments, and some consumers reported high satisfaction with primary care provider choices but low satisfaction with finding specialized healthcare providers and auxiliary care, such as physical therapy and mental health therapy. Because the results were mixed, the evaluation team was unable to provide clear results, but rather stated recommendations on ways to improve each of the three federally sponsored health insurance plans for consumers.

care unit, such as by ascertaining the average length of time working in the call center prior to leaving, the type of shifts (12-hour, 10-hour, 8-hour), education background, and years and type of experience; and 3) an assessment of case managers who left the call center, but remained employed at the health insurance company within a different division, versus those who resigned from the health insurance company. These data reveal case managers' job satisfaction by using a non-experimental design. However, it is noted that non-experimental design does not assess cause-and-effect relationships, but rather focuses on descriptive data, considers alternative explanations, and poses conclusions without causal relationships.[5]

SUMMARY

This chapter introduces quantitative evaluation designs. As discussed, quantitative evaluation uses numerical data and is analyzed using statistics. After developing the goals and objectives, the discussion moved to defining constructs, operations definitions, variables, and group assignments. Following this section, various types of designs were described, including non-experimental, quasi-experimental, and true experimental designs. It is important to remember that the purpose of the evaluation directs the type of design selected.

CASE STUDY

At North Central University, an evaluation team was hired to evaluate three nonmedical alternative practices used to lower hypertension. Group One (Greenfield Clinic staff) participated in yoga class a minimum of 60 minutes three times per week; Group Two (Banner Clinic staff) participated in mindful meditation for 20 minutes daily after attending a 90-minute introductory session to explain the components of mindful meditation; and Group Three (Main Street Clinic staff) participated in a 30-minute outdoor walking group three times per week at a time (before work, during lunch, or after work) agreed upon by the group members. Participants in all three groups are encouraged to maintain their usual exercise routine and only add yoga, mindful meditation, and walking/talking as per their group assignment.

Operational Definition

For this study, hypertension is defined as a clinical blood pressure reading of 140/90 mm Hg or higher during three consecutive clinic visits. Blood pressure is taken three times (beginning, middle, and end) per visit to verify blood pressure reading. The individual may not be taking any hypertensive medication at the time of study recruitment.

For this study, a participant is defined as any adult between 45 and 60 years of age, employed 40 hours per week at North Central University Hospital. All participants have the same health insurance plan offered by the university hospital.

Recruitment

Participants are recruited from the staff of the three university-based clinics located on the main university campus and the midtown university campus. A total of 150 (50 from each clinic) participants are recruited over a 6-month period from April to September. To receive the monthly $25 incentive (total $150), during the first week of each month, individuals stopped by the clinic to turn in their completed log sheets and have their blood pressure taken by the clinic nurse.

Study Design

Quasi-experimental design is used for this study. After IRB approval and informed consent forms were signed, the evaluators explained that the participating staff at the Greenfield Clinic would be involved in a yoga class a minimum of 60 minutes three times per week. The yoga classes would be offered before work, at noon, and after work for all clinic staff but required for those staff members participating in the evaluation. The Banner Clinic staff would have the opportunity to participate in mindful meditation for 20 minutes daily after attending a 90-minute introductory session to explain the components of mindful meditation. The mindful meditation introduction class would be open to all clinic staff, but required for those staff members participating in the evaluation. Last, the Main Street Clinic staff would have the opportunity to participate in a 30-minute outdoor walking group three times per week. Walking groups would be available before work, during lunch, and after work for all staff members, but required for the staff members participating in the evaluation. The independent variable is the nonmedical alternative practice and the dependent variable is blood pressure reading. For 6 months, each study participant stops by the clinic during the first week of each month to receive the $25 incentive, have his or her blood pressure taken twice, and turn in his or her log sheets.

Data Collection

At the end of the 6 months of data collection, the evaluation team will review the log sheets and clinic blood readings for each staff participant. The variables include gender, age, baseline blood pressure, monthly blood pressure readings, type of nonmedical alternative exercise, and log sheets.

Case Study Discussion Questions

1. What are the possible limitations of this study?
2. How could the study be improved?
3. What are the possible ethical issues?

STUDENT ACTIVITIES

Read the following peer-reviewed abstract summaries and answer the questions that follow each one.

Case 1

Data from Robitaille Y, Fournier M, Laforest S, Gauvin L, Filiatrault J, Corriveau H. Effect of a fall prevention program on balance maintenance using a quasi-experimental design in real-world settings. *J Aging Health*. Published online 15 March 2012. Epub ahead of print.

Researchers wanted to know if a community-based fall prevention program for the elderly named *Stand Up!* would have an effect on people's balance and would work under real-world conditions. The program promotes physical activity, home safety, and fall-safe behaviors among seniors in group settings like community centers. The 12-week program included biweekly group exercise sessions led by rehabilitation professionals; weekly home exercise modules; and weekly educational sessions on fall prevention. The regional health department invited community organizations to take part in the program, and some participants were very excited. For the first year, 10 organizations participated in the program and study assessment. During that time, 7 organizations participated in the assessment but did not immediately participate in the program. They would receive the program in the second year. Researchers gathered a lot of information from participants including age, sex, education, current frequency of physical activity, and current health information before they began the study. The year-long study collected data on balance tests and self-reported falls from participants before the program, immediately following the program, and 3 and 6 months later. During the study, only 10 people were lost to follow-up in the experimental group, and only 7 people in the control group. Researchers found that 9 months after the end of the program the intervention participants had higher balance scores and reported fewer falls.

Questions

1. Is this basic or applied research?
2. How were participants assigned?
3. What kind of research design did this study use?
4. How many observations were there?
5. What was the independent variable(s)?

6. What was the dependent variable(s)?

7. What are some variables that should be controlled by researchers?

8. What is one possible confounding variable?

9. What could be one possible mediating variable?

Answers

1. Applied. Because they are working in a real-world setting and not in a laboratory, these researchers want to know if a real health program has real effects in a real setting, with people with real need.

2. Ten organizations were assigned to receive the program (the experiment), and 7 organizations did not receive the program (control) in the first year, but would receive it after the study was over.

3. Quasi-experimental, because subjects were assigned to an experiment, but were not randomized into either the experimental or control groups.

4. There were four observations. There was a pretest, a posttest, and two follow-up tests.

5. The *Stand Up!* program.

6. Balance performance tests and the incidence of self-reported falls.

7. Researchers should be aware of participants' age, sex, education, current frequency of physical activity, and current health information, because they could all possibly affect the outcome of the study. For example, if the intervention group happens to have younger more active seniors and the control group happens to have seniors with more serious health problems that affect balance, it may be those factors that affect balance more than the intervention, unless they are controlled for in statistical analysis.

8. One possible confounding variable would be the number of people who dropped out of the study. If they left the study because they experienced a fall and hurt themselves, this would have an effect on whether the program was successful or not, and not just whether people randomly did not complete it. Researchers should always investigate why some people finish interventions and why others do not, to see if the reason they did not would have an effect of the efficacy of the program.

9. Some participants were very excited about the program. Therefore, it is possible that they were very motivated to integrate physical activity into their lifestyle, which had an outcome on intervention.

Case 2

Data from Turk V, Khattran S, Kerry S, Corney R, Painter K. Reporting of health problems and pain by adults with an intellectual disability and by their careers. *Journal of Applied Research in Intellectual Disabilities.* 2012; 25:155–165.

Information about the health of people with intellectual disabilities (ID) is normally obtained from the individuals who take care of them. A study in a major metropolitan city was undertaken to see if there was a difference between the health issues reported by the individual with ID and their caretakers (or "carers"). Participants were identified from the joint health/social services learning disability registers in a major city of all known adults with severe learning disabilities and adults with mild learning disabilities and additional complex needs. Participants were approached to provide their consent/assent after their doctors had agreed to take part in the research. Researchers used several measures: a health checklist devised for people with ID that could be read to them, another health problem checklist to measure the number and type of problems that people with ID and their caretakers knew to be treated in the past year, doctor visit recalls with medical record reviews, and a disability assessment. Interviews with participants to go over these measures took about an hour to an hour and a half, while interviews with their caretakers took an hour and a half to 2 hours. When answers were matched and analyzed, it appeared that participants reported different numbers and types of health problems than their caretakers reported. Knowing this information could lead health and caretaker staff to be trained on being more observant and responsive to the health needs reported by individuals with intellectual disabilities.

Questions

1. Is this basic or applied research?
2. How were participants assigned?
3. What kind of research design did this study use?
4. How many observations were there?
5. What were the independent and dependent variables?

Answers

1. Both. This study wanted to simply find out if people with ID reported their health problems differently from their caretakers. However, there are practical applications that could help caretakers better understand the needs of their charges and be more responsive to them.

2. All people who were listed on the learning disability register were eligible for the study as long as their physician agreed to it.

3. Non-experimental design. Random assignment was not used in this study, nor was there a control group used for comparison.

4. Even though participants were not interviewed on multiple occasions, there were still multiple observations because several different measures were taken. This is called triangulation.

5. There were no independent or dependent variables because no characteristic was being manipulated. This was an exploratory study that looked at different reporting practices among people with ID and their caretakers. If a training intervention was given to one group of caretakers on recognizing health problems and not given to another, then the intervention would be the independent variable, and differences in reported health problems would be the dependent variable.

Case 3

Data from Long JA, Jahnle EC, Richardson DM, Loewenstein G, Volpp KG. Peer mentoring and financial incentives to improve glucose control in African American veterans. *Ann Intern Med.* 2012; 156:416–424.

Compared with white persons, African Americans have a greater incidence of diabetes. A research group wanted to know whether peer mentors or a financial incentive was better than the usual care received among African American Veterans to decrease their blood glucose levels. Researchers chose a Veterans Affairs (VA) Medical Center as the location for their research study. Of 276 African American men between the ages of 50 and 70 who had poorly managed diabetes, only 192 could be contacted, of which 118 agreed to be in the study. Patients were randomly assigned to one of three groups: usual care, peer mentoring, or financial incentives. The participants were listed in an Excel file, and a group was assigned per every 40 participants. Using a random-number generator, each group was given a random number and put into ordered numbers in envelopes. The envelopes were sealed, shuffled, and stacked, and a research assistant took the top envelope after consent was obtained to determine group assignment. Neither study investigators nor laboratory personnel knew who was in which group. All patients were given a baseline survey, and their blood glucose was measured prior to starting the intervention. The mentoring group was assigned trained peer mentors of similar age, sex, and ethnic background, and was instructed to talk to their mentees at least once a week. Patients were called once a month to determine diabetic symptoms and intervention safety; blood glucose was tracked at participants' regular doctor's appointments. At the end of 6 months, the intervention was complete and data were analyzed. Researchers found that peer mentoring was statistically significant in reducing blood glucose levels over financial incentives and care as usual.

Questions

1. What was the research question of this study?
2. Was this basic or applied research?
3. How were participants assigned?
4. What kind of research design was this?
5. How many observations were there?
6. What was the independent variable(s)?
7. What was the dependent variable(s)?
8. Were there controlled variables?

Answers

1. Does a peer mentoring or financial incentive lower blood glucose levels among diabetic patients better than care as usual?
2. Applied. Researchers wanted to know which kind of care helped patients with diabetes lower their blood glucose best.
3. Randomly, because neither the study researchers nor the VA lab staff knew who was in which group.
4. True experimental design. This was a randomized controlled trial, the gold standard of research.
5. Many. There was a pretest and a posttest, which looked at blood glucose levels. Additionally, patients were surveyed monthly on whether they had experienced any diabetic symptoms.
6. Peer mentoring or financial incentive group assignment was the independent variable.
7. Blood glucose levels at the end of the study were the dependent variable.
8. Yes, all participants were male, of the same age group, and all were African American. This reduced the likelihood that any difference in the outcomes was confounded due to differences in gender, age, and race. Further, in the peer-mentoring group, all mentors were of similar gender, age, and racial background, limiting the likelihood that differences between groups were due to confounding variables.

Case 4

Data from Craciun C, Schuz N, Lippke S, Schwarzer R. Facilitating sunscreen use in women by a theory-based online intervention: A randomized controlled trial. *J Health Psychol.* 2012; 17:207–216.

Researchers wanted to know if there were differences between types of sunscreen use promotion. They wanted to know whether or not a motivational intervention was better or worse than a motivational plus planning intervention in increasing sunscreen use among women. Participants were recruited through announcements placed on university websites, blogs, and discussion forums worldwide. The intervention was available in English, German, Portuguese, and Romanian. Two hundred five women from the age of 18 to 66 years (average age of 25 years) gave their consent to participate in the study and were sent an online questionnaire about their sun protection habits. Each participant was randomized into one of three groups (control, motivational, and planning) using a computer-assisted, random number generator upon logging in to the website. Women in the control group were given information about their skin type. Women in the motivational intervention were given information about risks associated with sun exposure and the benefits of sunscreen use. Women in the planning intervention were also given information about the risk of sun exposure, the benefits of sunscreen use, and also were asked to generate an action and coping plan. All participants were assessed on their sunscreen use two more times before data were analyzed. The study found that only women who were in the planning intervention increased their sunscreen use, meaning that future interventions should not rely solely on motivating people about the risks of poor health behaviors and the benefits of good health behaviors.

Questions

1. What was the research question of this study?
2. Was this basic or applied research?
3. How were participants assigned?
4. What kind of research design was this?
5. How many observations were there?
6. What was the independent variable(s)?
7. What was the dependent variable(s)?
8. Were there controlled variables?
9. What are some possible confounding variables?
10. What is one mediating variable?

Answers

1. Does a difference in the type of sunscreen promotion affect actual sunscreen use?
2. Applied. Researchers want to know if an intervention will affect the real-world sunscreen use of individuals.
3. Randomly. The computer randomly assigned individuals to different groups upon logging in to the study website. Neither the individual nor the study participants knew who would be assigned to what intervention.

4. True experimental design. Because there was random assignment to groups with a manipulated characteristic, this study was a true experiment.
5. Three. This study had multiple observations; there was a pretest and two follow-up surveys.
6. The independent variable in this study was the type of sunscreen promotion used.
7. The dependent variable in this study was sunscreen usage.
8. The only controlled variable in this study was gender, as all participants were women. Therefore, if there are differences in the three different groups, they were not due to gender.
9. There are several possible confounding variables. First, participants were recruited from a number of websites including universities and blogs. There could be knowledge differences of sun exposure risks among these women based on educational differences. Second, women were recruited from different countries. There is no way of knowing if differences between the interventions were because of cultural differences. Finally, there was a wide range of ages in this study (18 to 66). The researchers did not discuss whether perhaps an older participant would be more likely to use sunscreen after learning about the risks and benefits than would a younger person.
10. The mediating variable in this research study was planning a sunscreen strategy. Both interventions were given motivational information. However, the added step of creating a plan to use sunscreen resulted in better future use.

REFERENCES

1. Johnson RB, Christensen LB. *Educational Research: Quantitative, Qualitative, and Mixed Approaches.* Thousand Oaks, CA: Sage Publications; 2008.
2. Trochim M. Construct Validity. Research Methods Knowledge Base. Available at: http://www.socialresearchmethods.net/kb/constval.php. Accessed May 3, 2012.
3. Colorado State University. Differences between Experimental and Quasi-Experimental Research. Available at: http://writing.colostate.edu/guides/research/experiment/pop3e.cfm. Accessed May 3, 2012.
4. Shadish WR, Cook TD, Campbell DT. *Experimental and Quasi-Experimental Designs for Generalized Causal Inference.* New York: Houghton Mifflin Company; 2002.
5. Crosby RS, DiClemente RJ, Salazar LF. *Research Methods in Health Promotion.* San Francisco, CA: Jossey-Bass; 2006.

CHAPTER **8**

Surveys

KEY TERMS

achievement tests
aptitude tests
Likert scales
performance tests
pilot test
pretest
readability score
semantic differential scales
subscales

INTRODUCTION

This chapter introduces survey selection, survey data collection, and types of surveys, as well as the differences among tests, inventories, and scales. Following the quantitative data survey discussion, the chapter moves to qualitative observational research methods and includes a consideration of ethical issues. The chapter ends with an exploration of cultural and diversity issues related to survey design. Lastly, reliability and validity are presented in terms of survey development.

SURVEY SELECTION

Let's begin by discussing the differences between selecting an existing survey versus creating a new survey. When evaluators determine that they will use a survey for data collection, they can use an existing survey or develop a new survey. It is useful to understand the advantages and disadvantages of using an existing survey (see **Table 8-1**).

If the decision is made to use an existing survey, then the evaluator needs to know where to find an existing survey that meets the goals and objectives of the evaluation. See **Table 8-2** for examples of where to locate a variety of existing surveys.

As with existing surveys, there are advantages and disadvantages to creating surveys. The major advantage is that survey questions created by the evaluation team may more closely address evaluators' goals and objectives than previously existing surveys. Other advantages include the ability to control survey length and literacy level. Disadvantages include the need to conduct several time-consuming pilot tests and revisions to establish reliability and validity and the high cost of development. After considering the advantages and disadvantages of using existing surveys or creating an original survey, some evaluators decide to use a combination—an existing survey to answer a few research questions and creating questions to answer the remaining objectives.

TABLE 8-1 Advantages and Disadvantages of Using Existing Surveys

Advantages	Disadvantages
Saves time	Costly if purchase is required
Saves money if available through open access	Trying to use with a different sample (e.g., adolescents instead of adults)
Pilot tested and revised	Questions do not exactly match research questions
Established reliability	Extraneous questions add length to survey
Established validity	Health literacy is too high or low for population
Previously used in at least one study	Evaluators do not have the statistical skills to perform data analysis required; costly to hire statistician
Established data analysis methodology	Must establish data analysis methodology

CREATING A SURVEY

This section provides an overview of survey development. Although the steps described are straightforward, new evaluators soon realize that each step involves numerous smaller steps to complete the task. The time spent in meticulous survey development is rewarded in high-quality results. Results are only as good as the survey.

Steps to create a survey include the following:

Step 1: Review the objectives with evaluation team members. Have each team member write possible survey questions on 3" × 5" cards that address the objectives. For example, if there are four objectives, evaluators label a card "Objectives: Question 1," then write a survey question pertaining to the first objective. They continue this with several cards, and after all the possible survey questions are written, the cards are sorted into one pile for each objective. At this point, evaluators review and edit survey questions written for Objective 1. Keep asking each other, "How does this question answer the objective?" Review and edit again until everyone agrees that each survey question addresses Objective 1. Repeat this process for each objective. Create the first draft of the survey from the selected questions.

Step 2: Ask only survey questions that address the objectives. Extra questions increase survey length and time required for respondents to complete the survey. Long surveys lead to respondent fatigue, which increases the possibility of inaccurate data.

Step 3: Organize survey questions from easy to difficult. The first question should be nonthreatening, such as

"How would you describe your health status today? (1) Excellent, (2) Very good, (3) Good, (4) Fair, (5) Poor." Leave plenty of white spaces, such as wide margins and space between questions, so that the survey is appealing. Dense text is intimidating and confusing.

Step 4: Write questions in a simple and concise manner. Use a vertical or horizontal format throughout the survey. Ensure the choices are distributed evenly. For example, uneven choices are (1) Good (2) Fair (3) Poor (4) Very Poor; these choices begin near the middle of the scale without listing Excellent and Very Good. If open-ended questions are used, limit the space on paper surveys or limit the number of characters in textboxes for online surveys. Avoid asking double questions. For example, "How satisfied are you with the quality of fruits and vegetables at this farmer's market?" or "Do you like swimming or surfing?" These questions should be two separate questions to lessen confusion. Suppose the survey respondent liked swimming very much, but did not enjoy surfing. How would he answer this question?

Step 5: Group similar questions. For example, all food intake questions are grouped together and all exercise questions are grouped together. Questions about sensitive issues (e.g., sexual behaviors, substance abuse, or other personal behaviors) are placed in the middle of the survey. Keep in mind that with long surveys, respondents get fatigued. Questions near the end may not receive the same attention from respondents. Place demographic questions at the end of the survey.

Step 6: Avoid skip patterns. Skip patterns on paper-and-pencil surveys are confusing. For example, "If

TABLE 8-2 Examples of Existing Surveys

Books of surveys	The *Mental Measurements Yearbook*[1] is a valuable resource that is published annually and provides extensive information about numerous existing surveys (e.g., survey questions, reliability, validity, methodology for data analysis, published studies that previously used the survey, how to gain permission to use the survey, and if applicable, the cost). Some scales have several different subscales. A scale measures and categorizes a variable. A subscale is just a smaller portion of a larger scale. For example, the National Health and Nutrition Examination Survey (NHANES) measures several dimensions of physical activity and fitness levels of children and adolescents in the United States through interviews and fitness tests.[2] All of the questions correspond to different physical fitness and nutrition subscales of the larger NHANES measure. If evaluators use a survey with multiple subscales, they must verify with survey authors if reliability and validity were established for each subscale or only for the entire survey. If reliability and validity were established for the entire survey, then evaluators selecting to use only one subscale need to establish reliability and validity for that one subscale. Some survey questions are available for free, but the score sheets that they use or data analysis that it requires is expensive. Other surveys are completely free.
Publications	While conducting the literature review, evaluators review which studies are published on the same topic. Within publications, authors refer to the survey they used for the study. Evaluators may decide to use the same study based on their evaluation objectives and the information provided in the journal article. If the survey is not shown as an appendix to the publication, then evaluators contact the authors for more information about how to obtain the survey.
Government websites	The Centers for Disease Control and Prevention (CDC) offers a variety of surveys that are available at no cost. Many of the surveys that are available through the government have been widely used and have been proven valid and reliable.
	Behavioral Risk Factor Surveillance System (BRFSS) is the world's largest ongoing telephone health survey system. This survey tracks health conditions, risk factors, and health behaviors. The 2013 version can be found at http://www.cdc.gov/brfss/questionnaires/pdf-ques/2013%20BRFSS_English.pdf.
	Measuring Intimate Partner Violence and Victimization and Perpetration is a set of surveys that measure partner violence on 20 different variables. It can be found at http://www.cdc.gov/ncipc/pub-res/IPV_Compendium.pdf.
	A growing public health concern, Measuring Bullying, Victimization, Perpetration, and Bystander Experiences is a set of surveys that measure a range of bullying and intimidation behaviors. It can be found at http://www.cdc.gov/ViolencePrevention/pdf/BullyCompendium-a.pdf.
	Youth Risk Behavior Surveillance System (YRBSS) is a survey similar to the BRFSS survey. The YRBSS measures many different risk behaviors among youth including smoking, drinking, drug use, and sexual activity. The YRBSS has been used since the 1990s and provides trend data over time among the U.S. youth population. It can be found at http://www.cdc.gov/healthyyouth/yrbs/questionnaire_rationale.htm.

you answer Yes to Question 16, then skip forward to Question 22." Such skip patterns lead to inaccurate responses and missing data. However, if a survey is administered online, skip patterns are invisible because the respondent does not realize they are being skipped based on an answer that they provided.

Step 7: Provide clear instructions for each transition. For example, if questions in one section use a 4-point Likert scale about quality of life and the next section is about exercise, then new instructions are needed. (For example, "The next six questions are about your exercise habits. Please select the response that best describes your behavior.")

Step 8: Check the readability score. Most word-processing software programs offer the ability to calculate readability scores. Generally, readability scores of seventh- to eight-grade reading levels are acceptable for adults. Lower reading levels are recommended for surveys completed by adolescents or adults with low literacy levels. Remember this simple rule: Avoid words with three or more syllables. For example, "daily medication" becomes "pills taken every day."

Step 9: Proofread the survey several times. Ask colleagues not involved in the survey development to proofread it. Remember that spell-check software only recognizes spelling errors, not inappropriate words. For example, "public" and "pubic" are both spelled correctly, but the letter "L" changes the meaning dramatically.

Step 10: Pretest the survey. For example, evaluators ask colleagues and students to review the survey and offer suggestions. From these comments, the survey is revised. A pretest differs from a pilot test in that a pretest is not asking individuals from the target population to complete the survey.

Step 11: Pilot-test the survey. Recruit 10–20 individuals similar to the target population to complete the survey. Respondents provide feedback to evaluators, either as a group or individually. Revise the survey based on their comments. A pilot test can also serve as the first step in establishing reliability. By testing and then retesting the same audience, evaluators calculate the consistency of the survey. In other words, did the respondents select the same choices for each question on the first and second administration of the survey? If necessary, researchers repeat pilot tests as needed.

Step 12: Finalize the survey format.

Although survey development is time consuming, if done correctly, well designed surveys become valuable evaluation tools and yield data for evaluating similar projects in the future. After data are collected, evaluators establish methodology for data analysis, including reliability, validity, cut-scores (which are discussed later in the chapter), and trends across samples from various target populations.[3,4]

After the survey question format is complete, evaluators write a cover letter to potential participants including a description of incentives. A short cover letter or opening statement on the computer screen describes the purpose of the evaluation but should also entice the potential respondent to complete the survey. The remaining portion of the letter states how long the survey takes to complete, potential benefits for participation (e.g., gift cards or incentives), and how their responses are kept confidential.[4] Keep in mind that evaluators are not present when a potential respondent opens the envelope or clicks on the emailed link, so the introduction needs to be concise and easy to read in a few seconds (see **Box 8-1**).

The closing statement thanks respondents for their participation, describes how incentives are retrieved (if applicable), and reassures them of the confidentiality of their responses. As previously mentioned, evaluators need to remember the audience (e.g., age, gender, reading level) when composing the cover letter and closing statement. The appropriateness of incentives is important to entice potential respondents. Most respondents will appreciate receiving gift cards to national discount stores. If the survey is collected in specific ZIP codes, verify that the national discount store is within the ZIP codes. Lastly, the value of incentives should be appropriate for time and effort. For example, a 25-question survey offers a $5 gift card, while a $50 gift card is appropriate for a 90-minute interview.[4]

SURVEY DATA COLLECTION

Whether the survey is conducted online, in person, or mailed, there are some common procedures used with all three methods of survey data collection.

Step 1: After developing the evaluation goals and objectives and obtaining approval from the institutional review board for human subject research, evaluators determine which survey data collection technique is appropriate.

Step 2: It is necessary to obtain access to the sample regardless of the survey data collection choice. First, for mailed surveys, evaluators must acquire the addresses, either email or postal, to which to send the survey. There are several ways to obtain postal addresses, including purchasing address lists from clearinghouse vendors or purchasing lists from professional organizations. As for email addresses, evaluators may contact professional organizations. If the evaluation is related to the mission of the professional organization, then email lists may be available. In some cases, email lists are available for purchase. If evaluators wish to email employees or students within a university or organization, then they contact administration for ways to send universal emails to the entire population of the organization. Second, if evaluators wish to conduct in-person surveys, they obtain names and contact information through key informants or snowball techniques. Key informants are individuals known to evaluators as being experts in a specific discipline. For example, evaluators request to conduct an in-person survey with current, former, and retired emergency responders within one

BOX 8-1 Example of a Cover Letter

Name of Company or University
on Official Letterhead

Date
Dear Participant:

You are being invited to participate in an evaluation called **<insert name of study>**. The study is being conducted by **<evaluator's name>** with **<insert institution, company, or university>**. The purpose of this evaluation is to **<insert purpose of evaluation>**.

You are being invited to participate in this evaluation by **<insert survey method (e.g., completing the attached surveys or completing the online survey)>**. This survey has been approved by the International Review Board of **<insert institution name>**. The following questionnaire will require approximately **<insert amount of time>** to complete, and there is no known risk. For completing this survey you are eligible for **<insert compensation stipulations>**. While you may not experience any benefits directly, information collected in this evaluation may benefit **<insert possible benefactors (e.g., a certain profession or a certain population)>** in the future by better understanding **<insert general purpose>**.

This survey collects no identifying information of any respondent, and responses are anonymous. In order to ensure that all information will remain confidential, please do not include your name. Copies of the project will be provided to **<insert appropriate information if applicable>**. If you choose to participate in this project, please answer all questions as honestly as possible and return the completed questionnaires promptly by **<insert method of return, such as interoffice mail, drop-box location, or provide stamped envelope>**. Participation is strictly voluntary and you may refuse to participate at any time.

Completion and return of the questionnaire will indicate your willingness to participate in this evaluation. If you have any questions concerning your rights as a participant, please contact **<insert IRB name>** at **<insert contact information>**. If you require any additional information or have questions, please contact **<insert evaluator's name>** at the number listed below.

Your participation is appreciated,
<Evaluator's name>
<Phone number and email address>
<Company/institution name and/or email address>

county. Snowball techniques involve interviewing one person and then asking if he or she is willing to give you the name of another person who might be interested in participating in the in-person survey. For example, evaluators conduct an in-person survey with an individual who is currently employed as a first responder in Jefferson County. Upon completion of the survey, the evaluator asks her if she knows another first responder who currently works in Jefferson County or worked in Jefferson County at some time in the past and who might be willing to answer the same questions. One individual connects to another and so on. The snowball technique has potential ethical issues if the first individual provides names and contact information without seeking permission from the referred individual.

Step 3: For in-person data collection, evaluators schedule appointments at the convenience of the respondents. If evaluators are using online or mailed surveys, they notify the potential respondents that they will be receiving a survey in a few days. This introduction notification (email or postal) allows the potential respondents to expect the survey in a few days. According to Dillman, Smyth, and Christian,[5] there are 7 days between each segment of the survey data collection. For example, there are 7 days between the introduction notification and the receipt of the survey. It is also recommended that online or mailed surveys arrive near the end of the week, when respondents are wrapping up their email or postal mail for the week.

Step 4: Surveys are received by potential respondents 7 days after the introduction notification. Mailed surveys are sent with a self-addressed stamped envelope (SASE), and the return address is also written on the survey in case the survey and SASE get separated.

Step 5: Seven days after surveys are received, evaluators send (via email or postal service) a thank you or reminder. If postal mail is used, the thank you or reminder is a postcard. The message is simple: "Thank you for responding to the <title of study> survey that was sent to you last Friday. If you have not had a chance to return it, please do so at your earliest convenience," then signed by the principal evaluator.

Step 6: Seven days after the thank you/reminder email or postcard, evaluators send a second survey. If postal mail is used, the second survey includes the SASE for return mail.[5]

There are advantages and disadvantages to each of the three (online, mailed, or in-person) survey data collection methods (see **Table 8-3**).

TYPES OF SURVEYS

Tests

Tests are defined as "a set of stimuli presented to an individual in order to elicit responses on the basis of which a numerical score can be assigned."[6] Let's look at each segment of the definition:

- *Set of stimuli:* This set may be written questions on a test (e.g., American College Testing [ACT] examination); demonstration of a specific skill, such as each step required to mix solutions in a laboratory; samples, such as a collection of soil and water samples to be tested for carcinogenic containments; or a verbal conversation assessment to verify proficiency in another language.
- *Elicit responses:* Responses are verbal, written, or kinetic as in a demonstration of a skill set.
- *Assigned numerical score:* Test results are recorded as a standardized number, so each individual is assessed using the same criteria.

The following discussion explores three types of tests: achievement, performance, and aptitude tests.

TABLE 8-3 Advantages and Disadvantages of Online, Mailed, and In-Person Surveys

	Advantages	Disadvantages
Online surveys	Fast way to collect data; inexpensive if email address lists are available for no cost; high number of potential respondents	Impersonal; no way of knowing who completed survey; no way for respondent to obtain clarification on any specific survey questions; no tracking system; no verifiable demographic information on respondents (e.g., not certain if respondent is providing accurate information); unable to predict number of respondents; difficult to receive email addresses for target population; expensive to purchase email addresses
Mailed surveys	Fast way to collect data; tracking system established by matching each survey	Impersonal; no way of knowing who completed survey; no way for respondent to obtain clarification on any specific survey questions; no tracking system; no verifiable demographic information on respondents; unable to predict number of respondents; difficult to receive mailing addresses for target population; expensive to purchase mailing addresses
In-person surveys	Able to clarify questions during survey interview; verify person responding to questions; in-depth information collected	Potentially difficult to recruit participants; expensive; time-intensive; data entry is time consuming

Achievement Tests

Achievement tests measure mastery, comprehension, or proficiency of acquired skills of individuals. Achievement tests compare one group of individuals to another group. There are two ways to interpret achievement tests: norm-referenced tests and criterion-referenced tests. Norm-referenced tests compare the test scores of each individual to the test scores of other individuals. For example, the Florida Comprehensive Assessment Test (FCAT) measures knowledge in different areas of education in elementary, middle, and high school.[7] The FCAT allows evaluators to calculate the mean or average scores of individuals for each grade level and subject area for all Florida public school students. The mean score becomes the norm by which all schools are compared. By using the norm for comparison, schools and students are ranked at various levels of achievement. In Florida, state funding is allocated by comparing the normative scores to each school. In norm-referenced tests, it is important that the difficulty of each question is close to equal, so the overall test yields consistent results (reliability) and measures what the tests claims to measure (validity).[6]

Criterion-referenced tests do not compare individuals, but rather describe the performance of one individual based on a set of criteria or level of mastery. In criterion-referenced tests, there is a predetermined required level of mastery used to assess the performance of each individual. For example, a state requires that all first-time drivers receive a minimum of 70% correct responses on the written driver's license examination. However, even though an individual passes the written driving test, there is no evidence that this individual knows how to drive a car.

Performance Tests

Performance tests measure what an individual can do rather than what an individual knows. Using the driving test example previously discussed, the achievement test determines that an individual knows the state laws pertaining to driving, but the performance test measures an individual's skill at actually operating a vehicle. When evaluators construct performance tests, they develop a checklist of skills that are assessed by individual performance. Performance testing has advantages because this type of testing cannot be assessed with paper-and-pencil examinations; however, the disadvantage is that performance testing is time consuming and expensive, and scoring is more subject to error or bias of the grader.[6]

Aptitude Tests

Aptitude tests measure general ability and knowledge, while achievement tests focus on specific subjects. It is easier to remember the difference by thinking that aptitude tests measure previously acquired knowledge. However, aptitude tests are not a measure of intelligence. Evaluators frequently use aptitude tests to predict future success. For example, the Graduate Record Examination (GRE) measures verbal reasoning, quantitative reasoning, and analytical writing skills acquired over a long period of time, but that can be related to any particular discipline.[8] The GRE measures general knowledge, but it is also used as a predictor of success in graduate school. Some universities use the GRE as one component of the graduate school admissions process along with the undergraduate grade point average, letters of recommendation, and personal statement.

Test performance range refers to the fluctuations in acceptable scores. All students know that their performance in a course determines their final grade. However, although students receive a wide range of scores, instructors determine the range of acceptable final scores needed to pass the course, such as 90–100% = A, 80–89% = B, 70–79% = C, 60–69% = D, and less than 60% = F.

Personality Inventories

Personality inventories assess certain patterns or trends. For example, the Myers-Briggs Type Indicator explores individuals' personality types and cognitive styles.[9] When evaluators select personality inventories, special attention toward validity and reliability is recommended. For example, some inventories only measure one personality trait (e.g., having an introverted or extroverted personality), while others are more comprehensive but limited in other ways. Generally, evaluators administer several personality inventories to determine trends. Administering several inventories strengthens the final inclination or tendency, even if several of the personality inventories have moderately weak validity. For example, in a criminal court case, the presiding judge may order that the court psychologist administer multiple personality inventories along with interviews to assist in the determination of whether a person is mentally fit to stand trial.

Scales

There are two kinds of scales: response scales and concept scales. Response scales assign an answer to a single question. For example, for the question, "How do you feel today?", the following responses are provided:

1. Excellent
2. Very good
3. Good
4. Fair
5. Poor

On the other hand, a concept scale is a collection of questions that measure a single subject or concept (e.g., self-esteem), while other scales measure several subjects. Single-dimension scales are like a number line. If self-esteem is measured, individuals respond to a series of questions related to the one topic. The responses from all questions are combined, so evaluators have one score for self-esteem. In the case of multiple subjects, evaluators select a scale that measures two or more topics (e.g., relationships between depression and self-esteem).[10] For example, the GRE measures several skills at once (e.g., quantitative, verbal, critical thinking, grammar, and reading comprehension). The following discussion focuses on one-dimension scales including Likert; Thurstone; sematic differential; and knowledge, attitude, and behavior scales.

Likert Scales

In Likert scales, evaluators may choose whether to have an even number of possible responses or an odd number of responses. Based on the results of the pilot study, this decision is different for each project. When an even number of responses are selected, the evaluator forces the respondent to provide either a positive or negative opinion, because the option would fall completely in the middle of positive or negative responses. So an "undecided" answer is removed. If the evaluator selects an odd number of choices, the "undecided" response is available. In either case, each response choice is assigned a numerical value. It is typical that low numbers are assigned to low-level responses (e.g., strongly disagree = 1 and strongly agree = 5) for ease in understanding data results. The following are examples of each response choice option.

Seven choices. Rate your level of satisfaction regarding the service that you received during your appointment with your academic advisor:

1. Very dissatisfied
2. Moderately dissatisfied
3. Dissatisfied
4. Undecided
5. Satisfied
6. Moderately satisfied
7. Strongly satisfied

Five choice. Rate your level of satisfaction regarding the service that you received during your appointment with your academic advisor:

1. Very dissatisfied
2. Dissatisfied
3. Undecided
4. Satisfied
5. Very satisfied

Four choices. Rate your level of satisfaction regarding the service that you received during your appointment with your academic advisor:

1. Very dissatisfied
2. Dissatisfied
3. Satisfied
4. Very satisfied

When evaluators reverse the wording of the survey questions to vary the selection choices, it is called item reversal. In the data analysis, evaluators must remember to reverse the coding scheme to achieve the correct results (see **Box 8-2**). The Rosenberg's self-esteem scale illustrates a 4-point Likert scale and reversal items.[11]

Lastly, Likert scale responses are summed to reach a final score for each responding individual. Evaluators develop a cut-score for the scale, or use the cut-score provided for established Likert scales.[12] Think of cut-scores as final grades in a course. If there are 500 possible points in a course, students receiving between 500 and 450 receive an A; 449 to 400 receive a B; 399 to 350 receive a C, and so on. Cut-scores are the same, but related to specific topics. For example, factory workers diagnosed with carpal tunnel syndrome from repetitive motion work on the assembly line are asked to complete a Likert scale survey related to their self-reported perceived daily degree of pain. Based on the summed scores of 10 questions, evaluators determine the cut-scores: Factory workers with a total score of 50 to 41 have severe pain, 40 to 31 have moderate pain, 30 to 21 have mild pain, and 20 to 0 have minimal pain. In this example, evaluators might use this type of Likert pain scale to more accurately determine what changes need to occur in the factory to reduce the occurrence of painful carpal tunnel syndrome among the factory workers. See Box 8-2 again. Note that Rosenberg's self-esteem scale does not offer a cut-score but rather merely states that the higher the score, the higher the respondent's self-esteem.

If evaluators decide to create an original Likert scale rather than use an existing scale, it is advisable to seek resources outside of this introductory text. The following description provides a brief overview of how scales are developed. Given that advice, the first step is to gather a group of experts to generate ideas related to the topic of interest. One method is to write each idea on separate 3' × 5' cards. After collecting at least 80 cards, the group sorts the ideas into piles for each subset subject area. From these piles, evaluators

BOX 8-2   Rosenberg's Self-Esteem Scale

The scale is a 10-item Likert questionnaire with items answered on a 4-point scale ranging from strongly agree to strongly disagree. The original sample for which the scale was developed consisted of 5,024 high school juniors and seniors from 10 randomly selected schools in New York State.

Instructions: Below is a list of statements dealing with your general feelings about yourself. If you strongly agree, circle **SA**. If you agree with the statement, circle **A**. If you disagree, circle **D**. If you strongly disagree, circle **SD**.

1.	On the whole, I am satisfied with myself.	SA	A	D	SD
2.*	At times, I think I am no good at all.	SA	A	D	SD
3.	I feel that I have a number of good qualities.	SA	A	D	SD
4.	I am able to do things as well as most other people.	SA	A	D	SD
5.*	I feel I do not have much to be proud of.	SA	A	D	SD
6.*	I certainly feel useless at times.	SA	A	D	SD
7.	I feel that I'm a person of worth, at least on an equal plane with others.	SA	A	D	SD
8.*	I wish I could have more respect for myself.	SA	A	D	SD
9.*	All in all, I am inclined to feel that I am a failure.	SA	A	D	SD
10.	I take a positive attitude toward myself.	SA	A	D	SD

Scoring: SA = 3, A = 2, D = 1, SD = 0. Items with an asterisk are reverse scored; that is, SA = 0, A = 1, D = 2, SD = 3. Sum the scores for the 10 items. The higher the score, the higher the self-esteem.

The scale may be used without explicit permission. The author's family, however, would like to be kept informed of its use:

The Morris Rosenberg Foundation
c/o Department of Sociology, Building 2112
University of Maryland
College Park, MD 20742-1315

Reproduced from Rosenberg M. *Society and the Adolescent Self-Image.* Princeton, NJ: Princeton University Press; 1965.

begin to create survey questions. Once the survey is finalized and approved by the evaluation experts within the group, it is time to conduct a pre-pilot test on the survey. A pre-pilot test involves asking other experts to review the survey and provide comments. These comments could indicate that you have left out an important subject area or that something should be left out. Again, changes are made based on suggestions. The next step is to conduct a pilot test with a group of individuals similar to those individuals who would be recruited for the actual study. The pilot test does not include individuals from the actual study sample. It is common for evaluators to employ statisticians as consultants to determine the psychometric properties and if the survey questions measure what the survey is intended to measure—in other words, to verify whether the survey is valid. In the last step, evaluators make final edits and then conduct the actual study using their Likert scale.

Thurstone Scales

Thurstone scales are similar to Likert scales, because both scales ask respondents about their attitudes. However, Likert scales ask the degree of agreement, while Thurstone scales list statements and ask respondents to pick the statements that match their attitude on the topic.[13] The following discussion presents how Thurston scales are developed.[6]

Step 1: A group of experts makes lists of about 50 to 100 statements related to a broad topic (e.g., coworkers with a substance abuse addiction).

Step 2: The original list is given to another group of individuals with some knowledge of the broad topic, such as first-year public health graduate students. The student groups read each statement and label it as positive, neutral, or negative. They are not providing their opinion or attitude, but rather their perception of the statement (see **Table 8-4**).[14]

Step 3: For each statement, evaluators create a table (see **Table 8-5**). Evaluators calculate the middle (median) score for each statement. The median score is defined as "50% are above and 50% are below that score." Next, evaluators calculate the first quartile. The first quartile is defined as "25% are below and 75% are above that score." In other words, the first quartile (Q1) is the value below which 25% of the cases fall and above which 75% of the cases fall—also called the 25th percentile. The median is the 50th percentile. The third quartile, Q3, is the 75th percentile. The interquartile range is the difference between third and first quartile, or Q3 – Q1.

Step 4: Evaluators select one statement for the median scores ranging from 1–11. Notice that in **Table 8-5**, not all 12 median scores are represented, but there is a representative sample of statements.

Step 5: In Table 8-5, look at the statements with median scores of 5 and 9. If several statements have the same median score, researchers select the statement with the smallest interquartile range. The smallest interquartile range shows the least amount of variability among the students ranking the statements.[14] Once all statements are selected, evaluators complete the final version of the Thurstone scale and pilot-test the scale with a representative sample. As with Likert scales, after the pilot study is complete, a few revisions are made prior to the actual data collection.

Semantic Differential Scales

Semantic differential scales measure an individual's attitude about a specific topic based on opposite adjectives. The middle of the scale is zero and both ends of the scale are opposites. The advantages of this scale include that it is simple to design, an inexpensive way to collect data, and easy to adapt to various uses with different age groups, cultures, and literacy levels.[15] For example, if evaluators wanted to know women's attitudes and knowledge about types of birth control, the semantic differential is shown in **Table 8-6**. Once individuals complete each of the semantic differential scales, evaluators analyze data by exploring each topic as well as the collective scores.

Knowledge, Attitude, and Behavior Scales

Scales of knowledge, attitude, and behavior are studied separately and collectively. When evaluators study the level of knowledge on a specific topic, results allow evaluators to develop health education programs based on the general knowledge known about a particular public health topic. Evaluators develop true/false questions or Likert scale–type responses depending on the type of data needed for the

---

TABLE 8-4 Example of Statement Labels

Negative	• Individuals with a substance abuse addiction deserve their health problems. • Substance abuse addictions control the population due to premature death. • I will never develop a substance abuse addiction.
Between negative and neutral	• I will not become addicted to a substance because none of my friends are addicted to a substance.
Neutral	• It's easy to become addicted to a substance. • Because substance abuse is preventable, resources should focus on prevention instead of curing. • People who are addicted to a substance are no different from other people I know.
Between neutral and positive	• People who are addicted to a substance can still have a normal life.
Positive	• Substance addiction is a disease that anyone can get if they are not careful. • Substance addiction affects us all. • People diagnosed with a substance addiction should be treated just like everybody else.

Data from Attitude scales: Rating scales to measure data. Management Study Guide. Available at: http://www.managementstudyguide.com/attitude-scales.htm

TABLE 8-5 Sample of Thurstone Statements

Statement	Median	Quartile 1 (25% below and 75% above)	Quartile 3 (75% below and 25% above)	Interquartile Range = Q3 – Q1
Individuals with a substance abuse addiction deserve their health problems.	1	1	2	1
Substance abuse addictions control the population due to premature death.	2	1	2.5	1.5
I will never develop a substance abuse addiction.	3	1.5	5	3.5
I will not become addicted to a substance because none of my friends are addicted to a substance.	4	2	4.5	2.5
It's easy to become addicted to a substance.	5	4	6.5	2.5
Because substance abuse is preventable, resources should focus on prevention instead of curing.	5	4	6	2
People who are addicted to a substance are no different from other people I know.	6	5	9.75	4.75
People who are addicted to a substance can still have a normal life.	8	5.5	11	5.5
Anyone can become addicted to a substance.	9	5.5	10.5	5
Substance addiction is a disease that anyone can get if they are not careful.	9	6	10	4
Substance addiction affects us all.	10	7.5	11	3.5
People diagnosed with a substance abuse addiction should be treated just like everybody else.	11	10	11	1

Data from Attitude scales: Rating scales to measure data. Management Study Guide. Available at: http://www.managementstudyguide.com/attitude-scales.htm

analysis. Of course, keep in mind that true/false data are nominal and Likert scales are ordinal. **Box 8-3** shows an example of a scale of knowledge, attitude, and behavior.[16]

Attitude scales measure opinions, values, attitudes, and other characteristics.[6] As with all evaluations, the first step is to develop the evaluation objectives, followed by creating operational definitions for each variable. For example, if evaluators are studying adolescents, they state the age range as the operational definition (e.g., 13–19 years of age, 12–20 years of age, or another range determined by researchers). At this point, evaluators determine whether a scale is needed to answer the evaluation objectives. This process begins by answering the question "What is being measured in this evaluation?"

Behavior questions ask about specific actions rather than about knowledge and attitudes. The following questions change the knowledge questions about diabetes into behavior questions about diabetes.[16]

Since I was diagnosed with diabetes, I follow the diabetic diet as prescribed by my physician.

1. Strongly disagree
2. Disagree
3. Agree
4. Strongly agree

I select baked salmon instead of a baked potato, because baked potatoes are high in carbohydrates.

1. Strongly disagree
2. Disagree
3. Agree
4. Strongly agree

I drink water, because some drinks (e.g., low-fat milk) are high in fat.

1. Strongly disagree
2. Disagree
3. Agree
4. Strongly agree

TABLE 8-6 Semantic Differential Scale About Attitudes and Knowledge of Birth Control Options

Daily Birth Control Pills											
Inexpensive	5	4	3	2	1	0	1	2	3	4	5	Expensive
Inconvenient	5	4	3	2	1	0	1	2	3	4	5	Convenient
Requires clinic visit	5	4	3	2	1	0	1	2	3	4	5	Does not require clinic visit
Not for spontaneous sex	5	4	3	2	1	0	1	2	3	4	5	Good for spontaneous sex
Requires partner cooperation	5	4	3	2	1	0	1	2	3	4	5	Partner cooperation not required
Protects against sexually transmitted infections	5	4	3	2	1	0	1	2	3	4	5	Does not protect against sexually transmitted infections
Not very effective for protection against pregnancy	5	4	3	2	1	0	1	2	3	4	5	Very effective for protection against pregnancy

Long-Term Reversible Contraception (IUDs and Vaginal Rings)											
Inexpensive	5	4	3	2	1	0	1	2	3	4	5	Expensive
Inconvenient	5	4	3	2	1	0	1	2	3	4	5	Convenient
Requires clinic visit	5	4	3	2	1	0	1	2	3	4	5	Does not require clinic visit
Not for spontaneous sex	5	4	3	2	1	0	1	2	3	4	5	Good for spontaneous sex
Requires partner cooperation	5	4	3	2	1	0	1	2	3	4	5	Partner cooperation not required
Protects against sexually transmitted infections	5	4	3	2	1	0	1	2	3	4	5	Does not protect against sexually transmitted infections
Unpleasant side effects (e.g., weight gain)	5	4	3	2	1	0	1	2	3	4	5	No unpleasant side effects (e.g., weight gain)
Dangerous side effects for women who smoke	5	4	3	2	1	0	1	2	3	4	5	Safe for women who smoke
Not safe for young women	5	4	3	2	1	0	1	2	3	4	5	Safe for young women
Not safe for older women	5	4	3	2	1	0	1	2	3	4	5	Safe for older women
Protects against HIV/AIDS	5	4	3	2	1	0	1	2	3	4	5	No protection against HIV/AIDS
Messy to use	5	4	3	2	1	0	1	2	3	4	5	Not messy to use
Requires skill to use properly	5	4	3	2	1	0	1	2	3	4	5	Does not require skill to use properly
Not very effective for protection against pregnancy	5	4	3	2	1	0	1	2	3	4	5	Very effective for protection against pregnancy

I go to the lab every 3 months to get my glycosylated hemoglobin (hemoglobin A1) levels checked, because it measures my average blood glucose level for the past 6 to 10 weeks.

1. Strongly disagree
2. Disagree
3. Agree
4. Strongly agree

I try to avoid letting my blood glucose level get too high, because high blood glucose levels might cause infections.

1. Strongly disagree
2. Disagree
3. Agree
4. Strongly agree

CULTURAL AND DIVERSITY INFLUENCES IN DATA COLLECTION

When developing surveys, it is important to keep in mind cultural and ethnic influences in data collection measurement decisions. Let's go over a few examples of how respondents may feel excluded by the question response choices. If individuals feel that questions or response choices disrespect them, they are less likely to complete the survey or interview. When evaluators lack cultural sensitivity in the interview or survey development phase, it results in missing

BOX 8-3 Example of a Knowledge Survey

The following five questions are a sample test related to knowledge about a diabetic diet.

The diabetes diet is:
  a. Not the way most people eat
  b.* A healthy diet
  c. High in carbohydrates
  d. Too high in protein for most people

Which of the following is highest in carbohydrates?
  a. Baked salmon
  b. Cheddar cheese
  c.* Baked potato
  d. Peanut butter

Which of the following is highest in fat?
  a.* Low-fat milk
  b. Apple juice
  c. Baked potato
  d. Honey

Glycosylated hemoglobin (hemoglobin A1) measures the average blood glucose level for the past:
  a. Day
  b. Week
  c.* 6–10 weeks
  d. 6 months

High blood glucose levels may be caused by:
  a.* An infection
  b. Vomiting
  c. Dehydration
  d. Excessive physical exercise

The asterisk (*) denotes correct response.

If evaluators wished to use the entire Michigan Diabetes Knowledge Test for their study, it would be necessary to obtain permission, use the complete survey, and score the test according to analysis described by the original authors.

Modified with permission from Diabetes Knowledge Test. University of Michigan Diabetes Research and Training Center. Available at: http://www.med.umich.edu/mdrtc/profs/survey.html#dkt.

---

data. In this case, evaluators are left wondering why data are missing, but never relate it back to lack of diversity and cultural sensitivity. Here are a few examples from survey questions:

Example 1
What is your race/ethnicity? (Select one)
  1. White
  2. Black
  3. Hispanic
  4. Other

This question eliminates many groups, for example, Native Americans, Asians, Pacific Islanders, and so on. It also does not allow multiracial individuals to select several choices. The best solution is to use the ethnicity choices offered on the U.S. Census (see **Box 8-4**).[17]

Example 2
What is your gender?
  1. Female
  2. Male

The responses for this question exclude transgender individuals.

BOX 8-4 Questions About Ethnicity and Race

What is this person's race? Mark one or more choices.

1. White
2. Black, African American, or Negro
3. American Indian or Alaska Native
4. Asian Indian
5. Japanese
6. Native Hawaiian
7. Chinese
8. Korean
9. Guamanian or Chamorro
10. Filipino
11. Vietnamese
12. Samoan
13. Other Asian
14. Other Pacific Islander
15. Some other race

Write response:_____

Is this person of Hispanic, Latino, or Spanish origin?

1. No, not of Hispanic, Latino, or Spanish origin
2. Yes, Mexican, Mexican American, Chicano
3. Yes, Puerto Rican
4. Yes, Cuban
5. Yes, another Hispanic, Latino, or Spanish origin

Write response: _____

Reproduced from The 2010 Census Questionnaire: Seven Questions for Everyone. Population Reference Bureau. Available at: http://www.prb.org/Articles/2009/questionnaire.aspx

Example 3

What is your annual income?
1. Less than $59,999
2. $60,000–$89,000
3. $90,000–$129,000
4. Over $130,000

The responses for this question classify individuals into a narrow range of choices. Because poverty in the United States for a family of four is set at $23,050[18] and the median U.S. income is $51,914,[19] the choices classify almost 50% of the population within the lowest choice. These choices limit data accuracy.

Example 4

Do you describe yourself as any of the following choices?
1. Cancer survivor
2. Disabled person
3. Domestic violence victim
4. HIV+ person

All of these choices list the adjective first, followed by the individual. It is always best to describe the individual first followed by the descriptive term: (1) Person who survived cancer, (2) Person with a disability, (3) Survivor of domestic violence, and (4) Person living with HIV+ health status.

These are just a few of many examples where individuals feel excluded and then choose not to complete survey questions.

For interview questions, the way the question is presented influences the honesty of the response. Here are two examples:

1. "You don't smoke, do you?" versus "About how many cigarettes do you smoke each day?"
2. "Have you had more than 10 sexual partners in the last 30 days?" versus "How many sexual partners would you estimate that you have had in the last 30 days?"

Whether evaluators develop survey questions or interview questions, the level of cultural and diversity awareness influences the data collection process. Pilot testing is critical in the development of culturally appropriate data collection. Evaluators ask a representative sample to read questions and provide honest feedback to ensure suitability of questions and response choices.

SURVEY: RELIABILITY AND VALIDITY

Before closing the discussion about surveys, it is essential to remind readers to review the concepts of reliability and validity. These two concepts are fundamental regardless of whether evaluators select an existing survey or develop a new survey. As a brief review, reliability is defined as the consistency of what is measured. For example, if an individual's time for a 1-mile run is measured using Brand A time monitor and then measured again several days later using Brand B monitor, the results should be approximately the same if the monitors are reliable. The same is true with data collection. If public health students are given an epidemiology exam on Wednesday and the same exam on Friday, the scores should be nearly the same if the exam is reliable. Validity is concerned about whether the test measures what it was intended to measure. There is external and internal validity. External validity deals with generalizability to other groups. Internal validity focuses on the rigor of the evaluation—for example, study design, precision in data collection, and consideration of all possible explanations for results. It is more important for a survey to be valid than reliable.

SUMMARY

This chapter covers survey selection, including whether evaluators decide to use an existing survey or develop a new survey. There are advantages and disadvantages to existing and new surveys, but decisions are made based on goals and objectives. Survey data collection can be conducted using online, mailed, and in-person surveys. The next section investigated various types of quantitative surveys including tests, inventories, and scales. Next, there was a discussion of cultural and diversity issues related to surveys. The final section provided a brief review of validity and reliability.

CASE STUDY

Research Questions

Evaluators wanted to evaluate a social media campaign to determine whether or not the social media campaign increased first-time student blood donors on the campus of Georgia State University.

Goal: Throughout January and February (8 weeks), this evaluation will determine which form of social media was most effective in increasing student blood donations on the campus of Georgia State University.

Objective One: By March 1, there will be a 50% increase in blood donations from students at Georgia State University.

Objective Two: By March 1, 100% of students who donate blood will complete a brief social media survey related to donating blood.

Objective Three: By March 1, an intercept survey will be conducted over 3 days in the student union to determine awareness of the social media campaign to increase blood donation on campus.

Operational Definitions

College student is defined as any individual enrolled in at least one 3-credit course at Georgia State University during the spring semester.

First-time blood donor is defined as any Georgia State University student who donates 1 pint of blood for the first time during the months of January or February.

Survey Development

After evaluators develop a final draft, (see **Box 8.5**), the survey is pretested with colleagues of the evaluation team and then revised as needed. After receiving approval from the institutional review board, the revised survey is pilot-tested with 20 students who self-identified as not eligible to donate blood due to medical conditions or religious beliefs.

Example of Survey Instructions

Thank you for participating in this survey. We appreciate that you are taking the time to complete this survey. The person that gave you the survey will come by and pick it up in a few minutes.

Thank you for completing this survey. You will be given a gift card when the completed survey is returned.

Data Collection and Data Entry Training

Undergraduate and graduate students are invited to participate in data collection. Each student completes a 1-hour course related to data collection and the purpose of this

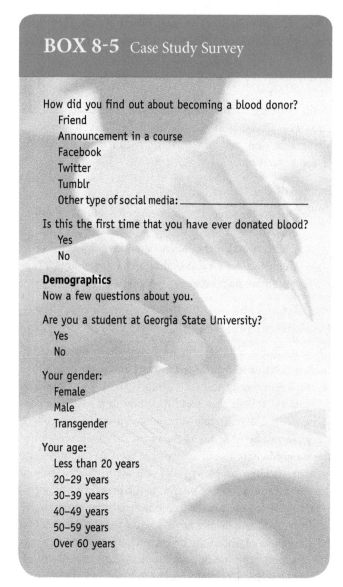

BOX 8-5 Case Study Survey

How did you find out about becoming a blood donor?
Friend
Announcement in a course
Facebook
Twitter
Tumblr
Other type of social media: _____

Is this the first time that you have ever donated blood?
Yes
No

Demographics
Now a few questions about you.

Are you a student at Georgia State University?
Yes
No

Your gender:
Female
Male
Transgender

Your age:
Less than 20 years
20–29 years
30–39 years
40–49 years
50–59 years
Over 60 years

evaluation. Data entry training includes tracking data, entering data, and basic data analysis (e.g., frequencies and histograms).

Data Collection

The student volunteers will be stationed outside the mobile blood donation bus on campus each time that the bus is serving blood donors on campus in January and February.

The first page of the survey is the informed consent form. Student volunteers answer any questions, provide a pencil, and ask the blood donors to complete the survey while they wait to donate blood. The blood donor receives a $5 gift card when the survey is completed and returned to the student volunteer.

Data Entry

When student volunteers are not collecting data, they enter data into an Excel spreadsheet on the laptop in the evaluation office.

Data Analysis

Upon entering survey data, the evaluation team analyzes data. The final report for the study includes frequencies, histograms, and statistical analyses required to answer the research questions.

Case Study Discussion Questions

1. Discuss the strengths and weaknesses of this proposed evaluation.
2. Discuss whether the survey questions address the goals and objectives for this evaluation. How would you suggest improving the survey questions?

STUDENT ACTIVITIES

Charlottesburg is a medium-sized college town in the Midwest. Historically, the town was a farming community. At the beginning of the 20th century, the town opened an agricultural college that steadily gained in size and importance. Now a 4-year state-supported university, the college has grown to become one of the major public universities of the state. Many of the town's citizens work at the university and live within a couple of miles of it. Recently, the issue of obesity became a topic of interest to the president of the college, Ms. Delcomb. Ms. Delcomb noticed that many of the students, staff, and faculty are less active than in the past and have a variety of unhealthy habits, such as smoking and eating fast food. After talking with local doctors, Ms. Delcomb has decided that Charlottesburg is just one more town that

must face the obesity epidemic. In order to help the town, Ms. Delcomb wants to start encouraging healthy practices at the university among the students, staff, and faculty.

Ms. Delcomb thinks it would be a good idea to see what the current situation is like at the university in Charlottesburg before she goes forward with plans for a health campaign for the entire town. Because diet and exercise are important parts of preventing obesity, Ms. Delcomb wants to ask a sample of students, staff, and faculty about their habits. She has prepared a list of questions she would like you, a work study student who works in her office, to help her turn into a survey.

Here are the questions that Ms. Delcomb gives to you:

Question 1: Do you consider yourself to be overweight, underweight, or "just about right"?

Question 2: Are you an unhealthy eater?

Question 3: Do you exercise regularly? (*Exercise* means any physical activity where you are moving your body for at least 30 minutes, *regularly* means most days a week.)

Question 4: What makes it hard for you to eat healthily?

Question 5: What makes it hard for you to exercise regularly?

Question 6: How many servings of vegetables and whole grains did you eat last week?

Question 7: How would a program that helped you eat better and exercise more make you happier in the future?

After looking at the questions, you think that they can be improved somewhat. Answer the following questions about what you would do to make this survey better and explain your answers.

Questions

1. You want to make sure all of the questions that Ms. Delcomb gave you answer the research question. In this case, the research question is "What are the current diet and exercise habits of students, staff, and faculty at the college in Charlottesburg?"
2. Is Question 1 the best question to start the survey with?
3. Are there any questions that are "double-barreled," meaning they ask about more than one thing?
4. Which question is most likely to elicit an untrue response?
5. Question 3 seems very long. Should we shorten it and just ask people if they exercise regularly?
6. Questions 5, 6, and 7 are open ended. Should we keep these?

Answers

1. While knowing if a program to help people make better food choices and exercise more would make them happier is a great idea, it doesn't answer our research question, which is to determine current diet and exercise habits. Question 7 will have to be removed.

2. Question 1 is probably not the best question to start the survey with, because some people may be sensitive about their weight. Placing it near the end of the survey might be a better idea.

3. Yes. Question 6 is a double-barreled question because it asks about vegetables and whole grains. While vegetables and whole grains are both foods, they are very different types of foods. If somebody answered "five servings," would we know if they were all vegetables, all whole grains, or some combination of the two?

4. Question 2 is probably most likely to illicit an untrue response because it implies some judgment about the answer that is likely to be given. If healthy is good, then unhealthy is bad. Most people don't want to be seen as bad, so they might be inclined to answer the question in a socially desirable way. You might consider changing this question to ask how many times a week they eat certain foods such as fast-food, sugary drinks, salty snacks, and so on. This way you are the one who can ascertain the healthiness of their diet.

5. You should not shorten Question 3. This question provides an operational definition of "regular exercise." If you didn't have this definition, someone who walks to the end of their driveway once a day might consider it regular exercise when it really isn't. Further, someone who went walking for half an hour every evening might not consider it exercise because it is not physically intense, when in fact it should be counted.

6. This is a trick question. The real answer is that it depends on what you want to know, how many people you are surveying, how many other questions there are, the environment you are surveying them in, and so on. However, we might consider leaving them in because open-ended questions can give us valuable information. If we were to have respondents check predetermined boxes, it might exclude some very important impediments to healthy eating and exercise that we failed to consider.

REFERENCES

1. Spies RA, Carlson JF, Geisinger KF, eds. *Mental Measurement Yearbook*, 18th ed. Lincoln, NE: Buros Institute of Mental Measurement; 2010.

2. Centers for Disease Control and Prevention. National Health and Nutrition Survey. Available at: http://www.cdc.gov/nchs/nhanes.htm; Accessed May 21, 2014.

3. U.S. Department of Justice, Office of Juvenile Justice and Delinquency Prevention. *Evaluating Juvenile Justice Programs: A Design Monograph for State Planner.* Washington, DC: Community Research Associates. Available at: https://www.bja.gov/evaluation/guide/documents/basic_guidelines_for_the_develop.htm. Published 1989. Accessed September 7, 2013.

4. eSurveysPro.com. Questionnaire Development. Available at: http://www.esurveyspro.com/article-questionnaire-development.aspx. Accessed May 17, 2014.

5. Dillman D, Smyth J, Christian L. *Internet, Mail, and Mixed-Mode Surveys: The Tailored Design Method*, 3rd ed. Hoboken, NJ: Wiley Publications; 2009.

6. Ary D, Jacobs L, Razavieh A, Sorenson C. *Introduction to Research in Education*, 8th ed. Belmont, CA: Wadsworth/Cengage Learning; 2010.

7. Florida Department of Education. The Florida Comprehensive Assessment Test. Available at: http://fcat.fldoe.org/fcat/. Accessed May 17, 2014.

8. Educational Testing Services. About the GRE Revised General Test. Available at: http://www.ets.org/gre/revised_general/about/. Accessed May 17, 2014.

9. Personality Pathways. Myers Briggs Test: What Is Your Personality Type? Available at: http://www.personalitypathways.com/type_inventory.html. Accessed May 17, 2014.

10. Trochim MK. General Issues in Scaling. Research Methods Knowledge Base. Available at: http://www.socialresearchmethods.net/kb/scalgen.php. Accessed May 17, 2014.

11. Rosenberg M. *Society and the Adolescent Self-Image.* Princeton, NJ: Princeton University Press; 1965.

12. Trochim MK. Likert Scaling. Research Knowledge Base. Available at: http://www.socialresearchmethods.net/kb/scallik.php. Accessed May 17, 2014.

13. Thurstone LL. Attitudes can be measured. *Am J Sociol.* 1928;33:529–554.

14. Management Study Guide. Attitude Scales: Rating Scales to Measure Data. Available at: http://www.managementstudyguide.com/attitude-scales.htm. Accessed May 17, 2014.

15. Heise, DR. The semantic differential and attitude research. In: Summers F, ed. *Attitude Measurement.* Chicago, IL: Rand McNally; 1970:235–253. Available at: http://www.indiana.edu/~socpsy/papers/AttMeasure/attitude.htm. Accessed September 7, 2013.

16. University of Michigan Diabetes Research and Training Center. Diabetes Knowledge Test. Available at: http://www.med.umich.edu/mdrtc/profs/survey.html#dkt. Accessed May 17, 2014.

17. Population Reference Bureau. The 2010 Census Questionnaire: Seven Questions for Everyone. Available at: http://www.prb.org/Articles/2009/questionnaire.aspx. Published April 2009. Accessed May 17, 2014.

18. Families USA. 2012 Annual Federal Poverty Guidelines. Available at: http://www.familiesusa.org/resources/tools-for-advocates/guides/federal-poverty-guidelines.html. Accessed May 17, 2014.

19. The United States Census Bureau. USA People QuickFacts. Available at: http://quickfacts.census.gov/qfd/states/00000.html. Accessed May 17, 2014.

Data Tools

CHAPTER OBJECTIVES

By the end of this chapter, students will be able to:

1. Describe the importance of operational definitions.
2. Evaluate the differences between categorical and continuous data.
3. Apply data organization skills to present data.
4. Describe measures of central tendency.
5. Evaluate the relationship between variance and standard deviation.
6. Define correlation coefficients when using continuous data.

KEY TERMS

categorical data
continuous data
frequency distributions
measure of central tendency
normal curve
standard deviation
variance

INTRODUCTION

This chapter describes how data tools are used by evaluators. Data are classified by scales of measurement including categorical data using nominal and ordinal scales and continuous data using interval and ratio scales. Next there is a discussion about how data are organized using frequency distributions and graphic presentations. The chapter concludes with a detailed explanation of the measures of central tendency (mean, median, and mode), the normal curve, and the concepts of variance and standard deviation. The information provided in this chapter serves as a foundation for understanding the basic concepts of inferential statistics.

DATA CLASSIFICATION

There are numerous ways to classify data, so this discussion begins with the most basic way and then moves into more detailed descriptions. As shown in **Figure 9-1**, the first way to classify data consists of categorical and continuous data.

Categorical Data

Categorical data are defined as variables that are named and placed into groups, classification, or categories. For example, if you wanted to group zoo animals by type, you could put them into different categories (e.g., mammals, birds, fish, reptiles, amphibians). Each animal belongs to only one category and not any other. There are two types of categorical data: nominal and ordinal.

Nominal Data

Nominal data are best remembered when you think of naming variables. For nominal data, there is no particular order and the codes are arbitrary. One example is if the evaluator wishes to know the residential ZIP code of the responding individual. Evaluators code the ZIP codes with arbitrary numbers: 1 = 33610, 2 = 33612, 3 = 33479, 4 = 33481, and 5 = 33509. It does not mean that individuals marking 5 have "more ZIP code" than individuals marking 1 on the survey.

FIGURE 9-1 Classifications of data.

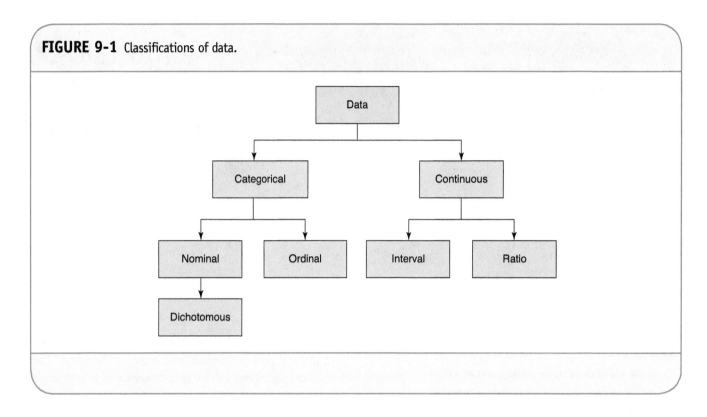

Each code number is merely an alternate code given to the ZIP codes (see **Table 9-1**).

Other examples of nominal data include ethnicity, place of employment, and geographic location. A subset of nominal data is dichotomous data. Dichotomous data consist of only two choices. For example, a survey question could ask, "Have you ever told a physician that you have chronic back pain?" The choices are "Yes" or "No" and no other choices are available. For coding purposes, No = 0 and Yes = 1. See **Table 9-2**

Ordinal Data

Ordinal data are best remembered by thinking about a marathon race. The winners are ranked as first, second, and third

TABLE 9-1 Sample of Nominal Data

Case Number	ZIP Code
1	33612
2	33479
3	33481
4	33610
5	33612
6	33509
7	33610
8	33612
9	33612
10	33509

TABLE 9-2 Sample of Dichotomous Data

Case Number	Reporting Chronic Back Pain to a Physician
1	0
2	0
3	1
4	0
5	1
6	1
7	0
8	1
9	0
10	0

place in the order that they cross the finish line. However, ordinal data do not assume that the distance between each runner as they cross the finish line is equal. There might be 3 seconds between the first-place runner and the second-place runner, but there may be 20 seconds between the second-place runner and the third-place runner. For example, the survey question asks:

Which choice describes your age?
1 = 20–29 years old
2 = 30–39 years old
3 = 40–49 years old
4 = 50–59 years old
5 = 60–69 years old
6 = 70–79 years old
7 = 80–89 years old
8 = over 90 years old

These choices allow the respondent to select a category of age rather than provide information about their exact age. The evaluator gains information related to the age range of respondents rather than their exact age. For example, if a respondent selects "4," the evaluator knows that the age of the individual is 50 to 59 years. See **Table 9-3.**

Ordinal data are also represented in satisfaction scales. A range from 0 (no satisfaction) to 10 (high satisfaction) allows satisfaction to vary among respondents The evaluator does not know the exact difference between a satisfaction response of 4 for one respondent and 6 for another respondent (see **Table 9-4**).

The ordinal data for satisfaction scale in Table 9-4 can be arranged from lowest to highest: 0, 1, 2, 3, 4, 5, 6, 6, 8, 9. Each

TABLE 9-4 Sample of Ordinal Data Satisfaction Scale

Case Number	Satisfaction Scale
1	2
2	8
3	1
4	6
5	4
6	5
7	0
8	6
9	9
10	3

respondent ranks his or her amount of satisfaction based on his or her perspective of satisfaction.

Continuous Data

Continuous data are defined as data that have equal space between each variable, much like a ruler or yardstick. A continuous variable is any variable between the two values. For example, height and weight are continuous variables. There are two common types of continuous data: interval and ratio.

Interval Data

Interval data are in rank order, like ordinal data, except that the space or intervals between the data are always equal. Think of a measuring tape. There is an equal distance of 1 inch between 10 and 11 inches and between 18 and 19 inches. The same is also true for days (24 hours), weeks (7 days), months (12 per year), or years (365 days, 52 weeks, or 12 months). One example is when the evaluator involves adolescents in a clinic, and the survey question asks:

What is the month and year of your birthday?
Month: _____
Year: _____

From this information, evaluators calculate the exact age in months for each respondent. This information is more accurate than asking an adolescent only their age in years, because one adolescent is 13 years and 1 month, while another adolescent is 13 years and 11 months. This additional information is valuable, because adolescents mature at different rates.

Another example is to ask employees to estimate how long they have experienced chronic back pain (see **Table 9-5**).

TABLE 9-3 Sample of Age (Ordinal Data)

Case Number	Age
1	2
2	3
3	2
4	4
5	2
6	5
7	6
8	3
9	5
10	4

TABLE 9-5 Sample Interval Data

Case Number	Time (in Weeks) of Chronic Back Pain Symptoms Prior to Seeking Health Care
1	6
2	4
3	12
4	10
5	4
6	6
7	8
8	14
9	9
10	6

Ratio Data

Ratio data are like interval data with even intervals, except ratio data have an absolute zero point. Absolute zero is defined as the absence of the variable measured. For example, when measuring height, the absolute zero is 0 inches, because you can't have a negative height. In an example using currency, a ratio is calculated to say that $20 dollars is four times as much as $5. Ratios are also used to describe election results; for example, when announcers state that the winner received twice as many votes as the losing candidate. In public health, evaluators use ratios to calculate the numbers of people in the population with a specific disease; for example, there are 195.2 deaths due to heart disease in the United States per 100,000 population per year.[1] An example survey question for ratio data is the following:

What was the cost of your pain medication prescription copayment when you obtained your prescription at the local pharmacy today?

1 = I did not pay a copayment today for my prescription.
2 = $5
3 = $10
4 = $15
5 = $20
6 = $25
7 = $30
8 = $35
9 = $40

Evaluators list these choices after investigating the amount of copayments collected prior to obtaining a medication prescription at the pharmacy. In this example, it is assumed that prescription copayments fall into $5 increments up to $40.

Another example of ratio data is when evaluators try to determine if the Healthy Back Program is effective 12 months after implementation. By retrieving data from employee medical records after institutional review board (IRB) approval, the evaluators gather data related to height, weight, and body mass index (BMI) of employees who participated in the Healthy Back Program over the past 12 months (see **Table 9-6**).

Now let's summarize the four types of data and explore how evaluators analyze and report data (see **Table 9-7**).

Now practice your skills using **Table 9-8**.

Now with an understanding of the four types of data, let's explore how evaluators can analyze and report data.

DATA ORGANIZATION

Evaluators organize data in a variety of ways depending on the purpose of reporting. This section includes descriptive data, graphic presentations, measures of central tendency, the normal curve, and standard deviation and variance.

Descriptive Data

After evaluators collect their data, they enter the data into a spreadsheet (e.g., Microsoft Excel) or directly into a statistical

TABLE 9-6 Sample of Ratio Data: Height, Weight, BMI

Case Number	Height	Weight	Body Mass Index
1	5'7"	156	24.4
2	5'4"	162	27.8
3	5'10"	209	30.0
4	5'5"	132	22.2
5	5'6"	147	23.7
6	5'11"	230	32.1
7	5'2"	136	24.9
8	5'8"	182	27.7
9	6'1"	197	26.0
10	5'8"	159	24.2

Category	BMI Score
Underweight	<18.5
Normal	18.5–24.9
Overweight	25–29.9
Obese	≥30

TABLE 9-7 Summary of the Data Types

Case Number	Reporting Chronic Back Pain to a Physician	Age	Height	Weight	Body Mass Index	Cost of Copayment for Prescription
1	0	2	5'7"	156	24.4	$5
2	0	3	5'4"	162	27.8	$10
3	1	2	5'10"	209	30.0	$20
4	0	4	5'5"	132	22.2	$10
5	1	2	5'6"	147	23.7	$20
6	1	5	5'11"	230	32.1	$30
7	0	6	5'2	136	24.9	$15
8	1	3	5'8"	182	27.7	$5
9	0	5	6'1"	197	26.0	$15
10	0	4	5'8"	159	24.2	$20

TABLE 9-8 Evaluation Practice: Data Classification

When evaluators develop surveys, they are aware of data created from each question. For the following questions, select the data classification that the responses yield.

Question	Data Classification			
	Nominal (a)	Ordinal (b)	Interval (c)	Ratio (d)
1. How old are you today?				
2. What is the highest level of education you have achieved? • High school diploma or GED • Trade or vocational training • Some college—no diploma • Associate degree • Bachelor degree • Graduate degree or higher				
3. Rate your health today: • Excellent • Very good • Good • Fair • Poor				
4. How many points did you receive on your midterm exam in Biology I?				
5. What letter grade did you receive on your Biology I midterm exam? • A • B • C • D • F				

(continues)

TABLE 9-8 Evaluation Practice: Data Classification (Continued)

Question	Data Classification			
	Nominal (a)	Ordinal (b)	Interval (c)	Ratio (d)
6. What was the temperature this morning when you stepped outside your home?				
7. How did you acquire an appointment to have your new flat-screen television delivered? • I made an appointment when I purchase the flat-screen television. • I went online to schedule an appointment for delivery. • I called to schedule an appointment for delivery.				
8. How many minutes did you wait in the store before a sales person assisted you with the purchase of your flat-screen television?				
9. Would you recommend this store to a friend? • Yes • No				
10. How would you rate the customer service from the sales-person in this store? • Excellent • Very Good • Good • Fair • Poor				

Answers: 1c, 2b, 3b, 4c, 5c, 6d, 7a, 8c, 9a, 10b

software program (e.g., SPSS or SAS). The first step allows evaluators to view the data and to identify missing data. For example, in **Figure 9-2**, Case 5 has missing data for the age of the respondent, and Case 16 has "7" entered under satisfaction, which is not a valid choice (1 = low and 5 = high). Because each survey was numbered when collected, evaluators locate surveys with errors and enter the corrected or missing data. In addition, evaluators randomly select 10% of the surveys and reenter the responses to verify the accuracy of the data-entry process. *Data cleaning* is the term used for the process of checking the data for accuracy and correcting errors.

Once descriptive data are cleaned, evaluators organize it in order to answer the objectives of the evaluation. For example, if the objective of the evaluation was to determine what percentage of adults over age 50 years responded to a satisfaction survey, evaluators could use Excel to sort the data and report concise results.

Step 1: Highlight all three columns.
Step 2: Click on the Data tab and click on "A to Z."
Yield the spreadsheet shown in **Figure 9-3**.

Report: Of the 20 responding adults, the age distribution is 6 adults (30%) age 50–59 years, 5 (25%) 60–69 years, 5 (25%) 70–79 years, 2 (10%) 80–89 years, and 2 (10%) 90+ years.

To sort by gender, highlight all three columns, click the Data tab, then in the A to Z drop-down menu click Custom Sort, and then add one level by clicking the plus (+) button (see **Figure 9-4**). This procedure provides the information shown in **Figure 9-5**.

Because there are only 20 respondents, evaluators calculate results by hand. However, Excel can be used for calculations on larger datasets.

Report: Of the 20 responding adults, the gender distribution is 12 (60%) females and 8 (40%) males.

The same sorting process is used if evaluators wished to report satisfaction of survey respondents.

Report: Of the 20 responding adults, the satisfaction is 2 (10%) poor, 7 (35%) fair, 6 (30%) good, 4 (20%) very good and 1 (5%) excellent.

FIGURE 9-2 Sample of Excel data spreadsheet.

	A	B	C
1	Age	Gender	Satisfaction
2	50	1	3
3	57	1	4
4	56	1	2
5		2	3
6	71	1	2
7	73	1	1
8	61	2	2
9	67	1	3
10	59	2	4
11	78	1	2
12	81	1	3
13	90	1	4
14	58	2	5
15	68	2	1
16	83	2	7
17	94	1	3
18	57	2	2
19	72	1	4
20	78	2	3
21	62	1	2
22			

Used with permission from Microsoft.

FIGURE 9-3 Sorting Excel spreadsheet.

	A	B	C
1	Age	Gender	Satisfaction
2	50	1	3
3	56	1	2
4	57	1	4
5	57	2	2
6	58	2	5
7	59	2	4
8	61	2	2
9	62	2	3
10	62	1	2
11	67	1	3
12	68	2	1
13	71	1	2
14	72	1	4
15	73	1	1
16	78	1	2
17	78	2	3
18	81	1	3
19	83	2	4
20	90	1	4
21	94	1	3
22			

Used with permission from Microsoft.

FIGURE 9-4 Sorting by level.

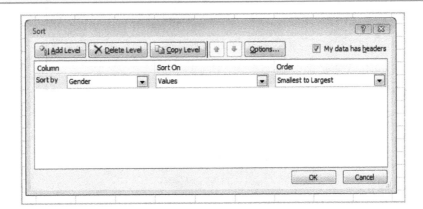

Used with permission from Microsoft.

FIGURE 9-5 Advanced Excel sorting.

	A	B	C
1	Age	Gender	Satisfaction
2	50	1	3
3	56	1	2
4	57	1	4
5	62	1	2
6	67	1	3
7	71	1	2
8	72	1	4
9	73	1	1
10	78	1	2
11	81	1	3
12	90	1	4
13	94	1	3
14	57	2	2
15	58	2	5
16	59	2	4
17	61	2	2
18	62	2	3
19	68	2	1
20	78	2	3
21	83	2	4

Used with permission from Microsoft.

Graphic Presentation

Although descriptive data are useful to organize information, evaluators usually use histograms and frequency polygons to provide a visual depiction of data. Histograms are generally used to display nominal data (see **Figure 9-6**), while frequency polygons display continuous data (see **Figure 9-7**).

Figure 9-7 shows a frequency polygon of continuous data collected on three patients who participated in a 12-week weight-loss program. Data show that Patient A lost the most weight, followed by Patient B, and then Patient C.

Now it is time to practice your skills using **Table 9-9**.

Measures of Central Tendency

Measures of central tendency are used to summarize data and make comparisons between data. Measures of central tendency include the mean, median, and mode.[2]

Mean

The mean is defined as the average score. To find the mean, evaluators add all the scores and divide by the total number of scores. Mean scores are used for interval and ratio data, but not for nominal and ordinal data. For example, if evaluators asked on a survey, "What is your age?" followed by a blank line, the respondents would fill in the blank.

This section presents two ways of calculating a mean. The first example is calculated by hand by merely adding up all of the ages and dividing by number of responses. This method

FIGURE 9-6 Histogram of ordinal data.

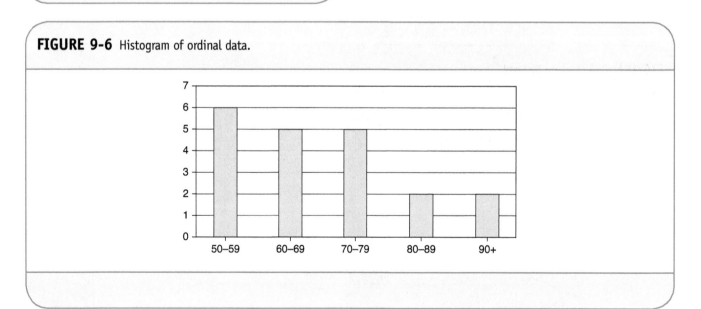

FIGURE 9-7 Frequency polygram.

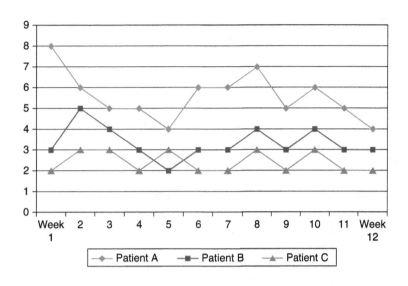

TABLE 9-9 Practice Descriptive Data Skills

Review collected data: Using the data table and the codebook, answer the following questions.
1. Are there any missing data?
2. Write a statement to summarize severity of injuries.
3. Write a statement to summarize the location of injuries on property.

Data of Injuries in Three Clinics

Case	Clinic	Number of Injuries in the Last Month	Severity of Injury	Blood Exposure	Description of Injured Person	Location of Injury on Property
1	2	6	1	0	1	3
2	3	4	1	0	1	4
3	1	7	1		1	2
4	2	1	1	1	2	1
5	3	2	2	0	1	4
6	1	1	4	1	3	5
7	2	3	1	0	1	1
8	1	2	1	1	1	3
9	1	5	2	1	2	3
10	3	2	1	0	1	4

(continues)

TABLE 9-9 Practice Descriptive Data Skills (Continued)

Codebook					
Variable	**Codes**				
Location of Factory	1 = Bradbury	2 = Graham	3 = Seffner		
Number of Injuries in the Last 3 Months	Numerical value				
Severity of Injury	1 = Basic first aid treatment (e.g., Band-Aid and ointment)	2 = Medical exam by healthcare provider	3 = Taken to hospital and released within 23 hours	4 = Transported by ambulance and admitted to hospital	
Blood Exposure	0 = No	1 = Yes			
Description of Injured Person	1 = Assembly line workers	2 = Office workers	3 = Administrator		
Location of Injury on Property	1 = Parking lot or surrounding landscaped area	2 = Factory floor	3 = Back office, file room, break room, exam room	4 = Lab or procedure room	5 = Maintenance and grounds building

1. In Case 3, the blood exposure data are missing.
2. Of the 10 injuries in the past month, 7 (70%) injuries were treated with basic first aid, 2 (20%) injuries required a medical examination by a healthcare provider, and 1 (10%) injury required that the injured individual be transported by ambulance to the hospital for admission.
3. Of the 10 injuries, 1 (10%) occurred in the maintenance and grounds building; 1 (10%) occurred in the waiting room; 2 (20%) injuries occurred in parking lot or surrounding landscaped area; 3 (30%) occurred in the back office, file room, break room, or exam room; and 3 (30%) occurred in the lab or procedure room.

FIGURE 9-8 Amount of weight lifted without pain after back injury at work.

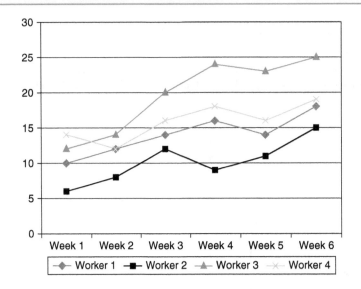

works fine if you have only a small number of responses, such as 20, in this example:

Mean = 13 + 18 + 14 + 19 + 15 + 14 + 17 + 18 + 13 + 17 + 14 + 16 + 13 + 19 + 16 + 14 + 17 + 13 + 19 + 15 = 314, then divide 314 by 20 = 15.7 = mean age.

The second example is for a larger number of responses and utilizes an Excel formula for the calculation.

The Excel formula to calculate the mean is fx = AVERAGE(A2:A21). See **Figure 9-9**.

On the other hand, suppose evaluators asked on a survey, "Select your age group," followed by these choices:

1. 13 or younger
2. 14–15
3. 16–17
4. 18–19

FIGURE 9-9 Age data.

	A
1	Age
2	13
3	13
4	13
5	13
6	14
7	14
8	14
9	14
10	15
11	15
12	16
13	16
14	17
15	17
16	17
17	18
18	18
19	19
20	19
21	19
22	

Used with permission from Microsoft.

Evaluators would not be able to calculate the mean age, because they are trying to calculate a mean by using nominal data. There are 4 in group 1 (13 or younger), 6 in group 2 (14–15), 5 in group 3 (16–17), and 5 in group 4 (18–19).

Mean score = 1 + 1 + 1 + 1 + 2 + 2 + 2 + 2 + 2 + 2 + 3 + 3 + 3 + 3 + 3 + 4 + 4 + 4 + 4 + 4 = 51

Then divide 51 by 20:

51 ÷ 20 = 2.55

This value shows that the average age is somewhere between 14 and 17, which is not accurate, and proves the point that means cannot be calculated on nominal or ordinal data. Because the mean is more accurate, it is used for interval and ratio data.

Median

The median is defined as the middle value of the data. When there are an even numbers of scores, the median is calculated by adding the two middle scores together and dividing by two. In **Figure 9-10** there are 20 age scores, so (15 + 16)/2 = 15.5 is the median. Generally, median is used for ordinal data. The Excel formula is fx =MEDIAN(A2:A31).

Mode

The mode is defined as the most frequently occurring score. In **Figure 9-10**, there are two modes because 13 and 14 were both picked the same number of times. When this happens, the data are called bimodal.[2] The mode is used for nominal data. The Excel formula is fx =MODE(A2:A21).

Normal Curve

In this section, several topics related to the normal curve are discussed, including skew, variance, and standard deviation. Let's begin with the normal curve, shown in **Figure 9-11**. If data are evenly distributed, Figure 9-11 shows that mean, median, and mode are the same. In the normal curve, there are equal numbers of variables above and below the mean, median, and mode. For example, if the annual income in one county was evenly distributed, the mean, median, and mode of income remain the same: $43,000 annually. In addition, half of the population has an income below $43,000 and half the population has an income above $43,000.

When the mean, median, and mode are not the same number, the curve is lopsided or skewed. The skew of the curve is positive or negative. In a positive skew, the mean is greater than the median[3] (see **Figure 9-12**).

In Figure 9-12, notice that the mode is not changed by the direction of the skew, because the mode is the most frequent

FIGURE 9-10 Summary of mean, median, and mode.

	A	B	C	D	E
	C25		▼	f_x =MODE(A2:A21)	
1	Age				
2	13				
3	13				
4	13				
5	13				
6	14				
7	14				
8	14				
9	14				
10	15				
11	15				
12	16				
13	16				
14	17				
15	17				
16	17				
17	18				
18	18				
19	19				
20	19				
21	19				
22					
23		Mean	15.7		
24		Median	15.5		
25		Mode	13		

Used with permission from Microsoft.

FIGURE 9-11 The normal curve.

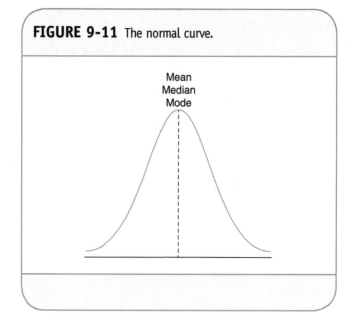

number. In a negative skew, the mean is smaller than the median. For example, if the county has a large proportion of low-income individuals, the mean is pulled in a negative direction. In a positive skew, the mean is larger than the median. For example, if the county has a large population of wealthy individuals, the mean is pulled in the positive direction.

Lastly, it is often possible to determine the skew by looking at the mean and median instead of constructing a histogram. Let's look at an example of skew. Salaries of personnel in the hospital lab are $280,000, $112,000, $80,000, $78,000, $61,000, $52,000, $39,000, $39,000, and $28,000. The median is $61,000. The mode is $39,000. The mean is $85,444. Without drawing a histogram, it is easy to determine these

FIGURE 9-12 Skewed distributions.

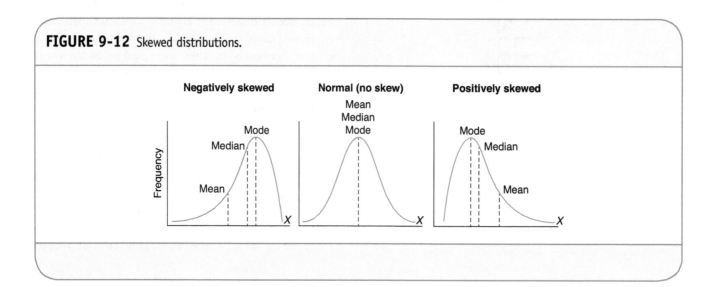

FIGURE 9-13 Standard deviations on the normal curve.

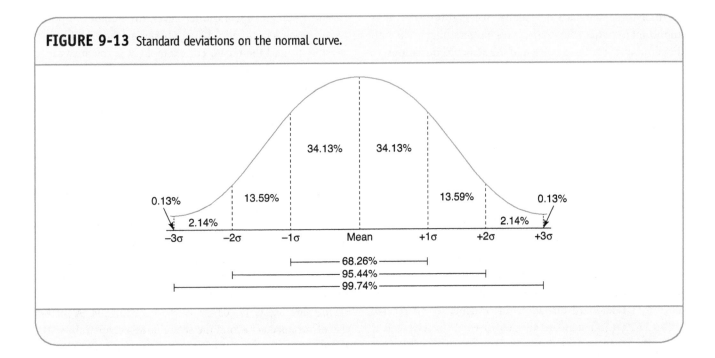

data have a positive distribution, because the mean ($85,444) is greater than the median ($61,000).

Standard Deviation and Variance

Standard deviation (Greek symbol sigma, σ) is defined as how much variation or "dispersion" exists from the mean or average. A low standard deviation shows that data are gathered tightly around the mean, whereas a high standard deviation shows that data are dispersed or spread out far from the mean. Look at the normal curve in **Figure 9-13**. The vertical line represents the mean score. The area shows one standard deviation from the mean or 68.26% of the population, with 34.13% above the mean and 34.13% below the mean. The second area represents about 28% (13.59% above the mean and 13.59% below the mean) for a total of two standard deviations, representing about 95.44% of the population. The third area represents about 4% (2.14% above the mean and 2.14% below the mean). By summing, the area of the three standard deviations equals nearly 99% of the population.[4]

Let's begin with an example of exam scores of students from Classes A, B, and C. There were 27 students in each class and 100 points possible on the exam (see **Figure 9-14**). The Excel formulas are fx =MEAN(A2:A28); fx =STDEV(A2:A28), and fx =VAR(A2:A28).

Notice that in Classes A, B, and C exam scores have a mean of 70.4, but let's suppose that the three instructors decided to assign student grades based on the normal curve. Using Figure 9-14, let's calculate how many students are in

FIGURE 9-14 Exam scores of class A, B, C.

	A	B	C	D	E	F
1	Class A		Class B		Class C	
2	24		24		63	
3	36		28		64	
4	50		52		65	
5	50		53		67	
6	51		58		67	
7	61		67		67	
8	61		68		67	
9	62		70		68	
10	62		72		68	
11	64		73		70	
12	70		73		70	
13	70		73		70	
14	70		74		70	
15	71		74		71	
16	71		74		71	
17	72		75		71	
18	80		76		72	
19	81		77		72	
20	83		77		72	
21	83		78		72	
22	86		79		72	
23	88		80		73	
24	90		81		74	
25	91		82		74	
26	91		86		76	
27	92		86		77	
28	92		91		79	
29	70.4	Mean	70.4	Mean	70.4	Mean
30	17.7034	St Dev	15.6236	St Dev	3.816294	St Dev
31	313.4103	Var	244.0969	Var	14.5641	Var

the first three standard deviations (see **Figure 9-15**). It is important to notice that exam scores have nothing to do with the number of students in each of the standard deviations.

1st standard deviation: 27 students × 34.13%
= 9 students below and 9 students above the mean.

2nd standard deviation: 27 students × 13.59%
= 4 students below and 4 students above the mean.

3rd standard deviation: 27 students × 2.14%
= 1 student below and 1 student above the mean.

Figure 9-15 shows that as long as the mean score is 70.4 in Classes A, B, and C, the distribution of students remains the same on the normal curve. Regardless of the exam scores, if the instructors used the normal curve to assign grades, 68.26% (1st standard deviation) of students would receive a C, 13.59% (2nd standard deviation) would receive a B if above the mean and a D if below the mean, and 2.14% (3rd standard deviation) would receive an A if above the mean and an F if below the mean.

Let's try one last comparison using the student grades. **Table 9-10** shows that when instructors use the normal curve and the first three standard deviations for distribution of grades, the percentage of students receiving A, B, C,

D, and F remains identical. However, the number of points to earn each letter grade changes based on the width of dispersion around the mean. For example, it is much easier to receive an A in Class C, because the exam scores are packed tightly around the mean of 70.4. However, students hoping to receive a C would rejoice about the wide dispersion (high standard deviation) in Class A (see Table 9-10).

When evaluators present frequency data, they also report standard deviations. This additional information allows the reader to know the spread of the data.[3] Using the previous example, if evaluators reported only mean scores, it appears that there are no differences among Class A, Class B, and Class C. However, by adding standard deviations, the differences among the classes are apparent.

Let's not forget to mention the term *variance*. Variance is defined as the square of the standard deviation.[3] For example, the standard deviation for Class A in Table 9-10 is 17.7034 so the variance is 17.7034 × 17.7034 = 313.4104. A further use of variance is beyond the scope of this chapter. In statistics courses, the concept of analysis of variance (ANOVA) is explained in greater detail.

SUMMARY

This chapter began by exploring how data are classified by scales of measurement, including categorical data using nominal and ordinal scales and continuous data using interval

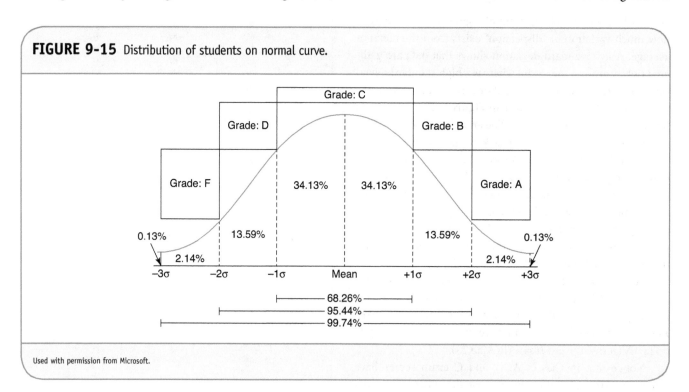

FIGURE 9-15 Distribution of students on normal curve.

Used with permission from Microsoft.

TABLE 9-10 Comparison of Grading Scale with Normal Curve

	Usual Grade Scale			Grades Using Normal Curve	
	Points	Number of Students (%)		Points	Number of Students (%)
Class A	A 90–100	5 (18.5%)		A 92–100	1 (2.14%)
	B 80–89	6 (22.25%)		B 90–91	4 (13.59%)
	C 70–79	6 (22.25%)		C 61–90	18 (68.26%)
	D 60–69	5 (18.5%)		D 36–60	3 (13.59%)
	F < 59	5 (18.5%)		F < 35	1 (2.14%)
Class B	A 100–90	1 (3.7%)		A 91–100	1 (2.14%)
	B 80–89	5 (18.5%)		B 81–90	4 (13.59%)
	C 70–79	14 (51.85%)		C 58–80	18 (68.26%)
	D 60–69	2 (7.4%)		D 28–57	3 (13.59%)
	F < 59	5 (18.5%)		F < 27	1 (2.14%)
Class C	A 100–90	0 (0%)		A 79–100	1 (2.14%)
	B 89–80	0 (0%)		B 74–78	4 (13.59%)
	C 70–79	18 (66.67%)		C 73–68	18 (68.26%)
	D 60–69	9 (33.33%)		D 64–67	3 (13.59%)
	F < 59	0 (0%)		F < 63	1 (2.14%)

and ratio scales. Once the data are collected, it is necessary to organize the data (e.g., frequency distributions and graphic presentations). The chapter ends with a discussion of concepts including measures of central tendency, components of the normal curve, variance, and standard deviation.

CASE STUDY

A national corporation of pharmacy stores hired an evaluation team to determine why some adults chose to receive annual flu vaccines, some adults occasionally receive flu vaccines, and other adults never receive flu vaccines. After a few meetings with the corporate office, the evaluation team members develop goals and objectives and strategize about the evaluation methods. Evaluators hire five public health graduate students to work 20 hours per week for 15 weeks. A convenience sample is used for survey data collection. Evaluators estimate they will need a response rate of approximately 1,000 individuals.

The Health Belief Model is utilized in this evaluation. The main components of the Health Belief Model are perceived benefits, barriers, risks, and severity for performing or not performing the specific health behavior of obtaining an annual flu vaccine.

Goal: By August 1, the public perception about flu vaccines will be evaluated based on the recent county social media campaign to increase the number of adults receiving the flu vaccine in Adams County.

Objective One: By August 1, 100% of the respondents will have shared their behavior patterns related to receipt of annual flu vaccines.

Objective Two: By August 1, 100% of respondents will have shared the behavior patterns of their friends related to receipt of annual flu vaccines.

Objective Three: By August 1, 100% of respondents will have shared their demographic data for determining relationship to behavior patterns of receipt of annual flu vaccines.

For 10 weeks prior to the peak of flu season, evaluators asked the five public health graduate students to sit in the waiting area of the local national chain pharmacies with a clipboard. As each person pays for his or her prescription, clerks invite each customer to participate in the national pharmaceutical chain research related to flu vaccines. If the response is positive, the clerk introduces the graduate student. A $10 store gift card is offered as an incentive. Prior to conducting the survey, graduate students explain the purpose of the evaluation, obtain consent signatures on the institutional review board–approved consent forms, and keep one copy and give a copy of the consent form to the participating individual. Using clipboards to hold surveys, the graduate student records each response verbatim.

Survey Questions

1. Have you ever received a flu vaccine?
   Yes
   No
   If "Yes," then ask, "Why do you receive flu vaccines each year?" If "Yes, but not every year," then ask, "Why not every year?"
   If "No," then ask, "What is the reason that you do not receive a flu vaccine?"

2. Do your family members receive flu vaccines?
   Yes
   No
   If "Yes," then ask, "Why do you think that your family members receive flu vaccines each year?" If "Yes, but not every year," then ask, "Why do you think that they do not receive the flu vaccine every year?"
   If "No," then ask, "What is the reason that your family members do not receive a flu vaccine?"

3. Do your friends receive flu vaccines?
   Yes
   No
   If "Yes,: then ask, "Why do your friends receive flu vaccines each year?" If "Yes, but not every year," then ask, "Why do you think that your friends do not receive the flu vaccine every year?"
   If "No," then ask, "What is the reason that your friends do not receive a flu vaccine?"
   Now a few questions about you:

4. What is your age? _____

5. What is your employment status? (Check all that apply)
   Full time
   Part time (less than 30 hours per week)
   Temporary
   Seasonal
   Active-duty military
   Retired

Because the evaluation is based on a convenience sample, the graduate students conduct as many interviews as possible during their assigned 4-hour shifts at the randomly selected national chain stores across various ZIP codes in their large county. The shift hours are randomly assigned as morning, afternoon, and evening during weekdays and weekends to ensure responses from a wide variety of customers.

Upon completion of data collection, a spreadsheet is created for entering the data. Graduate students enter the survey data. After checking the data to ensure accuracy, evaluators determine the measurements of central tendency and skew of the curve. Results are presented to the corporate executives of the national pharmaceutical chain that designed and implemented the social media campaign to increase receipt of flu vaccines. Based on the results, the evaluation team will make recommendations related to the success of the social media campaign. After flu season, evaluation teams repeat the survey to determine if the flu vaccine social media campaign increased the flu vaccine compliance.

Case Study Discussion Questions

1. What other survey questions could have been added to the survey to enhance the results?
2. What would have been the advantages of using a tablet for collecting the data?
3. Which measure of central tendency would most likely be used in the data analysis? Why?

STUDENT ACTIVITIES

Jamestown is a small rural town in the southeastern part of the United States. Historically, the town was mainly a farming community. However, a furniture factory has been the main source of income for most families for the last 50 years. The nearest major city is about 45 minutes away. Recently, the mayor of the town, Mr. Smith, returned from the annual National Conferences of Mayors meeting. Among the many topics that were discussed at the meeting was the growing obesity epidemic in the United States. Mr. Smith is very interested in this topic, because he has noticed that more and more people in Jamestown are overweight, including young children. Mayor Smith thought that doing something about the obesity problem in his town would benefit all its citizens. However, before he started working on programs and spending valuable community money and resources, he wanted to make sure that there was indeed a problem with obesity in his community. When he got back from the conference he went to the local clinic and met with the healthcare providers. Also at the meeting was the clerk from the county vital records department. Mayor Smith explained his concerns to them and asked for data that would prove or disprove his suspicions. He asked the healthcare providers how many people at the clinics were overweight (according to the body mass index for their height and weight). He also wanted to know their ages (grouped in 10-year increments) and who among them was diagnosed with an obesity-related illness like type 2 diabetes or chronic heart disease. From the vital records clerk, he wanted to know if obesity-related causes of death had grown over the last decade.

The healthcare providers and clerk gave Mayor Smith the requested statistics. However, the data were provided on long lists on paper. Because Mayor Smith is a very busy man, he hired you, a local community college student, to prepare all the data in an easy-to-understand and straightforward fashion that he can present to the city council.

To help you prepare the data, you will need to answer the following questions about the information sent to you by the doctor's office:

1. What data classification and measurement scale does age represent?
2. What data classification and measurement scale does obesity-related illness represent?
3. If you wanted to show the mayor how many men and women were overweight by their age group, what would be the best way to present this to the city council?
4. Now, suppose you wanted to show the city council which age groups and which genders had the highest numbers of overweight people, what would you do?
5. The clerk gives you the numbers of deaths that were related to obesity (such as type 2 diabetes and chronic heart disease) for each year over a 10-year period. What would be the best way to show the city council if obesity is better or worse than it used to be?

After assembling these data for the mayor, he tells you that you are not quite done. He would like for you to create some simple descriptive statistics that he can present to the city council. He would like to know the mean, median, and mode of the ages of those individuals who are overweight. The following table shows a representative sample of 20 people from the data.

25	13	67	7
33	42	11	18
28	31	36	47
52	73	80	15
23	14	44	36

6. What is the mean?
7. What is the median?
8. What is the mode?
9. Based on the information that you have, would the distribution curve be normal, positively skewed, or negatively skewed?

Answers

1. Age represents continuous data. Because age has an absolute zero, it is a ratio scale.
2. Obesity-related illness represents categorical data. Because it has no numerical value, this is a nominal scale.
3. You would present this information to the city council in a simple distribution frequency.
4. The easiest way would be to show this information with a histogram.
5. The best way to show a trend over time using continuous data would be to use a frequency polygon. Even though the types of obesity-related deaths are categorical data, the number of them from year to year represents continuous data. Because it is continuous data over the last 10 years, we can see whether or not there is a trend. The trend could be that obesity has gotten worse, has gotten better, or hasn't changed much over the last 10 years.
6. The mean is 34.75, almost 35 years of age.
7. The median age is 29.5.
8. The mode is 36, because there are two people who are 36 years of age.
9. This curve is only slightly positively skewed, because the mean age is slightly larger than the median age.

REFERENCES

1. The Centers for Disease Control and Prevention. Heart Disease. Available at: http://www.cdc.gov/nchs/fastats/heart.htm. Accessed May 18, 2014.
2. Johnson B, Christensen L. *Educational Research: Quantitative, Qualitative, and Mixed Approaches,* 4th ed. Thousand Oaks, CA: Sage; 2012. Available at: http://www.southalabama.edu/coe/bset/johnson/lectures/lec15.htm. Accessed May 18, 2014.
3. Ary D, Jacobs L, Razavieh A, Sorenson C. *Introduction to Research in Education,* 8th ed. Belmont, CA: Wadsworth/Cengage Learning; 2010.
4. Kalla S. Measurement of Uncertainty: Standard Deviation. Experiment Resources. Available at: http://www.experiment-resources.com/measurement-of-uncertainty-standard-deviation.html. Accessed May 18, 2014.

CHAPTER **10**

Populations and Samples

By the end of this chapter, students will be able to:

- Define population and sample.
- Discuss how probability relates to inferential statistics
- Discuss hypothesis testing and type I and II errors
- Analyze how each component of sample size determination influences the other components.
- Evaluate the differences between probability and nonprobability sampling.
- Discuss how sampling bias affects the study results.

KEY TERMS

margin of error
nonprobability sampling
nonresponse sampling bias
null hypothesis
population
probability sampling
sample size
type I and II errors

INTRODUCTION

Evaluators plan, implement, and evaluate programs, but they are not always able to study the entire population. For example, if the evaluation involves the entire community, evaluators must select a subset or sample of the population. This chapter introduces how probability and inferential statistics are used to make predictions from the random sample selected from the population. The next step involves making decisions that influence the sample size calculation. Once decisions are finalized, the chapter moves into how to recruit individuals. The recruitment process depends on probability or nonprobability sample designs. Probability sampling involves strict criteria in which every individual in the population has an equal chance of getting selected for the sample. Nonprobability sampling is more flexible, inclusive, and not based on chance procedures. With this overview in mind, let's begin the chapter with a discussion about populations and samples.

POPULATIONS AND SAMPLES

Let's step back and look closely at the relationship between populations and samples. In statistics, the word *population* is defined as the group or collection of interest for the research. Population does not necessarily indicate only humans. Populations may be soybean crop yields in Iowa, bacteria counts in culture dishes, or cancer clusters within brain tissue. Now let's focus on what a sample is. As previously stated, a sample is a subset of a population. The closer the sample is to representing the whole population, the more accurate the inferences or assumptions that evaluators can make about the population. If the sample does not represent the population, then the assumptions are less likely to be accurate. As discussed later in this chapter, it is important that the sample is randomly selected from the population to increase the chance that the characteristics match the population.[1]

PROBABILITY AND INFERENTIAL STATISTICS

Probability is defined as every single event being random. For example, the result of the coin toss at the beginning of a football game is a single and random event. However, if the same coin is tossed 100 times, an approximately equal pattern of heads and tails develops (e.g., 46 heads and 54 tails). If the same coin is tossed 1,000 times, the pattern becomes more accurate (e.g., 489 heads and 511 tails). Probability allows evaluators to predict the outcome based on repeating the process, which in this case is tossing a coin.[1]

The word *infer* is defined as to assume or understand. Inferential statistics are mathematical procedures used to assume or understand predictions about the whole population based on data collected from a random sample selected from the population.[2] These predictions are based on estimates or probabilities rather than absolute facts. Evaluators use characteristics of the sample (statistics) to estimate the characteristics of the population (parameters). When evaluators use inferential statistics, they assume a certain degree of error, because they are never 100% accurate in making assumptions about the population based on the sample. For example, if researchers at a global health pharmaceutical company develop a new highly effective prophylactic malaria drug with few side effects, even after completing laboratory and animal studies, they *infer* the medication's effectiveness for humans. If they knew the exact human reaction process to the medication, it would be like coin tossing: patients would either experience side effects or would not experience side effects after ingesting the new medication. Because it is not possible to give this new malaria medication to the entire global population of individuals taking prophylactic malaria medication, evaluators select a random sample of individuals taking prophylactic malaria medication to evaluate the extent of side effects. The evaluators conduct the evaluation, gather data, and use inferential statistics to estimate the degree of side effects of the new prophylactic for the population of individuals needing to take malaria medication. Because evaluators accept a certain degree of error regarding the effectiveness and possible side effects, the global health pharmaceutical company states in marketing materials that the side effects may vary among patients.

Null Hypothesis

Another component of inferential statistics is the development of a hypothesis. Keep in mind that not all evaluations utilize inferential statistics. However, when evaluators plan to use inferential statistics, it is helpful to develop hypothesis statements. A hypothesis is a statement of what the evaluator expects the relationships to be among the study variables.[2] The four parts of a hypothesis are described by the following questions:[2]

- Is the hypothesis aligned with the current knowledge available on the topic?
- What is the expected relationship between the study variables?
- Is the hypothesis able to be tested?
- Is the hypothesis clearly stated?

Let's look at examples of hypothesis statements that answer each of the previously stated questions:

- *Example 1*: Because 30 minutes of moderate exercise performed three times per week helps to control weight, it is hypothesized that adults who participate in a community-based, 30-minute aerobic exercise program three times per week will achieve greater weight control than adults who do not participate in the community-based exercise program.
- *Example 2*: Because outdoor air pollution is a risk factor for childhood asthma, it is hypothesized that more children living in a city with consistently high rates of outdoor air pollution will be diagnosed with asthma than children living in cities with low rates of outdoor air pollution.

In evaluations, the term *null hypothesis* is also used. The null hypothesis states that there is no relationship between the variables.[3] Furthermore, the null hypothesis assumes that *if* a relationship is found, it is only by chance. Using the first example, the null hypothesis would state that there is no relationship between the amount of aerobic exercise for adults participating in the 30-minute aerobic exercise program three times per week and their rate of weight control. When using the null hypothesis, evaluators want their data from the random sample to reject the null hypothesis. They want their data to show that more frequent participation in the exercise program is advantageous to greater weight control for adults.

Evaluators must reject or fail to reject the null hypothesis. However, keep in mind that evaluators are making this decision based on the sample that they have rather than the population, so their results are always based on incomplete information and are subject to error. If evaluators fail to reject the null hypothesis, they are saying there is a chance that there is no relationship. Using Example 1, consider the possibility that there is no relationship between aerobic exercise and weight control. It might be that the community-based aerobic exercise program has nothing to do with weight management but rather is related to the fact that the exercise program is offered at the same time as the community farmers' market held in the parking lot of the community center. The exercise participants are purchasing and consuming more fresh fruits and vegetables than they did prior to participating in the community-based exercise program. Nevertheless, evaluators reject or fail to reject the null hypothesis, and their decision may be correct or incorrect. Decisions made regarding the null hypothesis have consequences that are labeled type I and type II errors.

Type I errors occur when the null hypothesis is true (there is no relationship between variables), and evaluators reject it.[3] In Example 1, evaluators report that there is a relationship between aerobic exercise and weight control, thereby rejecting the null hypothesis (that there is no relationship). The community center acts on the evaluation report and begins to offer the 30-minute aerobic exercise program daily. However, 1 year later, the community center observes that the adults only participate in the aerobic exercise program on the days when the farmers' market is open. Another evaluation team repeats the evaluation and declares the first evaluation was incorrect because they made a costly type I error (rejection of a true null hypothesis).

Type II errors occur when the null hypothesis is false (there is a real relationship between variables), and evaluators fail to reject it.[3] From the previous example, evaluators report that there is no relationship between participation in aerobic exercise and weight control, thereby failing to reject the null hypothesis when they should have. Their report states that the evaluation found insufficient evidence to increase the number of days that the aerobic exercise is offered at the community center. However, 1 year later, the community center observes that the rate of weight control remains the same among the adults participating in the aerobic exercise program. Another evaluation team repeats the evaluation and declares the first study was incorrect because they made a type II error (retention of a false null hypothesis). See **Table 10-1**.

Level of Significance

Before leaving the topic of type I and type II errors, it is necessary to understand the concept of level of significance.

Evaluators in fear of making type I errors decide to always fail to reject the null hypothesis or always reject the null hypothesis to avoid type II errors. Because neither of these options is feasible, evaluators make decisions related to the level of significance. Level of significance is the statistical risk that evaluators are willing to accept when making the decision to accept or reject the null hypothesis. If evaluators set the level of significance at 0.01, they are willing to accept that 1 out of 100 times the null hypothesis will be rejected when it is true (type I error). If the level of significance is set at 0.001, the risk of a type I error is 1 in 1000. Evaluators select the level of significance based on the type of evaluation and the severity of type I and II errors.[4] In social science, level of significance is typically set at 0.05, because frequently such evaluations are based on human behaviors with numerous confounding variables (e.g., age, gender, race/ethnicity, geographical location, environment, education, income, behavior, culture). In natural science, the level of significance is typically set at 0.01 or 0.001, because the study is conducted in controlled environments (e.g., constant temperature, light, humidity, sound, vibration).

Let's recap this complex but important section before moving on to determining sample size. The reader should understand that a sample represents the population, and if the sample does not represent the population, then the assumptions made from that sample are less accurate. Evaluators use inferential statistics to estimate the characteristics of the population based on the characteristics of the sample. Because of this assumption, they assume a certain degree of error. Evaluators develop a statement to predict the expected relationship among the study variables, called a hypothesis. The null hypothesis states that there is no relationship among the variables. Based on data gathered from the sample, evaluators reject or fail to reject the null hypothesis at the conclusion of their evaluation. Evaluators make type I errors when the null hypothesis is true and rejected, or type II errors when evaluators do not reject the null hypothesis and it is false. The

TABLE 10-1 Summary of Type I and Type II Errors

		Truth in Population	
		Null hypothesis is true	Null hypothesis is false
Based on Sample Taken from Population	Rejects null hypothesis	Type I error	Correct
	Accepts null hypothesis	Correct	Type II error

level of significance allows evaluators to set the risk they are willing to accept when rejecting a null hypothesis when there is no actual relationship (type I error).

SAMPLE SIZE CONSIDERATIONS

Why should an evaluator be concerned about the number of individuals in the sample for their evaluation? Let's look at this question from several viewpoints. As previously stated in this chapter, evaluators need to select individuals for the sample who represent the population being studied. For example, if the whole population is 10,000, it does not seem logical for evaluators to select 10 individuals for the sample and expect these 10 individuals to represent the entire population. On the other hand, it does not seem necessary or feasible to select 9000 individuals for the sample from a population of 10,000. But then evaluators ask: If 10 are too few and 9000 are too many, how many individuals are needed to adequately represent the population? There are no easy answers to this question. The following discussion introduces different aspects of how to determine the appropriate sample size for various types of evaluations. However, it is important for readers to realize that the topics presented in this chapter interact with each other, so determining the ideal sample size is never simple. Let's begin with the topics covered in the discussion (note that it is not expected that the reader would be fully familiar with all of these topics). This section defines each of the following terms:

- Margin of error
- Population, sample, and variability
- Confidence level
- Budget and budget justification
- Timeline

Margin of Error

Margin of error is about precision. Generally, evaluators do not use a margin of error over 5%. The more precision required, the smaller the acceptable margin of error. For example, if evaluators wish to know the level of employee satisfaction within an organization, they need to know how many surveys to mail to a random sample of employees to represent all departments. Evaluators want the survey data to represent honest responses related to employee satisfaction from 95% of employees who return the completed surveys. This 5% margin of error is described as plus or minus 2.5%. In this scenario, evaluators are willing to accept that 5% of the employees will not be honest in their survey responses. The best way to think of this concept is to watch the evening news during a national election. Reporters say, "With 36% of the votes counted, we predict that Senator Jones is going to win the election for Colorado." At the bottom of the screen, networks post the margin of error as ±5%, which means that Senator Jones has from 33.5% to 38.5% of the votes based on the accuracy of the exit polls. Networks want to be correct 95% of the time, so they selected a 5% margin of error.[5]

In **Table 10-2**, under margin of error, there are four columns labeled with a percentage. Evaluators select the margin of error across the top and population size from the

TABLE 10-2 Calculation of Sample Size from the Population

Population Size	Margin of Error			
	5.0%	3.5%	2.5%	1.0%
50	44	47	48	50
100	80	89	94	99
500	217	306	377	475
1000	278	440	606	906
1500	306	515	759	1297
2000	322	563	869	1655
2500	333	597	952	1984
3500	346	641	1068	2565
5000	357	678	1176	3288
10,000	370	727	1332	4899
50,000	381	772	1491	8056
100,000	383	778	1513	8762

Modified from Sample Size Table. Paul Boyd, The Research Advisors. Available at: http://www.research-advisors.com/tools/SampleSize.htm. Reprinted with permission.

far-left column. For example, if evaluators accept a 5% margin of error and the population size is approximately 5000, the sample size needed is 357. If they wish to increase the level of precision to a 2.5% margin of error, the sample size increases to 1176. Note that decreasing the margin of error by half, from 5% to 2.5%, increased the sample size by almost three times, from 357 to 1176.

Population, Sample, and Variability

Let's go back and revisit how to use Table 10-2 to determine an adequate sample size. To understand Table 10-2, we begin by defining population size and referring back to the previous discussion on margin of error. Population is defined as the total number of individuals in the group or community from which the sample is drawn. For example, if there are approximately 3500 employees where the survey data are collected, the sample size ranges from 346 to 2565, depending on the margin of error. If population size is not listed, select the highest number that is close to population size. The value in the next column is the sample size based on the margin of error. It is worth noting that for small population sizes, the sample size includes the entire population. Of course, using the population (e.g., 200 or less) as the sample is only possible with the availability of adequate funding. For example, if evaluators wanted to interview all Hurricane Sandy first responders who were on the scene within the first 24 hours, they would determine the total number of individuals from personnel records and then attempt to contact all of them. Such interviews would provide in-depth and personal insights into how the evacuation efforts were perceived by the local first responders rather than individuals who arrived later from other states. Lastly, the sample size needs to be large enough so that the data analysis will be able to detect a change among the individuals in the sample. For example, evaluators are trying to determine if the new air filters placed in particular hybrid cars are decreasing the degree of traffic exhaust fume smells reported by drivers more than the currently installed air filters in the same hybrid cars. If the sample size of drivers is too small, the data analysis would not likely show that the new air filters are better, worse, or the same as the currently used air filters.

Variability is another aspect of populations. Variability is defined as the similarities and differences among the population. If the population is composed of diverse (heterogeneous) individuals, in order to conduct a community-based evaluation, for example, a larger sample size is required to obtain a higher level of precision. If the individuals are similar (homogeneous) in the population, such as African American females with doctoral degrees in epidemiology, a smaller sample size is needed to obtain a high level of precision.

Confidence Level

Confidence level is defined as how much certainty evaluators have that the sample is a true reflection of the population. In other words, evaluators are certain that if other evaluators conduct the same evaluation with a different sample from the same population, both evaluations would yield the same results. In social science, evaluators generally use a 95% confidence level, but in natural science, evaluators use a 99% level of confidence. Why the difference? Social science evaluators are studying behaviors of individuals, animals, communities, and populations, whereas in natural science, experiments are more likely conducted in a controlled (temperature, humidity, light, vibration, etc.) laboratory environment, so results are more precise. For evaluators to have a 95% confidence level, it means that 95 out of 100 samples of the same population would obtain the same results. In other words, evaluators are willing to accept the risk that 5 times out of 100, the results are different (see **Box 10-1**).

Budget and Budget Justification

When determining sample size, evaluators make decisions based on their available funding. Evaluators need to consider all costs associated with sample size prior to final decisions. Let's explore how data collection, data entry, and data analysis affect the costs of sample size and selection.

Data Collection

What type of quantitative data will be used in the evaluation? There are two types of quantitative data: primary and secondary data. Primary data (e.g., surveys) are collected by evaluators. Secondary data are data that were previously collected by someone else that evaluators analyze anew.

Evaluators gain permission to explore information within the existing data set. Quantitative secondary data include using existing large national data sets that are collected by federal organizations, such as the Centers for Disease Control and Prevention or the National Cancer Institute. Secondary data might also include personnel records or insurance claims within a large organization.

Evaluators also consider the availability of selected individuals. For easier data collection, evaluators have a convenient sample of easily assessable individuals. However, in more difficult cases individuals under study are limited in number or are more difficult to identify.

Data Entry

How will the data be entered for analysis? If the survey data were collected online, limited data entry costs will be involved. If the data were collected via paper surveys, there are costs associated with data entry.

BOX 10-1 Case Study: Confidence Level

The Newark Airport wants to know if they should increase the number of vendors offering a variety of caffeinated beverages in each of its concourses. An evaluation team is hired to evaluate the type and amount of caffeinated beverage purchases in each concourse. Evaluators hired five undergraduate students to stand near the check-out line at 10 different beverage vendor locations in the Newark Airport. After obtaining institutional review board approval (IRB), the undergraduate students randomly asked people to participate by simply telling the students what type of caffeinated beverages they purchased. Each participant received a $2 coupon for any vendor in the airport. Each undergraduate student collected 20 responses, so the sample size was a total of 100. Evaluators analyzed the data and found that one undergraduate student's data showed 5 out of 20 measurements yielded much higher rates of caffeine consumption than the mean (average) of the other 95 measurements. When questioning the data, the student reported that on her concourse two flights to Canada had been delayed for more than 8 hours and passengers were purchasing more caffeine beverages to stay awake to avoid missing their connecting flight to snowy Canada. The delayed passengers were bored and therefore willing to participate in the evaluation. Evaluators showed the undergraduate students that if the study were conducted 100 times, 95% of the time the amount of caffeinated beverage purchases would be approximately the same for the true population. Evaluators explained that they are willing to accept that 5 times out of 100 (5%), the sample contains a segment of the population that consumes more caffeinated beverages than 95% of the rest of the population.

Quantitative data require data cleaning, which involves looking at the data spreadsheet and determining what percentage of the data are entered incorrectly or missing from the survey. These errors are corrected by going back to the original survey and correcting the data-entry mistakes. Evaluators randomly select about 10–15% of the surveys to double-check the data entry for validation. Look at **Table 10-3** for a sample of a data spreadsheet used in quantitative analysis. Find the data-entry errors; there are eight data entry errors total. The answers are located at the end of the chapter.

Data Analysis

Evaluators need to consider the data analysis that they will be conducting when selecting the sample size. If descriptive statistics are used (e.g., frequencies and means) then nearly any sample size over 30 is generally sufficient. On the other hand, some complex statistical analyses require a larger sample size (e.g., 200–500). To save time and resources, evaluators consult biostatisticians prior to initiating any project to ensure that adequate sampling is achieved for appropriate data analyses. Finally, sample size formulas provide the minimum number of responses needed. However, many evaluators add 10–30% to the sample size to compensate for the inability to contact individuals and for missing data. Evaluators plan for this increase when calculating the research budget.[6]

The cost of data analysis is based on volume of data, the amount of data cleaning needed, complexity of the data analysis performed, and whether or not there is a need to hire a biostatistics consultant to assist with the analysis (see **Table 10-4**).

Timeline

In addition to the budget and budget justification, it is important to create a timeline for each evaluation. Although there are multiple types of timelines, each one serves the purpose of keeping the project or study on track (see **Table 10-5**).

PROBABILITY AND NONPROBABILITY SAMPLES

Now let's explore the two most common types of samples. Let's begin with the basic differences between probability and nonprobability samples. With probability samples, there is no bias in sample selection. The participants are selected based on a strict, objective, and limited criterion such as a random number list. With nonprobability, there is an element of judgment in the selection process. With these two basic differences in mind, let's delve deeper into how probability samples are selected. Keep in mind that prior to the initiation of any type of sampling, an approved IRB application is required.

Probability Sampling

The first step in probability sampling is to determine the population of interest. Evaluators make this decision based on the goals and objectives. For example, the population may be based on one or a combination of potential demographic

TABLE 10-3 Sample Spreadsheet for Quantitative Analysis

Case	v1	v2	v3	v4	v5	v6
	Age	Gender 1 = Female 2 = Male	ZIP code	Number of days missing due to work-related injuries	Satisfaction 1 = Excellent 2 = Very good 3 = Good 4 = Fair 5 = Poor	Recommend 0 = No 1 = Yes
1	45	1	33612	2	5	1
2	62	1	33611	3	5	1
3	57	2	32312	4	4	1
4	33	2	1278	2	4	1
5	47	1	33638	2	3	1
5	68	2	33937	3	4	1
6	71	2	32199	4	5	0
7	73	2	33618	2	3	
8	65	1	33629	1	2	10
9	3	2	32911	1	3	1
10	56	1	32833	3	4	1
11	42	2	33725	4	3	1
12	39	4	33219	38	3	0
13	28	1	34581	1	4	1
14	63	2	33409	3	5	1
15	218	1	33609	3	5	1
16	49	2	32199	3	5	0
17	63	1	33217	2	6	0
18	54	12	33021	1	3	1
19	68	2	93301	2	2	1
20	72	1	33217	3	1	1

or other specific variables, such as geographical location, gender, age group, ethnicity, religious affiliation, economic status, marital status, type of employment, or environmental exposures.

Once the population is framed, the second step is to determine the different layers within the subset of the population. For example, suppose we have an objective in the evaluation that looks at 10 years of toxic environmental exposure data and asks whether there are different survival rates beyond 12 months for patients with lung cancer based on three things: their years of occupational exposure at time of diagnosis, type of initial symptoms at diagnosis, and age at

diagnosis. The first step limits the population of study from *all* types of cancer patients with occupational exposure to just lung cancer patients. The second step involves limiting the dataset for patients who survived until at least 12 months after their diagnosis. Within the 12-month survivors, the third step would group the survivors by years of occupational exposure, then initial symptoms, and age at diagnosis. Each subsequent step adds another layer until the appropriate groups are formed for further data analyses. This type of probability sampling is systematic and objective. There are no vague decisions, because either the sample subject is in one group or the other group in the decision tree.[7]

TABLE 10-4 Simple Sample Budget: Quantitative Data

Personnel	Hourly Rate/Number Needed	Hours per Week/ Cost per Piece	Weeks	Total
Researcher	$80	20	50	$80,000
Student assistant	$20	25	50	$25,000
Data analysis consultant	$150	10	10	$15,000
Printing				
Recruitment flyers	2000	0.18		$360
Surveys	1000	2.15		$2150
Sample				
Incentives	1000	10		$10,000
Total				$132,510

Note: Personnel costs for this simple budget sample do not include fringe benefits, health insurance, or student tuition.

Budget Justification for Quantitative Data

Personnel:

An evaluator works 20 hours per week for 50 weeks at $80 per hour, for a total of $80,000.

One student works 25 hours per week for 50 weeks at $20 per hour, for a total of $25,000.

A biostatistics consultant works 10 hours for the last 10 weeks at $150 per hour, for a total of $15,000.

Sample:

Printing for 2000 recruitment flyers at $0.18 each will cost $360.

Printing and stapling 1000 copies of the survey at $2.15 will cost $2150.

Incentives for 1000 participants at $10 each will cost $10,000.

Total: $132,510

TABLE 10-5 Sample Timeline: Simple 12-Month Timeline for Quantitative Data

Month	Activity	Person Responsible
1st	Establish a funding account for the study; advertise for employment positions.	Principal investigator (PI)
2nd	Hire staff.	PI
3rd	Develop survey; submit application for institutional review board (IRB) approval for human subjects research.	PI
4th	Develop recruitment strategies for participants.	PI
5th	Establish a way to provide gift card incentives for participation.	PI and student
6th	Quantitative: Print surveys or post online.	PI and student
7th	Conduct pilot study.	PI and student
8th	Revise and submit revisions to the IRB for approval.	PI and student
9th	Quantitative: Collect survey data.	PI and student
10th	Continue to collect data until sample size is achieved.	PI and student
11th	Begin to clean data; begin data analysis.	PI, student, and data expert
12th	Finalize data analysis	PI, student, and data expert
Wrap-up	Write, edit, and submit final report.	PI, student, and data expert

There are several types of probability design, including simple random sampling, quota sampling, and proportionate stratified random sampling.

Simple Random Sampling

Simple random sampling is the most basic way of selecting a group of individuals from a population. The key to simple random sampling is that every individual has an equal chance of being selected from the population. For example, if college administrators want to randomly select a group of graduate students to interview, every active graduate student enrolled in that college must have an equal chance at getting selected. To perform simple random sampling, evaluators use a table of random numbers or a computerized random number generator to select the sample of individuals (see **Figure 10-1**).

Simple random sampling has several advantages. It is a straightforward procedure to perform, and evaluators may be unable to influence the sample selection (also called bias) because the procedure is controlled by the computer software. However, simple random sampling is not feasible for large populations, such as obtaining a list of names of every individual living in a city or county.

Quota Sampling

Quota sampling is a technique that uses a small sample that matches characteristics of the target population. For example, suppose the 2010 U.S. Census data show that the Greenville County population is composed of 62% White, 18% African American, 12% Hispanic, 6% Asian, and 2% Other racial and ethnic groups and has a gender breakdown that is 51% females and 49% males. Rather than survey the entire population, evaluators recruit a sample of individuals who resemble the racial and gender composition of Greenville County. See **Table 10-6** for an example of quota sampling using a sample size of 500.

Using the information in Table 10-6, once the evaluators had 158 white females, they stopped recruiting any additional white females even if more were interested in participating. In this situation, where they have "met the quota," the evaluators would continue to recruit individuals in the other cells.

Proportionate Stratified Random Sampling

With stratified random sampling, evaluators divide the entire population into different subgroups, such as age, gender, geographical location, which are called strata. Then the evaluators randomly select subjects from each stratum using the same fraction predetermined by evaluators. It is important that individuals in each stratum not overlap with other strata. For example, in **Table 10-7**, individuals could not be in the 70–79 age stratum and in the 80–89 stratum.[8,9] Individuals may only be in one stratum, so all individuals over age 70 have an equal chance of being randomly selected for study. Stratified random sampling is commonly used for demographic variables, such as age, income, educational attainment, gender, religion, and ethnicity. There are two advantages to using stratified random sampling: (1) evaluators obtain representation from subgroups in the given population; and (2) a smaller, but representative, sample size saves evaluators money, time, and effort. For example, if evaluators wish to study the elderly population in a retirement community with 1,000 residents, they might use proportionate stratified random sampling. It is essential to remember to use the same sampling fraction across the different population size strata, so that each group is proportionately represented. This sampling ensures no overlap within the sample.

Nonprobability Sampling

Unlike probability sampling, nonprobability sampling does not use random selection. With nonprobability sampling, evaluators do not know if the selected sample truly represents the population; therefore, it is less rigorous, less accurate, and less generalizable to the larger population. However, there are situations where evaluators desire to select samples of individuals who represent a specific expertise, demographic characteristic, or condition. This purposeful sampling would not be feasible or practical if evaluators used a random sampling design. The following discussion covers several types of nonprobability samples including accidental or convenience sampling, purposive sampling, nonproportional quota sampling, expert sampling, heterogeneity sampling, snowball sampling, and systematic sampling (see **Figure 10-2**).

Accidental or Convenience Sampling

Accidental or convenience sampling is also called intercept sampling or "person on the street" sampling. A few examples of convenience sampling include emailing an online survey to all undergraduate students, asking for personal opinions about a specific topic by interviewing students as they walk through the student union (hence, intercept sampling), mailing a paper survey to all public health directors in a state to gain their opinion about a new state policy on immunizations, and interviewing voters as they exit a polling precinct location. Of course, there are problems with this type of sampling, because it is not representative of the population. However, it gives evaluators a quick and convenient way to gather data. For example, if evaluators want to know the opinion of college students on U.S. healthcare reform, evaluators ask students a few questions as they pass through the student union at a

FIGURE 10-1 Directions for using Microsoft Excel to randomize individuals.

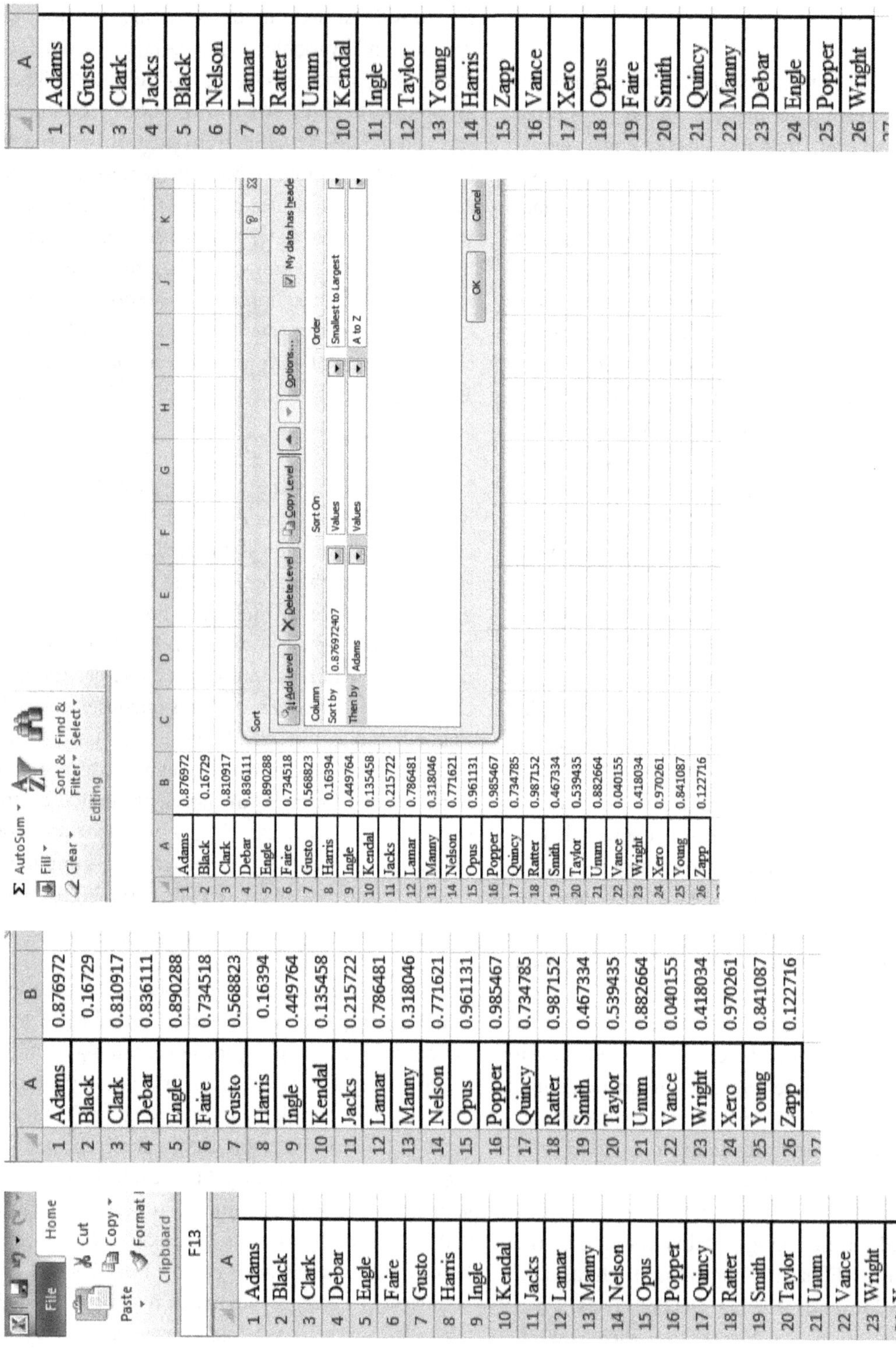

TABLE 10-6 Quota Sampling

	Female (**n = 255; 51%**)	**Male** (**n = 245; 49%**)
White	158	152
African American	46	44
Hispanic	31	29
Asian	15	15
Other races/ ethnicities	5	5

large public university. The sample is not representative of the entire student body, but it is convenient, fast, and relatively inexpensive and provides quick data collection.[2]

Purposive Sampling

With purposive sampling, evaluators select individuals with a specific *purpose* in mind. This type of sampling is commonly used by marketing or political advertisement agencies. For example, if marketing researchers want to know the opinion of African American males between the ages of 20 and 40 about a particular presidential candidate, evaluators might stand in the parking lot near a football stadium to recruit this specific, purposive sample. After approaching the prospective African American males, they verify their eligibility

TABLE 10-7 Example of Proportionate Stratified Random Sampling

Stratum	Individuals Age 70–79	Individuals Age 80–89	Individuals Over Age 90
Population size	600	280	120
Sampling fraction	½	½	½
Final sample size	300	140	60

FIGURE 10-2 Nonprobability sampling.

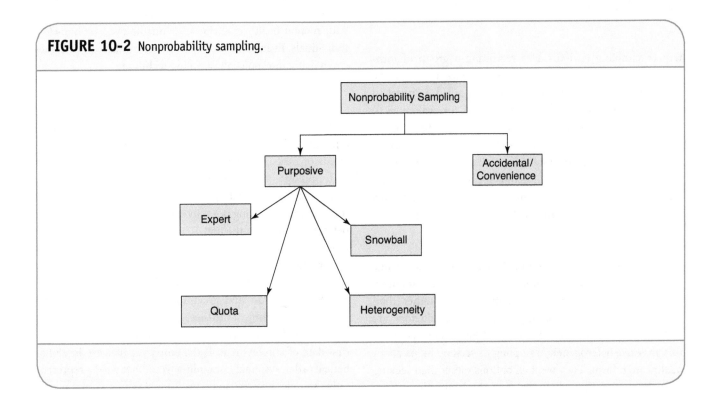

criteria and then quickly ask a few select questions.[10] In health studies, evaluators use purposive sampling to deliberately include individuals who may typically be excluded from the research.[11] For example, purposive sampling would be used if evaluators chose to include males who are the primary head of household and single parents with two or more children for a parenting evaluation.

Nonproportional Quota Sampling

Nonproportional quota sampling is similar, but less restrictive than quota sampling. With nonproportional sampling, evaluators specify the minimum number of individuals in each category, but these portions are not required to match proportions in the population. Evaluators want to ensure that all groups are represented in the study.[10] A 2007 study used nonproportional quota sampling to recruit women at risk for HIV based on their ethnicity and number of sexual partners. Evaluators used word of mouth, community organizations, and media sources to recruit equal percentages of White, Black, and Hispanic women, even though these ethnicity proportions were not representative of the demographics from the community they came from. Of the recruited women, 29% of the women were in single-partner relationships and the other 71% of the women were in multi-partner relationships. For this study, nonproportional quota sampling allowed adequate representation of women at risk for HIV.[12]

Expert Sampling

Expert sampling is defined as recruiting a group of individuals with known expertise or experience in a specific discipline. This type of sampling is also called a "panel of experts."[10] There are two common reasons for evaluators to use expert sampling. First, evaluators ask the experts about their opinion of the proposed evaluation to gain further insight into solutions or potential pitfalls. Second, evaluators ask the expert to support or refute specific topics of interest. This method allows evaluators to defend their decisions based on expert opinion rather than merely guessing.[13,14]

Heterogeneity Sampling

Heterogeneity sampling is defined as seeking a wide range of different and diverse opinions. In heterogeneity sampling, evaluators are recruiting a diversity of ideas rather than diversity among participating individuals. Evaluators are seeking unique and unusual opinions.[10] For example, evaluators may use heterogeneity sampling to seek opinions about healthcare reform. They want all options rather than seeking how the typical individual voted on the healthcare reform amendment on the ballot.

Snowball Sampling

Snowball sampling is when evaluators identify one individual who meets the inclusion criteria for the study and then ask that individual if he or she knows someone else meeting the inclusion criteria whom they could also ask to join the study or evaluation. With snowball sampling, the sample is not representative, but it can be valuable for specific studies.[10,15] For example, evaluators want to learn more about how county health departments transitioned from pre-HIV/AIDS procedures to post-HIV/AIDS procedures, so they plan to interview health department directors who worked in the health department from the mid-1980s into the mid-1990s. Snowball sampling poses some ethical issues that must be considered, such as revealing an individual's lifestyle choices or medical conditions without their expressed consent. For example, if the purpose of the evaluation is to determine the level of employment discrimination experienced by former prisoners, the evaluators would begin by interviewing a known former prisoner. After the interview, the evaluators would ask if the individual knew other former prisoners who might wish to participate in the interview to increase the sample size. This technique would pose ethical issues if the referred individual had not yet made the decision to be identified as a former prisoner. There are numerous other groups of individuals that may not wish to be identified, such as individuals living with HIV/AIDS or other diseases, individuals diagnosed with mental health challenges, or unemployed or homeless individuals. Evaluators need to be aware of such ethical issues when using the snowball sampling technique.

Systematic Sampling

Systematic sampling involves selecting every nth case from a population list (of course, the population list may be electronic or on paper). For example, if evaluators wish to draw 100 employee files from the list of 3000 employees, they would start by calculating 3000/100 = 30. Evaluators would then select the starting point by randomly selecting a number between 1 and 10 of the first 10 employee files. If the random number selected is 6, then evaluators begin by selecting the 6th employee file, then move through the 3000 employees by selecting every 30th employee file. They would select files 6, 36, 66, 96, 126, 156, and so on up to 3000. Prior to using this method of sampling, if the files are paper, the evaluators must know if the files are arranged in alphabetical order or by the first date of employment. If the employee files are in alphabetical order, systematic sampling would not yield a representative sample, because some traditional ethnic family names may be overrepresented in the sample, while other names are skipped. If the employee files are arranged by month, day, and year of first date of employment, systematic sampling is a good choice for selecting a sample from the population.[2]

SAMPLING BIAS

When evaluators choose a sampling design, they must be aware of potential bias. Bias is defined as an error caused by systematically selecting one individual or outcome over another.[16] Sampling bias occurs when the selected individuals do not represent the population. When sampling bias occurs, evaluators are not able to generalize their findings to the whole population that was supposed to be studied.[2] For example, evaluators wanted to study the effectiveness of e-cigarettes as a method for smoking cessation for adults. However, they recruited adults from a large inner-city Medicaid clinic. This type of sample results in sampling bias, because it is likely that adults receiving Medicaid are more likely to have different socioeconomic issues and smoking habits than adults not receiving Medicaid. Even when evaluators select the ideal sampling design, they may encounter bias after the data are collected. After evaluators recognize that data are missing, they determine if the missing data are cause for concern of a nonresponse bias. There are two types of nonresponse bias: item nonresponse and unit nonresponse.[17]

Item Nonresponse Bias

Item nonresponse is best described by thinking about when individuals complete a survey, but some people leave several survey questions blank (see **Table 10-8**).

When this situation happens, evaluators are faced with making a decision about what to do about the missing responses. In this situation, there are three common ways to handle the missing data: case deletion, mean replacement, and item deletion.

Case Deletion

With case deletion, evaluators determine what percentage of item nonresponse they are willing to tolerate. This percentage changes depending on the type of survey and sampling design. For example, if an individual completes only 50 out of the 100 survey questions, evaluators agree that the entire survey is removed from the data collection. However, if an individual leaves 2 out of 100 questions blank, evaluators would keep the other 98 responses. Prior to making the final decision on what percentage of blank survey questions are allowed in the data, evaluators calculate the overall response rate of survey questions. If the response rate is low, they are less likely to delete an entire survey with a few blank questions, because that would remove the completed responses as well.

Many problems related to item nonresponse are reduced or eliminated by conducting a pilot study. In the pilot study, the exact survey to be used in the study is given to a small sample of individuals to "test" the survey and note any errors. After the pilot study is complete, evaluators revise the survey as needed and print the final survey or post the survey online. Even after conducting several survey pilot-testing sessions, it is unlikely but still possible for errors to occur.

TABLE 10-8 Sample of Data Spreadsheet with Missing Data

Case	v1	v2	v3	v4	v5	v6
	Age	Gender	Marital Status	Health Status Today	Program Satisfaction	Recommend
		1 = Female 2 = Male	1 = Single 2 = Married 3 = Divorced 4 = Widowed	1 = Excellent 2 = Very good 3 = Fair 4 = Good 5 = Poor	1 = Excellent 2 = Very good 3 = Good 4 = Fair 5 = Poor	0 = No 1 = Yes
1	45	1	2	2	5	0
2	62	1	3	3	5	1
3	57		2	4	4	1
4	33	2		2	4	1
5	47	1	4		3	
6	68	2	1	3	4	1

If the survey is available online for 5 days, evaluators scan through the responses as data become available. Upon review, evaluators determine whether individuals complete every question, leave the same questions blank, or leave random questions blank. If many respondents leave the same question blank, then evaluators investigate the specific question and identify problems with inappropriate wording, response choices, or other possible errors. After the problem is identified, evaluators decide what they should do about it. If time and funding permit, evaluators correct the one question and repeat the survey online or, as a reprint for the remaining data-collection sites. As a last resort, evaluators simply delete the question from the survey.

Mean Replacement

Mean replacement is another way to handle item nonresponse. The word *mean* in statistics is defined as average. The mean is calculated by adding the responses and then dividing the sum total by the number of responses. In the mean replacement, evaluators calculate the mean response for each survey question, then each time that individuals leave a survey question blank, evaluators fill in the blank with the mean score of how the other individuals responded. For example, 179 out of 200 individuals answered the Likert-scale question "How would you rate your health today? 5 = excellent, 4 = very good, 3 = good, 2 = fair, and 1 = poor." The mean score (average) for the 179 respondents was 3.8 for this question. Evaluators would fill in 3.8 on the blank response for the 21 individuals who left this question blank. The same procedure is repeated for each missing response. The disadvantage of this solution is that it causes the survey response to be closer to the mean than it might have been if the individuals actually answered the question. For example, those individuals who left the question blank may have felt poorly and did not wish to complete the survey at all. Their actual response may have been quite different from the replacement mean score, but evaluators have no way to verify the information.

Item Deletion

Item deletion is defined as deleting only that one question. For example, 87 out of 200 college students answered the Likert-scale question "How many sexual partners have you had in the last 30 days? 7 = six or more sexual partners, 6 = five sexual partners, 5 = four sexual partners, 4 = three sexual partners, 3 = two sexual partners, 2 = one sexual partner, 1 = I did not have any sexual partners in the last 30 days, 0 = I prefer not to respond." If only 87 (43.5%) college students responded, mean replacement is not appropriate. A better choice is to report that 43.5% responded with a mean score of 2.8 (or between one and two sexual partners) in the last 30 days; however, 56.5% selected "I prefer not to respond."

Unit Nonresponse Bias

In unit nonresponse bias, the word *unit* is defined as if or when a type or group of individuals does not respond to a survey. The following examples illustrate several types of unit nonresponse bias.

Unit nonresponse bias occurs when the sampling design, such as quota sampling, is unable to obtain responses from certain segments of the samples. For example, unit nonresponse happens when evaluators are seeking 50 individuals in each of four different ZIP codes to represent different socioeconomic variations in the same county: 33611 (urban), 33647 (suburban), 33628 (rural), and 33690 (new development). In the rural ZIP code of 33628, only 18 of the 50 individuals completed the interview. The lack of respondents in one segment causes a bias to occur, because the 32 nonrespondents in the rural area may have provided responses different from the 18 individuals who did respond.

When evaluators collect survey data, they keep track of when each survey is returned. When paper copy surveys are returned, evaluators label each survey with the date it was received. In addition, each survey is numbered in consecutive order. For online surveys, the survey software assigns a date and time to each survey upon submission. During data analyses, evaluators determine if the early responders are different from the late responders. Because late responders are considered to be more like nonresponders, evaluators estimate how the nonresponders may have answered. This information provides an estimate of the unit nonresponse bias. For example, let's say that an online survey was emailed to all university employees. Evaluators found that administrative assistants responded first without any reminder emails, while administrators responded last and only after one or two reminder emails. Evaluators use these findings to make further predictions about the profile and reasons why some individuals respond early rather than late.

Instead of comparing early and late responders, evaluators investigate the demographic groups or profiles (e.g., gender, age, ethnicity, and income level) of survey respondents. In the data analysis, evaluators compare survey responses of various demographic characteristics. In some studies, evaluators compare survey response data to U.S. Census data. If data differ, there may be a nonresponse bias in the study data. For example, survey questions ask for respondents' ZIP code, annual household income, and mode of transportation used.

If the majority of respondents in the same ZIP code inflate their annual household income, evaluators would note this difference when compared to the U.S. Census. If 90% respondents in the same ZIP code respond that they drive a car as their mode of transportation, evaluators could verify the ZIP code and mode of transportation with the U.S. Census. If bias is noted, evaluators would need to question the accuracy of the other survey responses from the same respondents. This type of comparison is called database verification. Evaluators compare survey responses with data in a verifiable database, such U.S. Census data. This process allows evaluators to verify the accuracy of the data and to determine the accuracy and nonresponse bias. In another example, clinic patients are invited to complete a survey. In the survey, respondents are asked to provide their height and weight. Their responses are verified by the electronic medical record containing the respondents' actual height and weight. With community surveys, database verification is usually not possible.[12]

All of these techniques allow evaluators to presume when bias exists in their data. Discussion of how statisticians adjust the data analysis to account for unit nonresponse bias is beyond the scope of this chapter. However, it is noted that reducing nonresponse bias in the survey development phase saves time and data adjustment in the data analysis phase.[12]

SUMMARY

This chapter began by defining what a population and a sample was. It then discussed how populations and samples related to probability, hypothesis testing, and error within inferential statistics. Then it discussed sampling strategies, including important considerations for determining appropriate sampling sizes. Finally, the chapter focused on several types of nonresponse sampling bias as well as methods used to avoid sampling bias in research studies.

CASE STUDY

An evaluation team from a large Florida university was hired by the U.S. Federal Emergency Management Agency (FEMA) to conduct a post–BP oil spill evaluation. FEMA requested that the evaluation involve small business owners from Florida, Alabama, Mississippi and Louisiana affected by the 2009 massive oil spill in the Gulf of Mexico. The purpose of the evaluation is to determine the level of satisfaction regarding FEMA services during the oil spill, immediately after the oil well was capped, and a few years after the oil spill; the current rate of employment of affected small business owners; and the current perception of the water and beach sand quality along the Gulf of Mexico shoreline.

For this evaluation, evaluators selected a complex sample design. Because this evaluation involves qualitative and quantitative data collection, several different sample designs were used. Evaluators decided to begin the evaluation by contacting and interviewing gulf coast small business owners residing in the four affected states. However, the evaluation team was told by FEMA that due to privacy regulations and pending litigation, the list of small business owners is not available, so evaluators devised another recruitment strategy.

Phase 1: Prior to the initiation of phase 1, evaluators obtained IRB approval for this research. For phase 1, snowball sampling was selected to identify a few small business owners along the gulf coast in the four states. Evaluators asked those individuals for the names of other small business owners still living along the gulf coast. The disadvantage with this sampling technique is that the sample is not a representative sample of all gulf coast small business owners, but it remains valuable for the first phase of this research. During this phase, evaluators conducted in-depth interviews with small business owners to gain an overall snapshot of their perceptions of FEMA services during the oil spill and immediately after the oil spill and their current perceptions in relation to their small business. Identical questions were asked of each small business owner interviewed. The business owners were eager to participate in the interviews and gladly shared names of other small business owners along the gulf coast. The convenience of snowball sampling outweighed the disadvantages for phase 1 of the project. Upon completion of each digitally recorded interview, transcriptionists were available to transcribe the interviews for immediate review by the evaluation team. The general themes of the phase 1 interview paved the way for phase 2.

Phase 2: Before the BP oil spill, there was estimated to be approximately 25,500 small business owners along the coastline in the four affected states. However, after the BP oil spill, approximately 9000 small business owners remain. The required sample size is 370 with a 5% margin of error. However, researchers added 30% to the sample for possible missing data and inability to contact some small business owners due to inaccurate contact information.

Because demographic data for only coastline small business owners were not available, the evaluation team decided to oversample the small business owner population.

Number of small business owners:	9000
5% margin of error:	5%
Final sample size:	370
Additional 30% for missing data:	111
Total:	481

In phase 2, researchers contacted the Small Business Owner Association (SBOA) in each of the four states to purchase a list of their member mailing list. Because the SBOA is a private association, it is allowed to sell mailing lists of members. Although not all small business owners are members of SBOA, these lists serve as an adequate representative sample of all small business owners in the four gulf states. Because the survey will be mailed to SBOA members at their home addresses, the evaluation team can identify mailing addresses that reflect cities and small towns along the coastline in the four states. The small business owners may select to participate by completing and returning the survey or they may decline to participate.

Based on the general themes from phase 1, evaluators developed survey questions for phase 2. The 80-question survey questions included, but was not limited to, demographic information (e.g., age, ethnicity, marital status, gender), years of owning a small business on the coastline, location of small business, type of small business, reasons for staying or leaving the coastline after the BP oil spill, and how owning a small business has changed during their career. The last question in the survey asked respondents if they would be interested in participating in a 30-minute, follow-up telephone interview.

Phase 3: Assuming that the sample size of 481 was achieved in phase 2, researchers utilize random sampling and quota sampling (equal number from each state) in phase 3. Researchers had funding to conduct 100 thirty-minute telephone interviews. This process involved dividing the surveys into four piles based on location of the small business: Florida, Alabama, Mississippi, and Louisiana. The surveys in each pile were assigned consecutive numbers starting with 1. Using a random number generator, survey numbers were pulled until the quota was fulfilled (see **Table 10-9**).[18]

Interview questions for phase 3 were generated from survey responses in phase 2. Telephone interviews were conducted to verify if the survey data matched the actual perceptions of small business owners living on the coast who had been affected by the BP oil spill.

Case Study Discussion Questions

1. List the various types of sampling techniques combined in this case study.
2. Describe the process of how the researchers will coordinate and conduct 100 thirty-minute telephone interviews.

STUDENT ACTIVITY

Matthew is hired by the March of Dimes Foundation of Nevada to evaluate one of their programs. This educational program has been run in several cities in Nevada to lower the percentage of babies born prematurely and with low birth weight. It invites pregnant women to enroll into a prenatal health class at no charge; it has been in place for 2 years. The class is offered at local women's hospitals and allows women to schedule their prenatal checkups for the same day that they will attend the half-hour class. The class covers many issues, from eating healthy foods and exercising to the importance of stress reduction and social support. The class also offers important prenatal vitamins to the women. Over the last 2 years, 500 women have taken part in the educational classes in different cities. The March of Dimes Foundation of Nevada would like to see if this program is doing as good of a job at lowering rates of premature and low birth weight among women of poor physical and socioeconomic conditions as other groups endeavoring to lower these rates. Matthew decides to conduct a survey. To do this he must take a sample.

1. What does Matthew need to consider before he starts his research project?
2. What list does he need to have before he can select his sample?
3. What type of sampling method should Matthew use for this study? Why did you choose this method?
4. What is the appropriate sample size for this study if researchers want to have a 5% margin of error? (Use the following table.)
5. The following table lists one of the strata. Determine the number of individuals who will need to be included in the sample.

TABLE 10-9 Quota Sampling Based on Florida Demographics

	Florida 25%	Alabama 25%	Mississippi 25%	Louisiana 25%
Final sample size: 100	25	25	25	25

Data from How to measure variability in a dataset. Stat Trek. Available at: http://stattrek.com/sampling/variance.aspx

Stratum	Did Not Finish High School	Earned High School Diploma/GED	Some College Education	Earned College Diploma
Population size	63	246	74	117
Sampling fraction	50%	50%	50%	50%
Sample size				

Sampling fraction	50%	50%	50%	50%
Sample size	31	123	37	59

6. Suppose one of the clinics had a fire, and some of the patient files were lost. From talking to the prenatal educator, you know that this clinic regularly sees members from a nearby Native American community. You want to make sure that you are including an adequate number of Native Americans. Before completing your sampling frame and starting the research project, you ask a current participant in the program who is a member of this Native American community if she knows of other members who have gone through the program. She gives you the names of four other mothers, who then collectively give you an additional 17 names. What type of sampling is this?

Answers

1. Matthew needs to consider how many mothers he will investigate (the sample size).
2. Before he can select his sample, Matthew needs a list of all of the women who have attended the program over the last 2 years. This is called his sampling frame. Matthew will take the sample from the sampling frame.
3. The appropriate sampling method for Matthew to choose is stratified random sampling, because he would like to know more about the physical and socio-economic conditions of the mothers who have gone through the class in the last 2 years. Matthew could look at age, race, income, and education level as different strata.
4. The appropriate sample size for this study would be 217 participants.
5.

Stratum	Did Not Finish High School	Earned High School Diploma/GED	Some College Education	Earned College Diploma
Population size	63	246	74	117

6. This is called snowball sampling, where one person who met the criteria you were looking for informed you about others they knew who might also meet that criteria.

REFERENCES

1. Downing D, Clark J. *Statistics: The Easy Way*, 2nd ed. Hauppauge, NY: Barron's Educational Series, Inc.; 1989.

2. Ary D, Jacobs L, Razavieh A, Sorenson C. *Introduction to Research in Education*, 8th ed. Belmont, CA: Wadsworth/Cengage Learning; 2010.

3. Blair R, Taylor R. *Biostatistics for the Health Sciences*. Upper Saddle River, NJ: Pearson Prentice Hall; 2008.

4. Creative Research Systems. Significance in Statistics and Surveys. Available at: http://www.surveysystem.com/signif.htm. Accessed May 18, 2014.

5. The Research Advisors. Sample Size Table. Available at: http://www.research-advisors.com/tools/SampleSize.htm. Accessed May 18, 2014.

6. Israel G. Determining Sample Size. University of Florida, Institute of Food and Agricultural Studies Extension. Available at: http://edis.ifas.ufl.edu/pd006. Accessed May 18, 2014.

7. Doherty M. Probability versus non-probability sampling in sample surveys. *New Zeal Stat Rev*.1994;(7):21–28.

8. Castillo J. Stratified Sampling Method. Experiment Resources. Available at: http://www.experiment-resources.com/stratified-sampling.html. Accessed May 18, 2014.

9. Stat Trek. Stratified random sampling. Available at: http://stattrek.com/survey-research/stratified-sampling.aspx. Accessed May 18, 2014.

10. Trochim W. Nonprobability Sampling. Research Methods Knowledge Base. Available at: http://www.socialresearchmethods.net/kb/sampnon.php. Accessed May 18, 2014.

11. Barbour R. Checklists for improving rigor in qualitative research: A case of the tail wagging the dog? *Brit Med J*. 2001;322:115–17.

12. Morrow K, Vargas S, Rosen R, Christensen A, Salomon L, Shulman L, Barroso C, Fava J. The utility of non-proportional quota sampling for recruiting at-risk women for microbicide research. *AIDS Behav*. 2007;11:586–95.

13. Statistics Solutions. Sampling. Available at: http://www.statisticssolutions.com/academic-solutions/resources/dissertation-resources/sample-size-calculation-and-sample-size-justification/. Accessed September 26, 2013.

14. Stewart D, Strasser G. Expert role assignment and information sampling during collective recall and decision making. *J Pers Soc Psychol*, 1995;69(4):619–28.

15. Browne K. Snowball sampling: Using social networks to research non-heterosexual women. *Int J Soc Res Meth*. 2005;8(1):47–60.

16. Panzeri S, Magri C, Carraro L. Sampling Bias. Scholarpedia. Available at: http://www.scholarpedia.org/article/Sampling_bias. Accessed May 18, 2014.

17. Groves R. Nonresponse rates and nonresponse bias in household surveys. *Public Opin Q*. 2006;70(5):646–675.

18. Stat Trek. How to measure variability in a dataset. Available at: http://stattrek.com/sampling/variance.aspx. Accessed May 18, 2014.

ANSWERS to Table 10-3 Sample Spreadsheet for Quantitative Analysis

Case	v1	v2	v3	v4	v5	v6
	Age	Gender 1 = Female 2 = Male	ZIP code	Number of Days in Hospital	Satisfaction 1 = Excellent 2 = Very good 3 = Good 4 = Fair 5 = Poor	Recommend 0 = No 1 = Yes
1	45	1	33612	2	5	1
2	62	1	33611	3	5	1
3	57	2	32312	4	4	1
4	33	2	31278	2	4	1
5	47	1	33638	2	3	1
5	68	2	33937	3	4	1
6	71	2	32199	4	5	0
7	73	2	33618	2	3	No data
8	65	1	33629	1	2	10
9	3	2	32911	1	3	1
10	56	1	32833	3	4	1
11	42	2	33725	4	3	1
12	39	4	33219	38	3	0
13	28	1	34581	1	4	1
14	63	2	33409	3	5	1
15	218	1	33609	3	5	1
16	49	2	32199	3	5	0
17	63	1	33217	2	6	0
18	54	12	33021	1	3	1
19	68	2	93301	2	2	1
20	72	1	33217	3	1	1

CHAPTER **11**

Inferential Statistics

CHAPTER OBJECTIVES

By the end of this chapter, students will be able to:

1. Discuss the need for statistics to explain data.
2. Describe the differences between scientific hypothesis, research questions, null hypothesis, and alternative hypothesis.
3. Explain the difference between one-tailed and two-tailed inferential statistical tests.
4. Describe when it is appropriate to use an independent *t*-test and when it is appropriate to use a paired-samples *t*-test.
5. Explain the purpose of correlation coefficients.
6. Create a scenario to explain the benefits of confidence intervals.
7. Define type I and type II errors.

KEY TERMS

alternative hypothesis
chi-square
coefficients
confidence intervals
correlations
inferential statistics
null hypothesis
one-tailed tests
***t*-tests**
two-tailed tests
type I and type II errors

INTRODUCTION

This chapter begins with why we need to use statistics to understand data. The first section defines the concepts of the scientific hypothesis, null hypothesis, and alternative hypothesis. The next section explains the difference between one-tailed and two-tailed inferential statistical tests. Building upon this knowledge, various statistical tests are introduced using multiple examples. The chapter concludes by defining type I and type II errors. Because it is a common belief among students that learning statistics is difficult, this chapter attempts to present the new terms and definitions as clearly as possible with plenty of applied examples. If at any time, a concept is not understood, stop and review the previous section. Using this technique builds a foundation of basic definitions of statistics for future use.

TYPES OF STATISTICS

Statistics is a branch of mathematics used for data collection, analysis, and interpretation of data.[1] Statistics are used in evaluation and research across most disciplines, including natural science, social science, and business and government. Statistics are used to answer questions related to data. There are two basic types of statistics: descriptive and inferential. Descriptive statistics organize and summarize data without the use of complicated mathematical equations. In this chapter, inferential statistics are defined in detail. For now, think of inferential statistics as the study of determining associations about a population from a random sample of data taken from that population. For example, because it is impossible to study the driving habits of every driver in one county, evaluators survey a random sample of drivers and generalize about all drivers in that county based on the sample. Unlike descriptive statistics, inferential statistics use mathematical equations to generate probabilities about a population. These probabilities help program planners and evaluators make important decisions related to their proposed goals and objectives. By using Microsoft Excel, this chapter presents a few basic equations or statistical tests as a way to illustrate how inferential statistics are applied to data.

THE NEED FOR STATISTICS

Let's explore why statistics are important to use and understand. For evaluators, statistics are essential for understanding the data. Without using inferential statistics, it is not possible to determine patterns, make associations, and draw conclusions from the data collected from the sample. For example, without using inferential statistics, evaluators would have no way of knowing if one community-based participatory program was more effective in reducing obesity rates than another community-based participatory program. Evaluators could not see patterns in indoor air quality and asthma rates in a community. Evaluators would not know which type of smoking cessation programs was most effective in reducing smoking rates among young adults. Engineers would not know which model of automobile seatbelt was most effective in saving lives. Manufacturers would not know the level of sun protection factor (SPF) needed to provide adequate protection against sun exposure. The list goes on and on, but it is evident that inferential statistics are used to move science forward and thus improve quality of life. Lastly, it is important to note that statistics not only let us know if there are associations and patterns with which to draw conclusions, but also let us know that those associations and conclusions are not due to chance or random error within a particular sample. Although it involves more sophisticated statistical techniques than are discussed in this text, higher level statistics informs evaluators not only that a change took place, but also, sometimes, how the change took place.

INFERENTIAL STATISTICS

Now let's take the next step in describing inferential statistics in greater detail. As with all evaluations, it is necessary to begin with a question or a goal statement. Inferential statistics are no different in that each statistical project begins with a question. Think of the question as the road map. Travelers begin each trip by determining their destination. Whether traveling by car, train, bus, plane, or ship, travelers plot their journey by purchasing tickets or programming the GPS device. The same is true in evaluations. Evaluators do not collect data without first developing a question or roadmap for their study.

For example, suppose you were part of a team that wanted to ask, "Do university staff (nonfaculty or administration) employees who intentionally walk around the building every few hours report having improved concentration, improved productivity, less desire for caffeine, and less desire for snacks than those staff employees who remain at their desks for most of the day?" This university has two campus locations of approximately equal size: North Campus and South Campus. As previously stated, it is not feasible to study an entire population of university staff employees, so evaluators collect data from a randomly selected sample of the population. As the name implies, evaluators use inferential statistics to "infer" or understand how the sample data help to know the larger population. For example, let's suppose that there are about 4000 university staff employees on each of the two campus locations, and of that population approximately 1500 staff employees at each campus have job titles that imply that they sit at a desk most of the time. Because it is impossible to recruit all 3000 employees with desk job titles, the evaluators randomly recruit 300 staff employees with job titles that imply desk jobs. After signing the institutional review board (IRB)–approved informed consent documents, the 150 staff employees on the North Campus are asked to complete a monthly survey about their perceived concentration level at work, productivity level, desire for caffeine, and desire for snacks, and the 150 staff employees on the South Campus are encouraged to walk around the building for 15 minutes three times per day and complete the same monthly survey.

Prior to the initiation of the actual study, evaluators use inferential statistics to determine if the recruited staff employees have the same characteristics as most other non-recruited staff employees. For example, evaluators would compare the age, gender, weight and height, length of service, and job titles of both groups. This type of information allows evaluators to determine if their study sample is representative of the population of all university staff employees. It is important to make sure that the sample is representative of the entire population, because you want to discover whether walking for 15 minutes three times a day improves concentration and productivity and decreases desire for caffeine and snacks because it really is effective and is not due to the particular characteristics of the university staff employees included in the evaluation.

After the data are collected, the evaluators use inferential statistics to infer whether the walking: (1) improves concentration, (2) improves productivity, (3) decreases desire for caffeine, and (4) decreases desire for snacks as perceived by the staff employees. This simple example illustrates how evaluators move from asking the initial research question, to recruiting individuals, to collecting data, to using inferential statistics to determine if the staff employees at the large university perceive a change in work habits by simply walking for 15 minutes three times per day.

Before moving on to the next section, let's discuss a little more about statistical tests. Because there are hundreds of statistical tests, evaluators select the appropriate type of statistical test based on their questions and the type of data. By using inferential statistics, they draw conclusions related to the data. However, it is easy for inexperienced evaluators to use the drop-down menus available in complex statistical computer software programs, but this method does not ensure that the correct statistical test was chosen. Without thoroughly understanding the purpose of various statistical tests, it is easy to receive an incorrect computer-generated result due to choosing the wrong test. For this reason, it is important to consult with a statistician before choosing a test to ensure that the correct statistical test is chosen.

In this section, the discussion defines research questions, null hypothesis, and alternative hypothesis. All of these terms are useful in understanding inferential statistics.

Development of Research Questions

Because evaluation begins with goals and objectives, it is necessary for the evaluator to convert the objectives into research questions. Think of the research questions as defined by the question of interest in the evaluation project. Research questions provide a clear and concise roadmap on which to focus the study. When creating a research question, it is important to address the issue of what topic or evidence is being supported or refuted. Research questions need to be stated as testable questions that can be specifically studied in an investigation. Let's review how to convert objectives into research questions:

Objective: By May 2015, 100% of the 400 participating children younger than 14 years of age with asthma will report the day and time of their asthma episodes and the pollen index of their geographical location.
Research Question:
Weak: What is the relationship between asthma and air quality?
Strong: For 400 participating children younger than 14 years of age with asthma, is there a relationship between the day and time of their asthma episodes and the pollen index of their geographical location?
Objective: By January 2015, 100% of the 300 elderly residents over the age of 65 who completed the senior safe driving course offered by the State Department of Transportation will report receiving fewer driving citations over the next 12 months.

Weak: Does completing the senior driving course reduce the number of driving citations?
Strong: For the 300 participating elderly residents over the age of 65, is there a relationship between completing the senior safe driving course offered by the State Department of Transportation and the number of driving citations received over the next 12 months?

Null Hypothesis and Alternate Hypothesis

Let's begin by defining a hypothesis as an educated guess based on prior observation, knowledge, or experience that can be supported or refuted through observations or experiments. Hypotheses make predictions that can be duplicated with future research. After the same research is repeated multiple times, enough evidence is collected to support or disprove the scientific hypothesis.[2] For example, it took decades of research to gather enough evidence to link tobacco usage to lung cancer. Now let's apply the concept of research questions to the term null *hypothesis*. The word *null* means no difference or no association. The best way to remember the null hypothesis is to understand that the evaluator is trying to disprove or refute the statement that there is no difference or no association or no relationship. In other words, when using inferential statistics, the way that evaluators support their hypothesis is to refute the null hypothesis.

Remember that the evaluators study a representative sample from the population to find evidence to refute the null hypothesis. You may often hear another term used for the research question, called the alternate hypothesis, when evaluators are discussing the null hypothesis. For example, evaluators must assume their alternate hypothesis is wrong until they find sufficient evidence to the contrary.[3] By using inferential statistics, evaluators make a decision to reject or fail to reject the null hypothesis. However, what does that mean? Let's look at a few examples, so these concepts begin to make sense.

Example 1

Research question: For the 300 participating elderly residents over the age of 65, is there a relationship between completing the senior safe driving course offered by the State Department of Transportation and the number of driving citations received over the next 12 months?
Null hypothesis: There is no difference in the number of driving citations received over a 12-month period for elderly individuals who completed the safe driving course and those who did not complete the safe driving course.
Alternate hypothesis: There is a difference in the number of driving citations received over a-12 month period

for the elderly who completed the safe driving course and the elderly who did not complete the safe driving course.

Here is what you need to be thinking when you read this null hypothesis: Using inferential statistics to analyze the data collected from the two groups of elderly drivers, there is enough evidence to reject (or fail to reject) the null hypothesis.

Example 2
Research question: At the end of 3 months on the Lost-It weight management program, do women working the day shift or women working the night shift lose more weight?
Null hypothesis: At the end of 3 months on the Lost-It weight management program, there is no difference in weight between women working the day shift and women working the night shift.
Alternate hypothesis: At the end of 3 months on the Lost-It weight management program, there is a difference in weight between women working the day shift and women working the night shift.

Here is what you need to be thinking when you read this null hypothesis: Using inferential statistics to analyze the data collected from the day-shift women and night-shift women on the Lost-It weight management program, there is enough evidence to reject (or fail to reject) the null hypothesis.

Let's try one more example to verify your understanding of the concepts.

Research question: At the end of 3 months, do students using the Quick Learn System achieve higher Graduate Record Exam (GRE) practice test scores than students not using the Quick Learn System?
Null hypothesis: At the end of 3 months, there is no difference in the GRE practice test scores between students using the Quick Learn System and the students not using the Quick Learn System.
Alternate hypothesis: At the end of 3 months, there is a difference in the GRE practice test scores between students using the Quick Learn System and the students not using the Quick Learn System.

Here is what you need to be thinking when you read this null hypothesis: Using inferential statistics to analyze the data collected from the students using the Quick Learn System and students not using the Quick Learn System, there is enough evidence to reject (or fail to reject) the null hypothesis.

Why can't evaluators state that they "accept" or "reject" the null hypothesis? Why is the phrase "fail to reject" used instead of "accept"? It is easier to understand the answer to this question by looking at the previous example. Rejecting the null hypothesis means that the evaluation provided evidence to support the notion that there is a difference in weight loss among day-shift female workers and night-shift female workers that is not due to just chance alone at the end of 3 months on the Lost-It weight management program. Failing to reject the null hypothesis means that the research failed to provide evidence to support the notion that there is no difference in weight loss among day-shift female workers and night-shift female workers at the end of 3 months. Therefore, when the null hypothesis is rejected, the evidence from the data analysis does not support the null hypothesis.[4,5] Evaluators should never "accept" the null hypothesis. Doing so would say that they are 100% sure of the null hypothesis in all situations.

BASIC INFERENTIAL STATISTICAL TESTS

One-Tailed and Two-Tailed Statistical Tests

Now that you are starting to understand when to reject or fail to reject the null hypothesis, it is time to introduce the terms *one-tailed* and *two-tailed tests*. Let's begin with stating that evaluators determine whether to use a one-tailed or two-tailed test when they state the null hypothesis. Even though this discussion is placed in the independent *t*-test section, the majority of statistical tests allow evaluators to select the use of a one-tailed test or a two-tailed test. This discussion begins by defining a one-tailed test.

One-Tailed Test

Evaluators use a one-tailed test when their null hypothesis reflects a specific direction. See **Figure 11-1**. The white area shows 95% of all values that, if obtained, fail to reject the null hypothesis. The gray area shows the 5% of possible values that would reject the null hypothesis, also called the critical area. The critical value shown with an arrow is discussed in detail later in the chapter. One-tailed tests may have the critical value and area on either the far left side or the far right side, depending on the null hypothesis, but only on one side of the normal curve. If evaluators select a one-tailed test, the obtained or calculated value might fall on the extreme positive or extreme negative side, depending on what the researcher is studying. It is possible for evaluators to falsely reject the null hypothesis, thus evaluators select a one-tailed test only when they have reason to believe that the difference falls in a specific direction.

FIGURE 11-1 One-tailed statistical test.

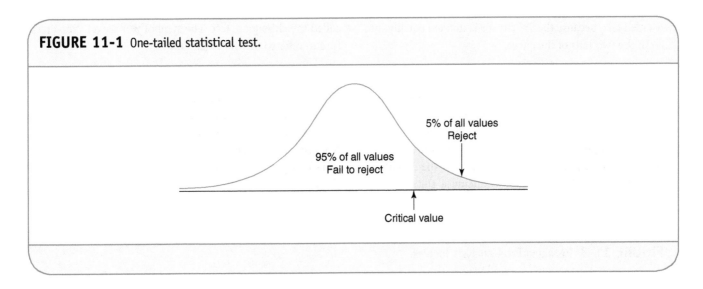

Null hypothesis: When using the Quick Learn System, there is no difference in the GRE practice test scores of the students.

Alternate hypothesis: When using the Quick Learn System, there is a difference in the GRE practice test scores of the students.

Evaluators stating this null hypothesis are interested in only the GRE practice test scores when using the Quick Learn System. Evaluators conducting this study are confident that the Quick Learn System improves the GRE practice test scores for students. In this example, evaluators must be so confident in the increased GRE practice test scores that they choose to ignore the possibility that some students using the Quick Learn System may get more confused and may actually decrease their GRE practice test scores and thus fall anywhere outside the critical area. Without high confidence based on previous evaluation results, using a one-tailed test results is a serious mistake. For example, when students may use the Quick Learn System and their test scores may decrease. Evaluators need to be certain that the Quick Learn System is not just based on sales hype and does not cause a decreased GRE practice test score prior to using a one-tailed test.

Two-Tailed Test

When using a two-tailed test, the normal curve is divided into three sections: the large middle section represents 95% of all possible values and each of the two side sections represents 2.5% of the possible values. The total of the possible values represented underneath the normal curve should be equal to 100%. **Figure 11-2** illustrates what is called a

FIGURE 11-2 Two-tailed statistical test.

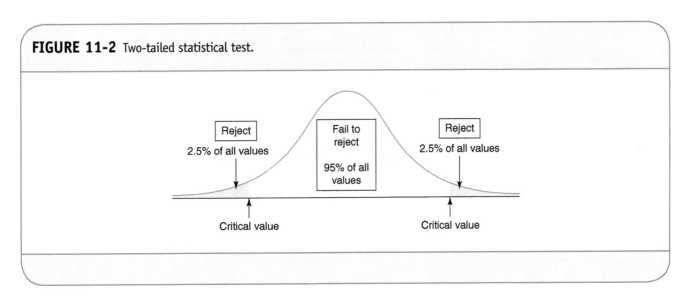

two-tailed test, because the 5% chance is divided equally into 2.5% in the two tails of the curve.

Using Excel for Statistics

Now it is time to use Microsoft Excel to learn a few basic statistical calculations. First, it is necessary to add the Excel Analysis ToolPak to your software by using the directions provided in **Figure 11-3**. Once you have added the Analysis ToolPak, it is easier to follow the examples in the remainder of this chapter. Let's begin by introducing a statistical test

called the chi-square test. The symbol χ^2 is used in the literature to refer to this statistical test.

Chi-Square Test

The type of data used for a chi-square test is called nominal, because it categorizes the data. Examples of nominal data are ZIP codes, gender, types of trees, names of cars, and so on. Nominal data are also called categorical data, because evaluators can place the data into categories. Evaluators use the chi-square test to analyze nominal data, such as frequencies.[5]

FIGURE 11-3 Installing Excel Analysis ToolPak.

Step One: Click the File tab, click Options, and then click the Add-Ins category.
Step Two: Select Analysis ToolPak. Click Go and then OK.

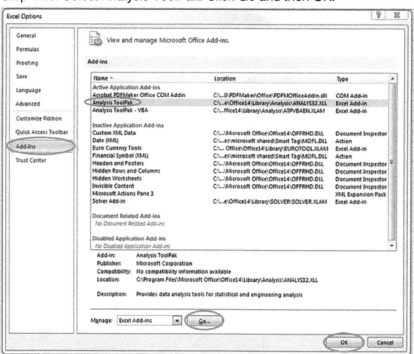

Step Three: Data Analysis appears in the Toolbar under the Data tab.

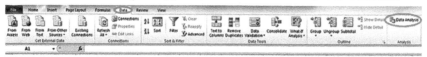

Used with permission from Microsoft.

There are several types of chi-square statistical tests. This discussion explains the one-sample chi-square or "goodness-of-fit" test. The one-sample chi-square test requires nominal or categorical data for two variables. Each variable has two, three, or four levels. For this example, one variable is dichotomous and offers only two responses: yes or no. The second variable is related to age. The categorical data must be independent. Independence is when there is no chance that one responding individual could correctly respond to two response choices for the same survey questions. Review the following survey questions:

1. At what age did your child complete the required series of immunizations?
   a. 6 months to 12 months
   b. 12 months to 24 months
   c. 24 months or later
2. Please mark the group that best describes your child's age:
   a. 6 months to 11 months
   b. 12 months to 23 months
   c. 24 months or older

The first example is not independent or mutually exclusive, because a responding individual could correctly mark (a) and (b) for completion of the required immunizations at 12 months or mark (b) and (c) for completion of the required immunizations at 24 months. The violation of independence does not allow evaluators to know how many respondents are incorrectly placed in the wrong category for analysis.[5] The second example shows no violation of independence because there is no overlap.

Before looking at the actual data, let's review the null hypothesis for this survey question:

Null hypothesis: There is no difference between the numbers of individuals in each of the three age groups. Alternate hypothesis: There is a difference between the numbers of individuals in each of the three age groups.

Note that the above alternate hypothesis does not state how big a difference there is between the three groups, just that there *is* a difference. Now let's look at some actual data

FIGURE 11-4 Survey codebook data.

	A			A
1	1		31	1
2	2		32	2
3	3		33	3
4	3		34	1
5	2		35	3
6	3		36	3
7	2		37	1
8	1		38	3
9	2		39	1
10	3		40	2
11	3		41	1
12	1		42	3
13	3		43	3
14	3		44	1
15	3		45	1
16	1		46	3
17	2		47	1
18	1		48	1
19	2		49	2
20	3		50	2
21	2		51	3
22	1		52	2
23	2		53	1
24	1		54	2
25	2		55	3
26	1		56	2
27	2		57	1
28	2		58	2
29	3		59	3
30	2		60	2

Used with permission from Microsoft.

entered into Excel for 60 individuals who responded to the survey question (see **Figure 11-4**). The codebook for this survey is as follows: 1 = 6 to 11 months; 2 = 12 to 23 months; and 3 = 24 months or older. **Table 11-1** shows the data in three groups.

TABLE 11-1 Actual Data Shown by Age

Age			
6–11 months	**12–23 months**	**24 months or older**	**Total**
19	24	17	60

TABLE 11-2 Calculation of Chi-Square

	Observed (O)	Expected (E)	Difference	$(O - E)^2$	$(O - E)^2/E$
6–11 months	19	20	1	1	0.05
12–23 months	24	20	4	16	0.8
24 months or older	17	20	3	9	0.45
Total	60	60			$\chi^2 = 1.23$

Using these data, evaluators want to know if the ages of responding individuals are equally distributed, so they conduct a chi-square test to answer this question. Of course, with this example, the reader can merely look at the numbers to see that the distribution is uneven. However, the purpose of the simple example is to explain the process. When using real datasets, the process is the same, but the datasets are much larger, and it is not as evident if there is a difference. The first column matches the actual or observed data from **Table 11-2**. The second column shows what the evaluators expect, or 20 individuals evenly distributed in each category. Conduct the calculations shown in the last column to verify that you understand the equations.

The next step is a bit confusing, so read this section carefully. Most statistical textbooks have an appendix that provides a variety of tables called critical value tables that correspond to specific types of statistical tests. Although how the critical values are calculated is beyond the scope of this chapter, these values are percentage points used in inferential statistics to reject or fail to reject the null hypothesis.[6] The critical value tables are provided in this chapter for ease of understanding. Critical value tables may also be easily found on the Internet. For the chi-square test, evaluators refer to the Table of Critical Chi-Square Values (see **Table 11-3**).[7]

To use Table 11-3, follow these steps:

1. The first step in reading Table 11-3 is to determine the degrees of freedom. This concept is based on a mathematical formula that is beyond the scope of this introductory chapter. For this chapter, degrees of freedom are defined as the number of choices (e.g., 18–23, 24–29, and 30+ years in this example) minus 1 for the overall category of age. In this example, there are three age group choices and one group called the age variable, so we have 2 degrees of freedom because $3 - 1 = 2$.[8]

2. Look at the far left column and locate 2 degrees of freedom. The critical chi-square value is 5.9915.

3. Decision: Look back at Table 11-2 to find the obtained χ^2 value of 1.23.

4. Compare the obtained χ^2 to the critical χ^2 value of 5.9915. The obtained value is less than the critical value. Therefore, evaluators fail to reject the null hypothesis. In other words, there is no statistically significant difference between the numbers of individuals in each of the three age groups. In chi-square tests, you want the obtained value to be larger than the critical value.

Let's try another example to confirm your understanding of chi-square tests. The following example asks the same survey question, but yields different responses from the different participating individuals (see **Table 11-4** and **Table 11-5**).

Once again, calculate the degrees of freedom as $3 - 1 = 2$. Look back at Table 11-3 at 2 degrees of freedom and find the critical chi-square value of 5.9915.

Decision: Compare the obtained χ^2 value of 30.14 to the critical χ^2 value of 5.9915. The obtained value is greater than the critical value. Therefore, evaluators reject the null hypothesis. There is a statistically significant difference in the age group of individuals who answer the survey.

t-Tests

t-tests are used to determine if the mean scores between two groups are statistically different. There are two types of t-tests: independent and paired samples. Independent t-tests look at two groups of individuals (or any other data being measured) examined only once in time. For example, two groups of categorical data (public high school seniors and private school seniors) take the SAT (continuous data) one time. The evaluators conduct an independent t-test to determine if there is a statistical difference between the mean scores of the public school seniors compared to the mean score of the private school seniors.

Paired-samples t-tests look at one group of individuals tested twice, such as with a pretest and posttest. For example, high school students are given the written driving test on the

TABLE 11-3 Table of Critical Chi-Square Values

Degrees of Freedom (df)	Critical Chi-Square Values	Degrees of Freedom (df)	Critical Chi-Square Values
1	3.8415	21	32.6708
2	5.9915	22	33.9223
3	7.8147	23	35.1703
4	9.4876	24	36.4144
5	11.0706	25	37.6501
6	12.5914	26	38.885
7	14.067	27	40.111
8	15.5073	28	41.3393
9	16.9189	29	42.5564
10	18.3072	30	43.7765
11	19.6746	31	44.9861
12	21.0261	32	46.1949
13	22.363	33	47.3973
14	23.6852	34	48.6062
15	24.9947	35	49.7982
16	26.2967	36	50.9972
17	27.5887	37	52.1894
18	28.8689	38	53.3811
19	30.1427	39	54.5684
20	31.4095	40	55.7596

TABLE 11-4 Actual Data Shown by Age

Age			
18–23 years	24–29 years	30 years and older	Total
34	67	19	120

TABLE 11-5 Calculation of Chi-Square

	Observed	Expected	Difference	$(O - E)^2$	$(O - E)^2/E$
18–23 years	34	40	6	36	0.9
24–29 years	67	40	27	729	18.23
30+ years	19	40	21	441	11.03
Total	120	120			$\chi^2 = 30.14$

first day of the driver's education course to determine their knowledge. A pretest mean score is calculated for the group of high school students. The high school students attend the 6-week driver's education course, after which they complete a posttest to determine how much information was learned during the driver's education course. For a paired-samples *t*-test, the pretest mean score is compared to the posttest mean score to determine if there is a statistically significant difference between the two mean scores. Now let's explore each of the two types of *t*-tests in more detail.

Independent t-Test

Independent *t*-tests determine if there is a statistical difference between the mean scores for two groups examined only one time. For example, let's say that evaluators want to know if the Lost-It weight management plan enabled women who work the day shift or women who work the night shift to lose more weight in 12 weeks. As always in inferential statistics, evaluators begin by stating the null hypothesis.

> Null hypothesis: There is no difference in weight between female day-shift workers and female night-shift workers at baseline prior to starting the 12-week Lost-It weight management program.
>
> Alternate hypothesis: There is a difference in weight between female day-shift workers and female night-shift workers at baseline prior to starting the 12-week Lost-It weight management program.

Look at **Figure 11-5** to review the baseline weight for all the participants in the program. In Excel, look at the top line to locate the formula for calculating the baseline mean score for all participants: *fx* =SUM(C2:C21)/20. After entering the formula, it is necessary to place the cursor where you wish the mean score to appear prior to hitting Enter. Now look at line 22 to see that the mean score for all participants is 188.6 pounds at baseline. Although Figure 11-5 familiarizes the reader with Excel formulas, it does not provide a baseline mean score by day shift and night shift. Note that in Figure 11-5, the codebook denotes column A as the case number and column B as their work shift, with 1 = day-shift female workers and 2 = night-shift female workers.

To calculate the baseline mean weight by work shift, it is necessary to sort the data. To sort in Excel, go to the toolbar and click on Data, then click on Sort. Highlight columns A, B, and C and then sort by adding levels as shown in **Figure 11-6**. Click OK.

Figure 11-6 shows that the evaluators sorted the data, so all the female day-shift workers' data are grouped first, followed by the female night-shift workers' data. From here,

FIGURE 11-5 Mean baseline weight for all participants.

	C22	▾	*fx*	=SUM(C2:C21)/20	
	A	B	C	D	E
1		Shift	Baseline		
2	1	1	152		
3	2	2	147		
4	3	2	210		
5	4	1	187		
6	5	2	164		
7	6	2	155		
8	7	2	149		
9	8	2	245		
10	9	1	213		
11	10	1	190		
12	11	1	175		
13	12	2	153		
14	13	1	201		
15	14	2	217		
16	15	1	199		
17	16	2	204		
18	17	2	258		
19	18	1	152		
20	19	1	167		
21	20	1	234		
22			188.6		

evaluators use the formula to calculate the mean score provided in **Figure 11-7**. The female day-shift workers' mean baseline weight is 187 pounds and female nigh-shift workers' mean baseline weight is 190.2 pounds. The female day-shift workers had a lower baseline weight than the female night-shift workers. However, this may be due to simple change. Evaluators want to know if the difference between the baseline weight mean scores are statistically significant, so evaluators conduct an independent *t*-test to reject or fail to reject the null hypothesis.

To calculate the independent *t*-test, go to Formulas on the toolbar, then click on More Functions, then Statistical, then TTEST. The box shown in **Figure 11-8** appears. In the box, enter B2:B11 in Variable 1 Range (day-shift workers) and B12:B21 (night-shift workers) in Variable Range 2. When you click OK, the results are as shown in **Figure 11-9**.

FIGURE 11-6 Sorting data in Excel.

Used with permission from Microsoft.

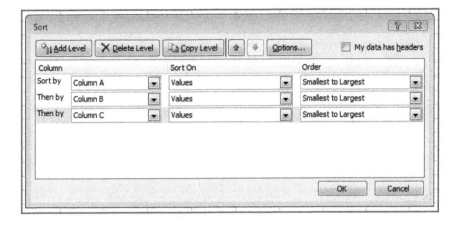

FIGURE 11-7 Baseline mean weight female day- and night-shift workers.

C21 f_x =AVERAGE(B12:B21)

	A	B	C	D	E
1	Shift	Baseline	Mean		
2	1	152			
3	1	152			
4	1	167			
5	1	175			
6	1	187			
7	1	190			
8	1	199			
9	1	201			
10	1	213			
11	1	234	187		
12	2	147			
13	2	149			
14	2	153			
15	2	155			
16	2	164			
17	2	204			
18	2	210			
19	2	217			
20	2	245			
21	2	258	190.2		

Used with permission from Microsoft.

FIGURE 11-8 Excel and independent *t*-tests.

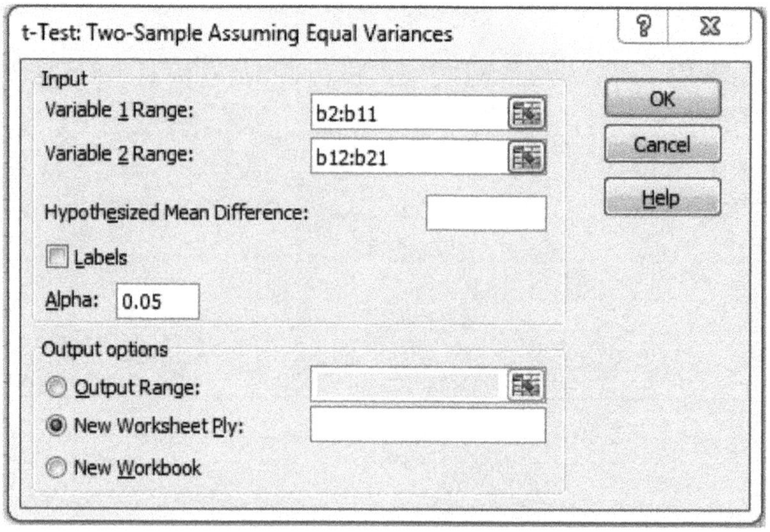

t-Test: Two-Sample Assuming Equal Variances

Input
Variable 1 Range: b2:b11
Variable 2 Range: b12:b21

Hypothesized Mean Difference:

☐ Labels

Alpha: 0.05

Output options
○ Output Range:
● New Worksheet Ply:
○ New Workbook

OK
Cancel
Help

FIGURE 11-9 Results of independent *t*-test.

	A	B	C
1	t-Test: Two-Sample Assuming Equal Variances		
2			
3		*Variable 1*	*Variable 2*
4	Mean	187	190.2
5	Variance	692	1752.622222
6	Observations	10	10
7	Pooled Variance	1222.311111	
8	Hypothesized Mean Differen	0	
9	df	18	
10	t Stat	-0.204665245	
11	P(T<=t) one-tail	0.420065063	
12	t Critical one-tail	1.734063607	
13	P(T<=t) two-tail	0.840130126	
14	t Critical two-tail	2.10092204	

To help the reader understand Figure 11-9, most lines are explained. The lines without explanation are beyond the scope of this chapter.

Line 1: *t*-Test: Two-Sample Assuming Equal Variance.
Line 3: Variable 1 = day-shift worker data; Variable 2 = night-shift worker data.
Line 4: Mean is the average baseline weight for day-shift workers as calculated in Figure 11-7.
Line 5: Variance.
Line 6: Observations: 10 day-shift and 10 night-shift workers.
Line 7: Pooled Variance.
Line 8: Hypothesized Mean Difference.
Line 9: *df* (degrees of freedom) is 20 (10 day-shift workers + 10 night-shift workers) observations – 2 groups (day-shift workers and night-shift workers) = 18.
Line 10: *t*-Stat is –0.2046 and is called the obtained *t*-value. It is calculated by Excel using a formula. (Note:

It is possible to calculate a *t*-test by hand, but the formula is beyond the scope of this introductory chapter, so the Excel formula is illustrated.)
Line 11: *p*-value (one tail).
Line 12: *t*-critical (one tail).
Line 13: *p*-value (two tail): Calculated by Excel; probability of *t*-value happening by chance is 0.84013.
Line 14: *t*-critical (two tail): Look at **Table 11-6**.

Note: Before proceeding to making a decision about the null hypothesis, it is important to become familiar with Table 11-6. As previously mentioned, there are critical value tables for most types of inferential statistic calculations.

Now let's follow the steps to make a decision regarding the null hypothesis for the *t*-test:

1. The first step in reading Table 11-6 is to determine the number of cases. In this example, there are 20 cases or participants. As previously stated, the statistical term *degrees of freedom (df)* for the *t*-test is calculated by

TABLE 11-6 Table of Critical *t*-Values

Degrees of Freedom (*df*)	One-tailed 0.05	Two-tailed 0.05 (0.025 in each tail)	Degrees of Freedom (*df*)	One-tailed 0.05	Two-tailed 0.05 (0.025 in each tail)
1	6.3138	12.707	21	1.721	2.08
2	2.9200	4.3026	22	1.717	2.074
3	2.3534	3.1824	23	1.714	2.069
4	2.1319	2.7764	24	1.711	2.064
5	2.0150	2.5706	25	1.708	2.06
6	1.9432	2.4469	26	1.706	2.056
7	1.8946	2.3646	27	1.704	2.052
8	1.8595	2.3060	28	1.701	2.049
9	1.8331	2.2621	29	1.699	2.045
10	1.8124	2.2282	30	1.698	2.043
11	1.7959	2.2010	35	1.69	2.03
12	1.7823	2.1788	40	1.684	2.021
13	1.7709	2.1604	45	1.68	2.014
14	1.7613	2.1448	50	1.676	2.009
15	1.7530	2.1314	55	1.673	2.004
16	1.7459	2.1199	60	1.671	2.001
17	1.7396	2.1098	65	1.669	1.997
18	1.7341	2.1009	70	1.667	1.995
19	1.7291	2.0930	75	1.666	1.992
20	1.7247	2.0860	80	1.664	1.99

Adapted with permission from https://www.statstodo.com/TTest_Tab.php.

subtracting 1 for each group from the total number of groups. In this example, there are two groups (day- and night-shift workers), so 20 – 2 = 18 degrees of freedom.

2. Locate 18 degrees of freedom on Table 11-6. The critical *t*-test value is 2.1009.

3. Look back at Figure 11-9 to find the calculated or obtained *t*-value of –0.2046.

4. Compare the obtained *t*-value of –0.2046 to the critical *t*-value of 2.1009.

5. If the obtained *t*-value does not exceed the critical value, the evaluators fail to reject the null hypothesis. Evaluators report that the null hypothesis is the best explanation and there is no difference in weight between female day-shift and night-shift workers at baseline prior to starting the 12-week Lost-It weight management program. In other words, the decision is that there is no significant difference between the baseline weight of day- and night-shift workers.

The mean is 187 pounds for day-shift workers and 190.2 pounds for night-shift workers. Because the obtained *t*-test value of –0.2046 is between –2.1009 and +2.1009, evaluators *fail to reject* the null hypothesis. There is no statistically significant difference between the baseline weight of the female day-shift and night-shift workers.

Now let's return to the example, using **Figure 11-10**. An alternative way to determine whether or not to reject or fail to reject the null hypothesis is to look at line 13 in Figure 11-9, $p(T \leq t)$ two-tail = 0.8401. The *p* stands for probability value. To determine whether to reject or fail to reject the null

hypothesis, the *p*-value must be less than 5%, or 0.05. In this example $p = 0.8401$, which is larger than 0.05, and therefore evaluators fail to reject the null hypothesis due to lack of evidence to reject the null hypothesis.

This second example of an independent *t*-test uses the same null hypothesis with a different dataset.

Null hypothesis: There is no difference in weight between day- and night-shift workers at baseline prior to starting the 12-week Lost-It weight management program.
Alternate hypothesis: There is a difference between day- and night-shift workers at baseline prior to starting the 12-week Lost-It weight management program.

Figure 11-11 shows the data. The baseline mean score for 20 day-shift workers is 149.6 pounds and the baseline mean score for 20 night-shift workers is 200.8 pounds.

As with the pervious example, in Excel, select the *t*-Test: Two-Sample Assuming Equal Variance (see **Figure 11-12**). When you click OK, the results are as shown in **Figure 11-13**.

To help the reader understand Figure 11-13, each line of interest is explained here:

Line 1: *t*-Test: Two-Sample Assuming Equal Variance was selected by the researcher.
Line 3: Variable 1 = day-shift female worker data; Variable 2 = night-shift female worker data.
Line 4: Mean is the average baseline weight for day-shift female workers (149.6 pounds) and night-shift female workers (200.75 pounds).
Line 6: Observations: 20 female day-shift workers and 20 female night-shift workers.

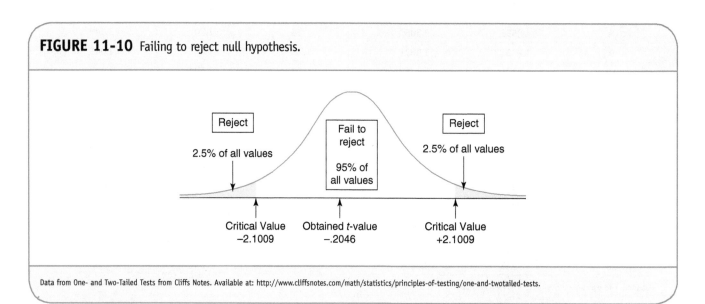

FIGURE 11-10 Failing to reject null hypothesis.

Reject
2.5% of all values

Fail to reject
95% of all values

Reject
2.5% of all values

Critical Value
–2.1009

Obtained *t*-value
–.2046

Critical Value
+2.1009

Data from One- and Two-Tailed Tests from Cliffs Notes. Available at: http://www.cliffsnotes.com/math/statistics/principles-of-testing/one-and-twotailed-tests.

FIGURE 11-11 Mean baseline weight for female day- and night-shift workers.

	A	B	C	D
1	1	97		
2	1	109		
3	1	117		
4	1	118		
5	1	118		
6	1	123		
7	1	124		
8	1	139		
9	1	145		
10	1	145		
11	1	149		
12	1	156		
13	1	157		
14	1	158		
15	1	163		
16	1	189		
17	1	193		
18	1	194		
19	1	197		
20	1	201	Mean	149.6
21	2	156		
22	2	158		
23	2	165		
24	2	168		
25	2	172		
26	2	173		
27	2	173		
28	2	180		
29	2	184		
30	2	190		
31	2	194		
32	2	195		
33	2	201		
34	2	210		
35	2	212		
36	2	231		
37	2	252		
38	2	260		
39	2	261		
40	2	280	Mean	200.8

Used with permission from Microsoft.

Line 8: Hypothesized Mean Difference.

Line 9: df (degrees of freedom) is 40 observations (20 day-shift female workers + 20 night-shift female workers) − 2 groups had their weight measured one time (female day-shift workers and female night-shift workers) = 38.

Line 10: t-Stat is −4.636, calculated by Excel, and is called the obtained t-value.

Line 11: p-value (one tail).

Line 12: t-critical (one tail).

Line 13: p-value (two tail): Calculated by Excel is 0.000004113 and is the probability of the t-value happening by chance. (Hint: In Excel, E-05 equals placing five zeros in front of the first number.)

Line 14: t-critical (two tail): Look at Table 11-6. The critical t-value is 2.024.

Compare the obtained t-value of −4.636 to the critical t-value of 2.024. If the obtained t-value is more extreme than the critical t-value, the evaluators reject the null hypothesis. Evaluators report that there is a significant difference in weight between female day-shift workers and female night-shift workers at baseline prior to starting the 12-week Lost-It weight management program. In other words, evaluators can say that the difference is not due to chance.

The mean is 149.6 pounds for female day-shift workers and 200.75 pounds for female night-shift workers. Because the t-test value of −4.636 is outside the range between −2.02439 and +2.02439, evaluators reject the null hypothesis (see **Figure 11-14**). Because the t-value is in the gray critical area, evaluators have enough evidence to *reject* the null hypothesis. There is a statistically significant difference between the baseline weight of the female day-shift workers and female night-shift workers.[5]

Now it is time for you to practice this new skill with another set of data. It is important to practice using Excel.

Null hypothesis: There is no difference in satisfaction survey scores between the online (online = 1) and telephone (telephone = 2) methods of how individuals purchased Affordable Care Act (ACA) health insurance. Alternate hypothesis: There is a difference in satisfaction survey scores between the online and telephone methods of how individuals purchased Affordable Care Act (ACA) health insurance.

Let's test your skills. Using the dataset in **Figures 11-15** and **11-16**, answer the following questions:

1. Given that online = 1 and telephone = 2, what is the satisfaction mean score for using the online method and the satisfaction mean score for the telephone method? (Answer: online = 4.4 mean score and telephone = 6.06 mean score.)

2. Because there are 15 online observations and 15 telephone observations, what is the degree of freedom for this independent t-test? (Answer: 28 degrees of freedom.)

FIGURE 11-12 *t*-test: Two-sample assuming equal variances.

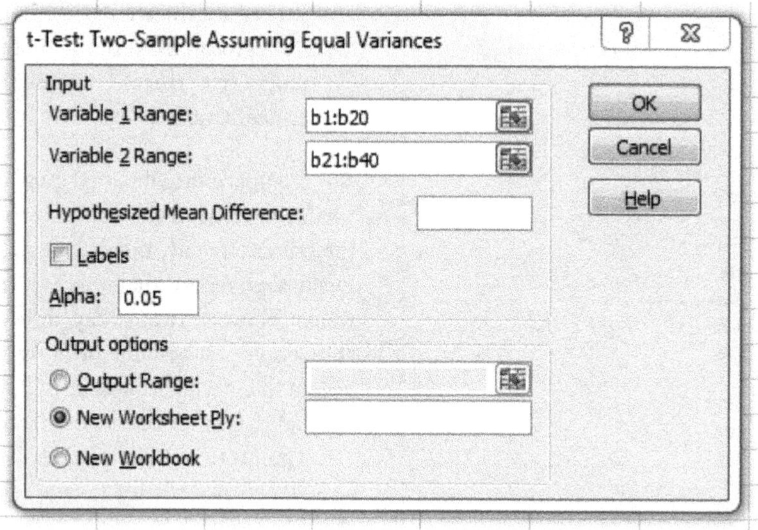

t-Test: Two-Sample Assuming Equal Variances

Input
Variable 1 Range: b1:b20
Variable 2 Range: b21:b40

Hypothesized Mean Difference:

☐ Labels

Alpha: 0.05

Output options
○ Output Range:
● New Worksheet Ply:
○ New Workbook

OK
Cancel
Help

FIGURE 11-13 Results of Example Two independent *t*-test.

	A	B	C
1	t-Test: Two-Sample Assuming Equal Variances		
2			
3		Variable 1	Variable 2
4	Mean	149.6	200.75
5	Variance	1033.410526	1401.460526
6	Observations	20	20
7	Pooled Variance	1217.435526	
8	Hypothesized Mean Difference	0	
9	df	38	
10	t Stat	-4.63577824	
11	P(T<=t) one-tail	2.05658E-05	
12	t Critical one-tail	1.68595446	
13	P(T<=t) two-tail	4.11315E-05	
14	t Critical two-tail	2.024394164	
15			

FIGURE 11-14 Illustration of rejecting the null hypothesis.

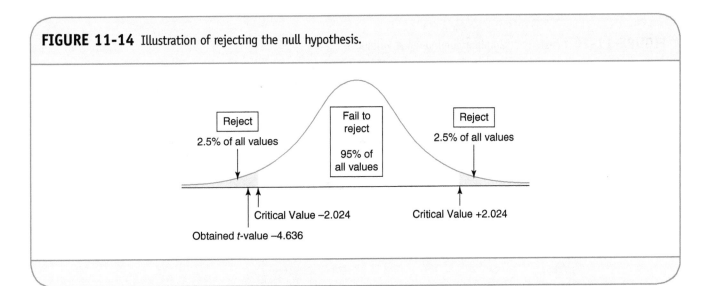

FIGURE 11-15 Method/satisfaction.

	A	B
1	Method	Satisfaction
2	1	7
3	2	6
4	2	7
5	2	8
6	2	4
7	1	5
8	1	6
9	2	7
10	1	5
11	2	6
12	1	6
13	2	4
14	1	6
15	2	5
16	1	6
17	2	7
18	1	5
19	2	8
20	1	9
21	2	3
22	1	5
23	2	7
24	1	9
25	2	4
26	1	5
27	2	3
28	1	6
29	1	5
30	1	7
31	2	6

3. For this independent t-test, assume a two-sample with equal variances. What is the t statistic? (Answer: t-Stat = −2.797.)
4. For this independent t-test, assume a two-sample with equal variances, what is the t-critical two-tail? (Answer: t-critical two-tail = 2.048.)
5. For this independent t-test, do you reject or fail to reject the null hypothesis? (Answer: Reject the null hypothesis.)

Paired-Samples t-Test

Paired-samples t-tests compare the mean scores of one group twice. For example, let's say that evaluators want to know if the Lost-It weight management program was effective in helping day-shift females (column A) lose weight between their initial weigh-in (column B) and at the end of the program after 12 weeks (column C). See **Figure 11-17**.

> Null hypothesis: There is no difference in weight between the baseline weight and the 12th week weight for day-shift workers participating in the Lost-It weight management program.
>
> Alternate hypothesis: There is a difference in weight between the baseline weight and the 12th week weight for day shift workers participating in the Lost-It weight management program.

To help the reader understand **Figure 11-18**, each line of interest is explained here:

Line 1: t-Test: Paired Two Sample for Means was selected by the researcher.

FIGURE 11-16 *t*-test: Two-sample assuming equal variances.

	A	B	C
1	t-Test: Two-Sample Assuming Equal Variances		
2			
3		*Variable 1*	*Variable 2*
4	Mean	4.4	6.066666667
5	Variance	2.257142857	3.066666667
6	Observations	15	15
7	Pooled Variance	2.661904762	
8	Hypothesized Mean Difference	0	
9	df	28	
10	t Stat	-2.797583931	
11	P(T<=t) one-tail	0.004604289	
12	t Critical one-tail	1.701130934	
13	P(T<=t) two-tail	0.009208578	
14	t Critical two-tail	2.048407142	

FIGURE 11-17 Comparison of baseline and 12-week data.

	A	B	C
1	1	152	142
2	1	152	140
3	1	167	160
4	1	175	158
5	1	187	180
6	1	190	173
7	1	199	187
8	1	201	189
9	1	213	201
10	1	234	209

Line 3: Variable 1 = female pre-weight data; Variable 2 = female post-weight data.

Line 4: Mean is the average pre-weight for day-shift workers (187 pounds) and post-weight (173.9 pounds).

Line 6: Observations: 10.

Line 8: Hypothesized Mean Difference.

Line 9: *df* (degrees of freedom) is 10 observations (one group of female day-shift workers with their weight measured twice) – 1 group of female day-shift workers had their weight measured two times (pretest and post-test weights) = 9.

Line 10: *t*-Stat is 7.604, calculated by Excel, and is called the obtained *t*-value.

Line 11: *p*-value (one tail).

Line 12: *t*-critical (one tail).

Line 13: *p*-value (two tail): Calculated by Excel as 0.00000301 and is the probability of the *t*-value happening by chance. (Hint: In Excel, E-05 equals placing five zeros in front of the first number.)

Line 14: *t*-critical (two tail): Look at Table 11-6. The critical *t*-value is 2.2621.

FIGURE 11-18 Results of paired-samples *t*-test.

	A	B	C
1	t-Test: Paired Two Sample for Means		
2			
3		*Variable 1*	*Variable 2*
4	Mean	187	173.9
5	Variance	692	557.4333333
6	Observations	10	10
7	Pearson Correlation	0.98251345	
8	Hypothesized Mean Difference	0	
9	df	9	
10	t Stat	7.694058975	
11	P(T<=t) one-tail	1.50919E-05	
12	t Critical one-tail	1.833112933	
13	P(T<=t) two-tail	3.01838E-05	
14	t Critical two-tail	2.262157163	

For females, the average baseline weight is 187 pounds and the average weight at the 12th week is 173.9 pounds. The paired-samples *t*-test yields a *t*-value of 7.6940. With 9 degrees of freedom, the critical *t*-value is 2.2621. Look at **Figure 11-19** to determine the decision. Because the obtained *t*-value is in the gray critical area, evaluators reject the null hypothesis. In other words, there is a statistically significant difference between the pre-weight and post-weight for day-shift workers who participated in the Lost-It weight management program.[5]

FIGURE 11-19 Illustration of paired-samples *t*-test.

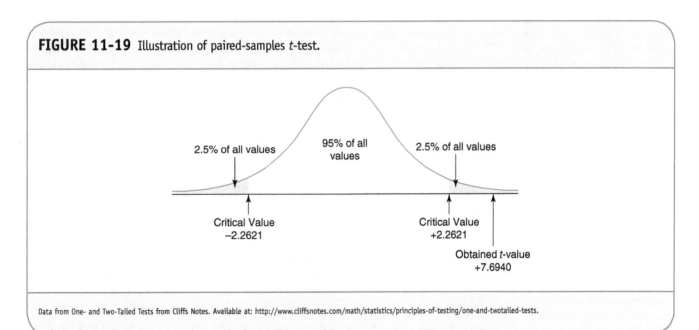

Data from One- and Two-Tailed Tests from Cliffs Notes. Available at: http://www.cliffsnotes.com/math/statistics/principles-of-testing/one-and-twotailed-tests.

Lastly, let's determine whether to reject or fail to reject the null hypothesis based on the *p*-value. Look at Figure 11-13 and see that the two-tailed *p*-value is 0.000003018. Knowing the *p*-value must be less than 0.05, evaluators decided to reject the null hypothesis.

Let's practice your skills with the paired-samples *t*-test, using the following example:

Null hypothesis: There is no difference in the 20-question knowledge survey pretest mean score for individuals attending a 6-week diabetic course and the identical 20-question knowledge survey posttest mean score upon completion of the 6-week diabetic course.

Alternate hypothesis: There is a difference in the 20-question survey pretest mean score for individuals attending a 6-week diabetic course and the identical 20-question survey posttest mean score upon completion of the 6-week diabetic course.

Now let's see if you can correctly answer a few questions related to the dataset (see **Figure 11-20**):

1. If the pretest = 1 and the posttest = 2, what is the mean score for both variables? (Answer: Pretest mean score is 12.2 and posttest mean score is 14.8.)

FIGURE 11-20 Pretest/posttest.

	A	B
1	Prestest Score	Posttest Score
2	12	15
3	14	15
4	10	14
5	17	18
6	11	14
7	13	17
8	15	18
9	13	14
10	9	13
11	10	14
12	11	16
13	17	18
14	12	14
15	8	10
16	11	12
17		

Used with permission from Microsoft.

2. Because there are 15 pretest scores and 15 posttest scores, how many degrees of freedom are used? (Answer: 14. It is 14 because for paired-samples *t*-tests, there is only one variable [knowledge survey] observed twice [pretest and posttest].)

3. For this paired two samples for mean *t*-test, what is the *t*-statistic? (Answer: *t*-Stat = −7.171.)

4. For this paired two samples for mean *t*-test, what is the *t*-critical two-tail statistic? (Answer: *t*-Critical two tail = 2.1447.)

5. Would you reject or fail to reject the null hypothesis? (Answer: Reject the null hypothesis.)

Correlation Coefficients

Statistical tests help tell evaluators if there are relationships or associations between two variables that are measured. For example, does a new type of treadmill affect the leg strength of marathon runners as compared to older models? Is there a relationship between wearing ear-buds daily for a minimum of 4 hours per day during work and the amount of hearing loss after 1 year? Though very important, statistical tests can only tell us if there is or is not a relationship. Correlation coefficients provide more information, such as the strength of the association or whether it has a positive or negative effect on the variables.

Correlation coefficients define a numerical relationship between two continuous variables (also called a Pearson product-moment correlation). There are other types of correlations, but this chapter introduces bivariate correlations that show the relationship between two continuous variables. Let's begin this discussion by providing a simple example of how correlations are used in everyday life. When parents take their child to the pediatrician, the child is weighed and measured. These data are plotted on the child's growth chart in his medical records. The pediatrician is interested in knowing if the child is proportional for his age for height and weight. This would help tell the doctor if the child is growing normally as compared to other children of the same age group. If the plot on the growth chart shows the child in the 90th percentile for height and the 40th percentile for weight, pediatricians recommend healthy choices of food in order to add calories to the child's diet because he is somewhat underweight. If, on the other hand, the percentiles were reversed, pediatricians recommend a reduction in calories because the child's weight exceeds the recommended weight for the child's height. At each visit, pediatricians plot the height and weight trends for each child. Pediatricians are more concerned about the child following a consistent pattern over time (e.g., 40th percentile for height and weight or

90th percentile for height and weight). Pediatricians become concerned when children's growth patterns are inconsistent. Keep in mind that growth charts are one of several criteria used by pediatricians to determine the overall health of a child (see **Figure 11-21**).[9]

The numerical value of a correlation is called a correlation coefficient and depicts two concepts: direction and strength. Direction is depicted as positive or negative. Positive direction occurs when variables on the x-axis increase as variables on the y-axis increase. For example, pediatric growth charts

FIGURE 11-21 Birth to 36 months growth chart for girls.

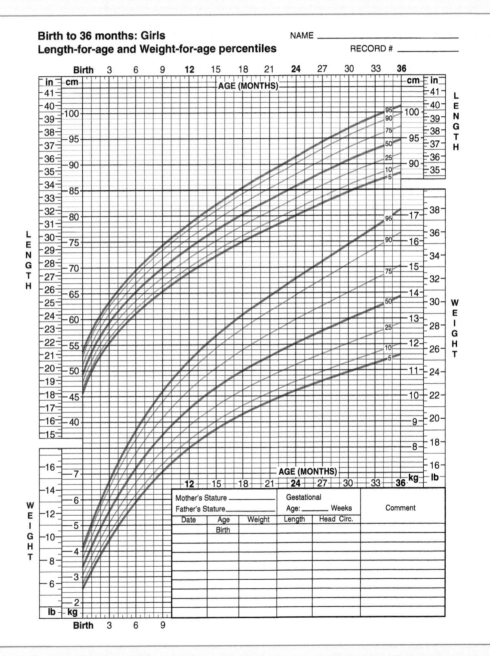

show height and weight, both of which are continuous data. Negative direction occurs when variables on the *x*-axis increase as variables on the *y*-axis decrease. For example, data show that as duration of exercise increases, weight decreases. Strength is described as how dispersed the dots are on the scatter plot. Wide dispersion means less strength and narrow dispersion shows greater strength. Scatter plots describe the

direction and strength of the correlations shown on a graph (see **Figure 11-22**). If the scatter plot dots are closer together, the strength is strong (−1.00 to +1.00), which means that for every unit of increase on the *x*-axis there is an equal increase in every unit on the *y*-axis. The reverse is also true for negative correlations. As the scatter plot dots become more widely dispersed, the strength weakens to close to 0. For example, in

FIGURE 11-22 Six scatter plots of continuous data showing strength and direction of correlations.

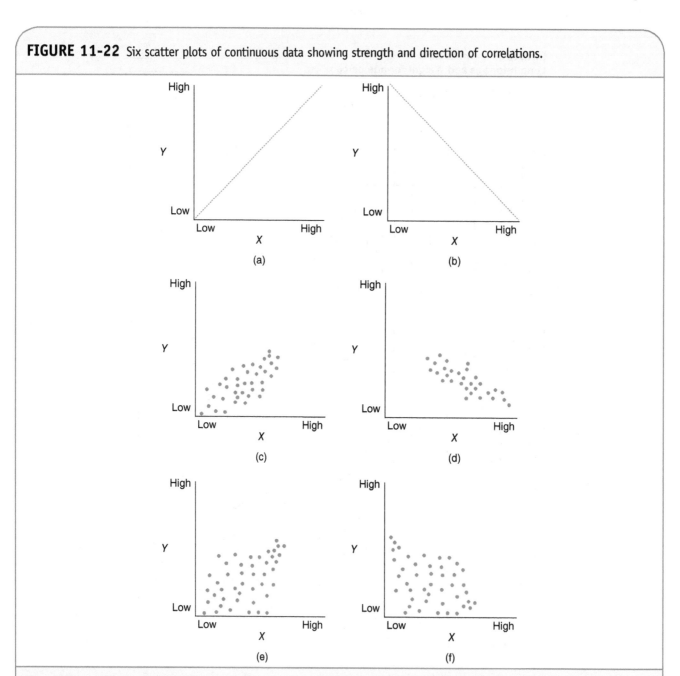

BOX 11-1 Practice Your Skills

Answer the following questions by referring to Figure 11-22.

1. Which correlation is the strongest?
- **a.** −0.75
- **b.** +0.48
- **c.** −0.20
- **d.** +0.65

2. Which correlation is the strongest?
- **a.** +0.18
- **b.** +0.20
- **c.** −0.30
- **d.** −0.18

Answers: 1. (a), −0.75 is the strongest correlation of the choices. See Figure 11-22 Example D.
2. (b), +0.30 is the strongest correlation of the choices. See Figure 11-22 Example E.

FIGURE 11-23 Data for height, weight, and BMI.

	A	B	C
1	Height	Weight	BMI
2	72	230	29.5
3	61	210	39.7
4	64	170	29.2
5	67	154	24.1
6	71	189	26.4
7	68	149	22.7
8	66	156	25.2
9	59	114	23
10	73	256	35.7
11	61	108	20.4
12	71	224	31.2
13	78	305	35.2
14	64	142	24.4
15	65	126	21
16	67	136	21.3
17	62	118	21.6
18	70	208	29.8
19	67	129	20.2
20	58	97	20.3

Used with permission from Microsoft.

Figure 11-22A, the dots line up in a straight line perfectly.[10] The direction is positive and the strength is +1.00. Now turn to **Box 11-1**.

Computing Correlation Coefficients

When determining a correlation, the result of the calculation is called a correlation coefficient and is reported in statistical writing as r. Let's begin with a null hypothesis using the data in **Figure 11-23**.

> Null hypothesis: There is no correlation ($r = 0$) between height and weight for female day- and night-shift workers.
> Alternate hypothesis: There is a correlation between height and weight for female day- and night-shift workers.

Next, enter the formula to calculate a correlation coefficient in the function (fx) toolbar in Microsoft Excel. The formula on the left is the correlation coefficient for height and weight. The formula on the right is the correlation coefficient for weight and BMI (see **Figure 11-24**). Information on how to calculate BMI can be found in **Box 11-2**.

When the CORREL formula is entered into the fx toolbar, the box shown in **Figure 11-25** appears. Enter Array 1 for height and Array 2 for weight. Repeat the same process for CORREL for weight and body mass index (BMI; see Figure 11-25).

Let's explore Figure 11-22 further:

1. Look at **Table 11-7**.[12]
2. The degrees of freedom are calculated: 19 (number of individuals in the data) − 2 (number of variables: height and weight) = 17.
3. Using 17 degrees of freedom, locate the critical value of 0.4555.

From Figure 11-22, the formula result (obtained r value) is +0.8303. The obtained value is more extreme than the critical value and therefore falls in the critical area for rejecting the null hypothesis (see **Figure 11-26**). Evaluators reject the null hypothesis. There is a statistically significant correlation between height and weight for adult females and males.

It is essential to remember that with correlations, one variable does not mean that it *causes* another variable to change, it simply means that two things are numerically related or associated. For example, gaining weight does not cause the individual to grow taller. In another example, more people drown when the temperature is over 90 degrees. In this case, the high temperature has nothing to do with tests, t-tests, and correlation coefficients, it is time to present the topic of confidence intervals. The confidence interval provides more information than simply rejecting or failing to reject the null hypothesis. By using the null hypothesis, evaluators know that there is a statistically significant difference between the mean scores, while the confidence interval calculates an estimate of the magnitude of the difference.

Let's explore this definition in greater detail for improved understanding. Remember back at the beginning of this chapter, you learned that in inferential statistics, evaluators are generally unable to gather data from the whole population, so they select a representative sample of individuals to participate in their study. Evaluators collect and analyze their data. If they use a t-test in the analysis, they would calculate a mean score. This mean score is derived from the sample, not from the whole population. Because evaluators cannot study the whole population, they are always left wondering how well the mean score for the sample estimates the actual mean score for the whole population. To ease their speculation, they calculate a confidence interval. Confidence intervals provide a range, including a lower and upper limit, of where the mean score of the population is likely to be contained.[13] Because evaluators only have data from the sample, they estimate the confidence interval range from the data collected from the sample representing the population.[14]

So, how do the evaluators decide their level of certainty in the calculated confidence interval? Good question. First, evaluators set the desired level of their "confidence," and this value is represented by a percentage. In most cases, evaluators set the level of confidence at 95%, so they can state that they are 95% certain that the lower and upper range of the calculated confidence interval captures the mean score of the population. In other words, the 95% confidence interval indicates the range of values within which the mean score

---

FIGURE 11-24 Formulas to calculate correlation coefficient.

	A	B	C	D	E	F
	Height	Weight	BMI			
1	Height	Weight	BMI			
2	72	230	29.5			
3	61	210	39.7			
4	64	170	29.2			
5	67	154	24.1			
6	71	189	26.4			
7	68	149	22.7			
8	66	156	25.2			
9	59	114	23			
10	73	256	35.7			
11	61	108	20.4			
12	71	224	31.2			
13	78	305	35.2			
14	64	142	24.4			
15	65	126	21			
16	67	136	21.3			
17	62	118	21.6			
18	70	208	29.8			
19	67	129	20.2			
20	58	97	20.3			
21		0.830357				

B21 = CORREL(A2:A20,B2:B20)

Used with permission from Microsoft.

---

drowning, but rather more people swim when the weather is warm. In reverse, just because more people are swimming does not make the temperature rise.

Confidence Intervals

Now that you have been introduced to the concept of rejecting and failing to reject the null hypothesis with chi-square

---

BOX 11-2 BMI Calculator and Information

The National Heart, Lung, and Blood Institute (http://nhlbisupport.com/bmi/bminojs.htm)[11] provides a free BMI calculator, if you wish to calculate your own BMI. BMI is the correlation of body fat based on height and weight.
BMI categories:

- Normal weight = 18.5–24.9
- Overweight = 25–29.9
- Obesity = BMI of 30 or greater

Courtesy of The National Heart, Lung and Blood Institute (http://nhlbisupport.com/bmi/bminojs.htm)

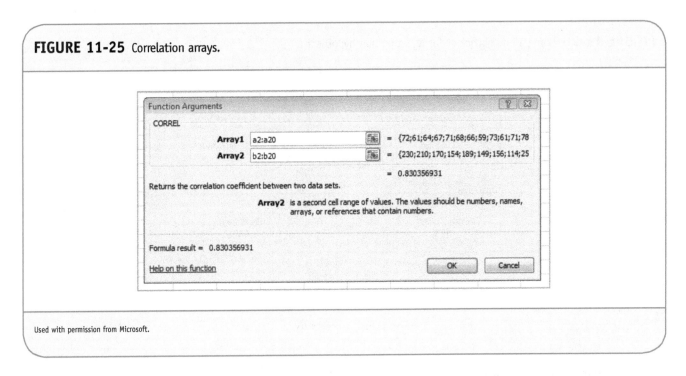

FIGURE 11-25 Correlation arrays.

would fall 95% of the time if evaluators repeated the study with an infinite number of sample size samples taken from the same population.[15]

For this example, the data from the second example for the independent *t*-test (Figure 11-13) are used to present the basic equation to introduce confidence intervals. Because Excel does not provide a simple formula for confidence intervals, this example uses a combination of Excel data and an equation that can be calculated by hand. (Note: Most specialized statistical software programs provide drop-down menus for ease of calculating confidence intervals.)

The following steps explain the equation used to calculate a confidence interval:

1. To calculate a confidence interval, you need to use Excel formulas to determine the values for mean scores, standard deviation, sample size, degrees of freedom, and the critical *t*-value.

TABLE 11-7 Critical Values for Correlation Coefficients

Degrees of Freedom (*df*)	One-tailed 0.05	Two-tailed 0.05 (0.025 in each tail)	Degrees of Freedom (*df*)	One-tailed 0.05	Two-tailed 0.05 (0.025 in each tail)
1	0.9877	0.9969	11	0.4762	0.5529
2	0.9000	0.9500	12	0.4575	0.5324
3	0.8054	0.8783	13	0.4409	0.5139
4	0.7293	0.8114	14	0.4259	0.4973
5	0.6694	0.7545	15	0.4120	0.4821
6	0.6215	0.7067	16	0.4000	0.4683
7	0.5822	0.6664	17	0.3887	0.4555
8	0.5494	0.6319	18	0.3783	0.4438
9	0.5214	0.6021	19	0.3687	0.4329
10	0.4973	0.5760	20	0.3598	0.4227

Data from Quantitative Psychology at Middle Tennesee State University. Available at: http://capone.mtsu.edu/dkfuller/tables/correlationtable.pdf.

FIGURE 11-26 Correlation coefficient for rejecting null hypothesis.

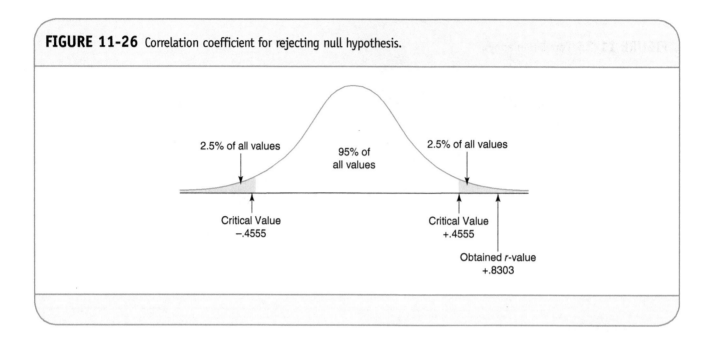

2.5% of all values

95% of all values

2.5% of all values

Critical Value −.4555

Critical Value +.4555

Obtained *r*-value +.8303

Mean scores: Day-shift female workers: 149.6 pounds

Excel: f_x =AVERAGE(B1:B20)

Night-shift female workers: 200.75 pounds

Excel: f_x =AVERAGE(B21:B40)

Standard deviation: Day-shift female workers: 32.14

Excel: f_x =STDEV(B1:B20)

Night-shift female workers: 37.43

Excel: f_x =STDEV(B21:B40)

Sample size: Day-shift workers: 20 and night-shift workers: 20

Degrees of freedom: 40 − 2 = 38

Critical *t*-value: 2.0243

2. To understand the confidence interval formula, it is necessary to know the meaning of each symbol:

$\bar{X}_1$ = Mean score 1 (night-shift workers: 200.75 pounds)

$\bar{X}_2$ = Mean score 2 (day-shift workers: 149.6 pounds)

s_1^2 = Standard deviation of night-shift workers (37.43) squared = 1,401

s_2^2 = Standard deviation of day-shift workers (32.14) squared = 1,033

n_1 = Number of night-shift workers = 20

n_2 = Number of day-shift workers = 20

Decision: Evaluators are 95% confident that the mean difference between day-shift worker baseline weight and night-shift worker baseline weight is between −73.48 pounds and −28.81 pounds (see **Figure 11-27**). Why are these

numbers negative? The answer is because the female day-shift workers started the Lost-It weight management programs weighing between 28.81 and 73.48 pounds less than the female night-shift workers.[16]

If program evaluators were aware of this weight difference, they could conduct the evaluation with a specific focus on the weight-loss challenges faced by the female night-shift workers that are different from those of the female day-shift workers.

Now let's compare the limited information received from conducting an independent *t*-test (Figure 11-9) and the expanded information received from adding the confidence interval (Figures 11-24 and 11-25). As shown in **Figure 11-28**, evaluators have enough evidence to *reject* the null hypothesis

FIGURE 11-27 Confidence interval lower level/confidence interval upper level.

$$(\bar{X}_1 - \bar{X}_2) - \begin{array}{c} \text{Critical} \\ t\text{-value} \end{array} \times \sqrt{\frac{S_1^2}{n_1} + \frac{S_2^2}{n_2}}$$

$$(\bar{X}_1 - \bar{X}_2) + \begin{array}{c} \text{Critical} \\ t\text{-value} \end{array} \times \sqrt{\frac{S_1^2}{n_1} + \frac{S_2^2}{n_2}}$$

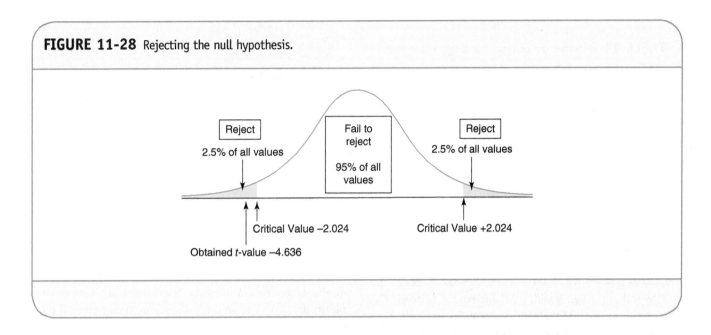

FIGURE 11-28 Rejecting the null hypothesis.

and to state that there is a statistically significant difference between the baseline weight of the day-shift and night-shift workers.[5]

However, **Figure 11-29** gives us the same information, plus it includes added information about the magnitude of the difference between the female day-shift workers' baseline weight and the female night-shift workers' baseline weight with the inclusion of the confidence intervals. Now evaluators have enough evidence to reject the null hypothesis and to state with 95% confidence that the mean weight difference between day-shift and night-shift workers for the population is between 21.81 pounds and 73.48 pounds.

Now let's consider two last important concepts about confidence intervals. First, if the lower and upper values include 0, the evaluators fail to reject the hypothesis. For example, if the lower value is –1.89 and the upper value is +3.73, the spread includes 0, so "fail to reject" is correct. Second, when the confidence interval is extremely wide (e.g., –6.79 to –218.09), the sample size is too small and needs to be increased for a more accurate representation of the population.

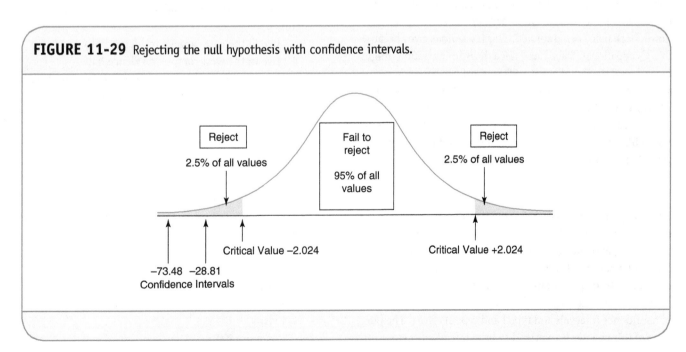

FIGURE 11-29 Rejecting the null hypothesis with confidence intervals.

TABLE 11-8 Summary of Type I and Type II errors

		Actual Situation	
		Null hypothesis is really true.	Null hypothesis is really false.
Researcher's Decision	Reject the null hypothesis.	Type I error	Correct
	Fail to reject the null hypothesis.	Correct	Type II

Adapted from Ary D, Jacobs LC, Razavieh A. Introduction to Research in Education, 6th ed. Belmont, CA: Wadsworth/Thompson Learning; 2002; and Salkind NJ; 2010. Statistics for People Who Think They Hate Statistics, 2nd ed. Thousand Oaks, CA: Sage; 2010.

TYPE I AND TYPE II ERRORS

Type I and type II errors build on the concepts of statistical significance level and rejecting the null hypothesis. Evaluators make a type I error when they falsely reject the null hypothesis when looking at differences between the intervention group and the control group. For example, suppose the null hypothesis is "For factory workers with lower back pain, there is no difference between wearing the usual narrow foam back support belt and the improved, wider and flexible back support belt for treating their chronic lower back pain." Evaluators commit a type I error when they report that there is a difference between the foam belt and the wide belt, when in fact there is no difference.[5,17]

It is helpful to think of type II errors as the opposite of type I errors. Type II errors occur when evaluators *fail to reject* the null hypothesis when there is a difference between the control and study groups. For example, evaluators commit a type II error when they report that there is no difference between the narrow foam belt and the wide belt on the outcome variable (lower back pain) being studied. This is a serious error because the Occupational Safety and Health Administration might recommend the use of either back support belt based on evaluators' conclusions that both back support belts are the same, when in fact the back support belts are different.[5,17] Type II errors are also defined as failing to reject a false null hypothesis. See **Table 11-8** for a summary of these definitions.[18] Practice your skills with **Box 11-3**. See **Box 11-4** for more resources.

SUMMARY

This chapter introduces inferential statistics. It begins by defining scientific hypothesis, research questions, null hypothesis, and alternative hypothesis. How to conduct basic inferential statistical tests using Excel was introduced using chi-square tests and *t*-tests as examples. After defining correlation coefficients, the chapter concluded with a discussion of confidence intervals and type I and type II errors. The purpose of this chapter is to provide a brief introduction to using

this technique and build a foundation of basic definitions of statistics for future use.

CASE STUDY

At the large State University Student Health Center, the administration hired an evaluation team to determine if they should install instant hand sanitizer dispensers near the elevators in the student residence halls as a way to decrease the spread of upper respiratory infections (URIs) and flu symptoms among students. At the beginning of the fall semester, instant hand sanitizers were installed in three of the high-rise student residence halls on the east side of campus and not in the three high-rise student residence halls on the west side of campus. Each time a student came into the student health center with flu or URI symptoms, while waiting to be seen, they were asked to complete a brief survey.

The survey questions were:

1. Do you live in the east residence halls or west residence halls?
    a. I live in the east campus residence halls.
    b. I live in the west campus residence halls.
2. In the past 2 weeks, how many times have you visited friends in the east campus residence halls?
    a. 0 visits
    b. 1 visit
    c. 2 visits
    d. 3 visits
    e. 4 visits
    f. 5 or more visits
3. In the past 2 weeks, how many times have you visited friends in the west campus residence halls?
    a. 0 visits
    b. 1 visit
    c. 2 visits
    d. 3 visits
    e. 4 visits
    f. 5 or more visits

BOX 11-3 Type I and Type II Errors Practice Problems

Practice with a few more examples.

Example 1

Null hypothesis: There is no difference between the Scholastic Assessment Test (SAT) scores of 1st-year university freshmen and 1st-year community college freshmen.

Data report: The SAT scores of the 1st-year university freshmen are higher than the SAT scores of the 1st-year community college freshmen.

Evaluators' decision: Reject the null hypothesis, because the null hypothesis is false.

Choose one of the following options to describe the evaluators' decision:

   a. Correct decision
   b. Type I error
   c. Type II error

Example 2

Null hypothesis: There is no difference between the indoor air quality in homes before and after the new air filter systems are installed in the attic of each home.

Data report: The indoor air quality is decreased after the installation of the attic air filters.

Evaluators' decision: The evaluator fails to reject the null hypothesis.

Choose one of the following options to describe the evaluators' decision:

   a. Correct decision
   b. Type I error
   c. Type II error

Example 3

Null hypothesis: There is no difference in job satisfaction between the night-shift factory workers and the day-shift factory workers.

Data report: The job satisfaction is the same between night-shift and day-shift factory workers.

Evaluators' decision: Evaluators reject the null hypothesis when the null hypothesis is really true.

Choose one of the following options to describe the evaluators' decision:

   a. Correct decision
   b. Type I error
   c. Type II error

Answers: Example 1 = a, Example 2 = c, Example 3 = b.

BOX 11-4 Websites Providing Free Confidence Interval and Sample Size Calculators

http://www.surveysystem.com/sscalc.htm
http://www.dssresearch.com/KnowledgeCenter/toolkitcalculators/samplesizecalculators.aspx
http://www.raosoft.com/samplesize.html
http://www.nss.gov.au/nss/home.nsf/NSS/0A4A642C712719DCCA2571AB00243DC6?opendocument
http://www.gifted.uconn.edu/siegle/research/samples/samplecalculator.htm
http://www.macorr.com/sample-size-calculator.htm
http://www.custominsight.com/articles/random-sample-calculator.asp

4. If you notice an instant hand sanitizer dispenser at an elevator, how likely are you to use it?
   a. I always reach out and apply the hand sanitizer when I see a dispenser.
   b. I sometimes reach out and apply the hand sanitizer when I see a dispenser.
   c. I never apply the hand sanitizer when I see a dispenser.
5. Since August, how many times have you come to the student health center because you had cold or flu symptoms?
   a. Today is my first visit for cold or flu symptoms.
   b. 2 times

   c. 3 times
   d. 4 times
   e. 5 times
   f. 6 times
6. What is your age?
   a. Younger than 18 years
   b. 18 years old
   c. 19 years old
   d. 20 years old
   e. Older than 20 years

Null hypothesis: There is no difference between the number of student health center visits for cold and flu

FIGURE 11-30 Pilot study data.

	A	B	C	D	E	F
1	East or West	Visit East	Visit West	Use	Visits	Age
2	1	0	5	2	1	1
3	1	2	4	3	1	3
4	1	3	2	1	2	3
5	1	1	`1	2	1	2
6	1	6	1	2	4	4
7	1	3	3	1	1	2
8	1	1	2	2	1	4
9	1	1	3	2	2	1
10	1	1	4	1	1	4
11	1	2	0	2	1	3
12	1	1	2	3	2	2
13	1	3	2	2	1	3
14	1	6	1	1	1	1
15	1	3	3	1	2	3
16	2	1	6	1	1	2
17	2	3	3	2	2	4
18	2	1	4	2	2	2
19	2	2	3	1	3	2
20	2	5	2	1	2	3
21	2	2	2	3	1	2
22	2	2	1	1	2	3
23	2	2	3	1	2	5
24	2	4	0	1	2	2
25	2	2	2	2	3	3
26	2	3	1	3	1	2
27	2	2	2	1	2	3
28	2	2	1	2	1	2
29	2	2	1	1	3	2
30	2	4	3	1	5	2
31	2	2	2	2	1	2

symptoms between the students living in the east campus residence halls and the students living in the west campus residence halls. See **Figure 11-30**.

Case Study Discussion Questions

1. What is the mean for number of student health clinic visits? (Answer: 1.8.)
2. What is the mode for age? (Answer: 2 or 18 years old.)
3. Using an independent *t*-test, what is the mean number of clinic visits for east residence hall students and for west residence hall students? (Answer: east mean = 1.5 visits and west mean = 2.06 visits.)
4. Using the independent *t*-test, do you reject or fail to reject the null hypothesis? (Answer: fail to reject—there is no difference.)
5. Create three more null hypotheses to test using this dataset.

STUDENT ACTIVITIES

This section provides some practice questions to help familiarize yourself with the concepts you have learned in this chapter.

Turn the following problem statements into an appropriate research question, a null hypothesis, and an alternate hypothesis.

1. Leila is a community organizer in a low-income urban center. She believes that there are much fewer grocery stores that offer fresh fruits and vegetables in her neighborhood than in other, wealthier neighborhoods in the same city. If this is true, she would like to try to encourage local grocers to carry more fruits and vegetables.

   Research question:

   Null hypothesis:

   Alternate hypothesis:

2. Carl is a nursing administrator in the emergency room of a busy hospital. He thinks that patients have better satisfaction with their care and nurses make fewer mistakes when nurses are allowed to take a nap when they are on the night shift. If this is true, he would like to allow nurses to take naps on long breaks.

   Research question:

   Null hypothesis:

   Alternate hypothesis:

3. Samuel works for the local YMCA. He believes that retired adults who participate in group exercises at

the YMCA have lower blood pressure than those who participate in exercise on their own. He thinks that not only does the exercise help them physically, but socializing with others helps lower their stress. If this is so, he would like to institute more group classes for retirees.

Research question:

Null hypothesis:

Alternate hypothesis:

Based on the following alternate hypotheses, should the researcher use a one- or two-tailed statistical test?

4. Alternate hypothesis: There are fewer grocery stores that provide fresh fruits and vegetables in District A than in District B.
5. Alternate hypothesis: There is a significant difference in patient satisfaction when nurses are allowed to take a nap while on night shift.
6. Alternate hypothesis: Retired adults who participate in exercise on their own at the YMCA have higher blood pressure than those who participate in group exercise.

   After running the appropriate statistical tests for several research questions, decide which null hypothesis to reject, which to fail to reject, and which to accept.

7. After running a chi-square statistical test you find that the obtained chi-square value is 6.0123 and the critical chi-square value is 5.9915. What is your judgment?
8. After running a two-tailed *t*-test, you obtain a *p*-value of 0.035. What is your judgment?
9. Based on a visual inspection of the normal curve in **Figure 11-31**, what is your judgment?
10. Evaluators have run a confidence interval. Their upper limit was 0.75 and their lower limit was –1.03. What is your judgment?

Answers

1. Research question: Are there significantly fewer grocery stores that offer fresh fruits and vegetables in Leila's neighborhood than in a wealthier neighborhood within the city?

   Null hypothesis: There is no difference in the number of grocery stores that offer fresh fruits and vegetables.

   Alternate hypothesis: There is a significant difference in the number of grocery stores that offer fresh fruits and vegetables.

2. Research question: Do nurses provide better care to emergency room patients if they are allowed to take a nap on night shift?

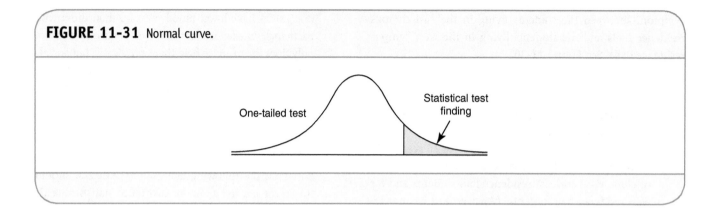

FIGURE 11-31 Normal curve.

Null hypothesis: There is no difference in patient satisfaction and number of mistakes when nurses are allowed to take a nap while on night shift.

Alternate hypothesis: There is a significant difference in patient satisfaction and the number of mistakes when nurses are allowed to take a nap while on night shift.

3. Research question: Do retired adults participating in group exercise classes at the YMCA have lower blood pressure than those retired adults who only participate in solo exercise at the YMCA?

Null hypothesis: There is no difference in blood pressure between retired adults who participate in group exercise and those who do their exercises on their own.

Alternate hypothesis: There is a difference in blood pressure between retired adults who participate in group exercise and those who do their exercises on their own.

4. One-tailed statistical test. This is because we are asking if there is directionality in the difference (i.e., that there are less stores in one neighborhood than in another).

5. Two-tailed statistical test. This is because we are not assuming that there are better or worse patient satisfaction outcomes, only that there are different outcomes. Therefore, we would expect that any extreme differences could be on either end of the normal curve.

6. One-tailed statistical test. This is because we are asking if there is directionality in the difference (i.e., that solo exercisers have higher blood pressure than those who participate in group exercise).

7. Reject the null hypothesis. The obtained chi-square value is larger than the critical chi-square value.

8. Fail to reject the null hypothesis. Normally, if you were running a one-tailed *t*-test, 0.035 would be statistically significant if you had an alpha level of 0.05. However, because we split the alpha level in two (for each side of the normal curve) in a two-tailed *t*-test, a significant result would be a *p*-value of less than 0.025. Because 0.035 is greater than 0.025, we fail to reject the null hypothesis.

9. Reject the null hypothesis. Because the obtained statistical test is in the critical area of the normal curve, we would reject the null hypothesis.

10. Fail to reject the null hypothesis. Because the confidence interval includes 0, we must fail to reject the null hypothesis.

REFERENCES

1. Lincoln LM. *Think and Explain with Statistics*. Boston, MA: Addison-Wesley Publications; 1986.

2. Zimmerman KA. What Is a Scientific Hypothesis. Live Science. Available at: http://www.livescience.com/21490-what-is-a-scientific-hypothesis-definition-of-hypothesis.html. Accessed May 19, 2014.

3. Lane DM. HyperStat Online. Rice University. Available at: http://davidmlane.com/hyperstat/A29337.html. Accessed May 19, 2014.

4. Durham College. Statistics: The Null and Alternate Hypotheses. A Student Academic Learning Services Guide. Available at: http://www.durhamcollege.ca/wp-content/uploads/STAT_nullalternate_hypothesis.pdf; Accessed on May 29, 2014.

5. Salkind NJ. *Statistics for People Who Think They Hate Statistics*, 2nd ed. Thousand Oaks, CA: Sage Publications; 2010.

6. Stockburger DW. One and Two-tailed t Tests. Psychological Statistics at Missouri State. Available at: http://www.psychstat.missouristate.edu/introbook/sbk25m.htm; Accessed on May 29, 2014.

7. Statistics Mentor. The T-Table Critical Values. Available at: http://www.statisticsmentor.com/tables/table_t.htm. Accessed November 3, 2012.

8. Blair RC, Taylor RA. *Biostatistics for the Health Sciences*. 1st ed. Upper Saddle River, NJ: Pearson Prentice Hall; 2008.

9. Dallal GE. *The Little Handbook of Statistical Practice*. Seattle, WA: Amazon Digital Services; 2012.

10. Centers for Disease Control and Prevention. Growth Charts. Available at: http://www.cdc.gov/growthcharts/. Accessed on May 19, 2014.

11. Weathington BL, Cunningham CJL, Pettinger DJ. *Understanding Business Research*. New York, NY: John Wiley & Sons, Inc.; 2012.

12. The National Heart, Lung, and Blood Institute. Calculate Your Body Mass Index. Available at: http://nhlbisupport.com/bmi/bminojs.htm. Accessed May 19, 2014.

13. National Institute of Standards and Technology. What Are Confidence Intervals? Available at: http://www.itl.nist.gov/div898/handbook/prc/section1/prc14.htm; Accessed November 3, 2012.

14. Yale University. Confidence Intervals. Available at: http://www.stat.yale.edu/Courses/1997-98/101/confint.htm. Accessed May 19, 2014.

15. Utah Office of Public Health Assessment. Confidence Intervals in Public Health. Available at: http://health.utah.gov/opha/IBIShelp/ConfInts.pdf. Accessed November 3, 2012.

16. Statistics Lectures. Confidence Intervals for Independent Samples t-Test. Available at: http://www.statisticslectures.com/topics/ciindependent-samplest/. Accessed May 19, 2014.

17. Campbell RB. University of Northern Iowa. Type I and II Error. Available at: http://www.cs.uni.edu/~campbell/stat/inf5.html#TI. Accessed May 19, 2014.

18. Ary D, Jacobs LC, Razavieh A. *Introduction to Research in Education*, 6th ed. Belmont, CA: Wadsworth/Thompson Learning; 2002.

CHAPTER 12

Budgets and Cost Analyses

CHAPTER OBJECTIVES

By the end of this chapter, students will be able to:

- Demonstrate how to create a personal budget.
- Describe the components of a research budget.
- Identify key areas in a profit and loss statement.
- Define the four types of cost analyses: benefits, effectiveness, utility, and feasibility.

KEY TERMS

cost-benefit analysis
cost-effectiveness analysis
cost-utility analysis
feasibility analysis
personal budgets

INTRODUCTION

This chapter begins by describing different types of budgets including personal budgets, evaluation budgets, and budget summaries. Once the basic components of budgets are explained, the next section links the budget concepts to the various types of cost analyses. Evaluators use cost-analysis techniques to determine the most effective and efficient health procedures, treatments, and programs.

BUDGETS

This section describes different types of budgets, beginning with personal budgets. If a student does not understand his or her own budget, it can be difficult to develop budgets for other purposes. Our first example of a budget utilizes the concept of the federal poverty level in the United States. Why do evaluators need to be concerned about the income of participants? For example, if evaluators use income as a variable in their study, they should take the concept of poverty level into consideration when interpreting the final results or making recommendations to stakeholders. After that, a sample budget for evaluation is examined along with a budget justification. Lastly, profit and loss statements for a small company are shown. For this chapter, Microsoft Excel is used to show examples of various types of budgets.

Personal Budgets

Let's begin with developing a simple budget for an individual who recently graduated from a 4-year university with an undergraduate degree and is now working full time. This exercise introduces the basics of using an Excel spreadsheet for budgets. When using Excel, it is essential to use the function (*fx*) toolbar located in the toolbar ribbon. For example, in **Figure 12-1** the required federal taxes are 7.65% and income taxes are about 10%, so the taxes that are subtracted from the gross income every paycheck amount to 17.65%. Note that cell G3 is the recent graduate's pay before taxes and G4 are the taxes (see the function [*fx*] toolbar). The equation for the graduate's take-home pay in cell H4 is cell G4 subtracted from cell G3 (G3 − G4 = $1841). You should also remember that months are calculated as 4.3 weeks equal 52 weeks in a year, reflecting the number in column E. This individual has a monthly excess of $6. Note that the annual income is $21,196 and the annual expenses are $21,114.

To practice Excel skills, try creating your own monthly budget in an Excel spreadsheet. Using the function (*fx*)

FIGURE 12-1 Example of a sample budget.

	A	B	C	D	E	F	G	H	I
	G4		▼	f_x =G3*F4					
1								Monthly	Annual
2	Income		Hours	Pay/Hour	Weeks				
3		Job	40	$ 13	4.3		$ 2,236		
4		Income Tax				17.65%	$ 395	$ 1,841	
5		Health Insurance					$ 75	$ 1,766	$ 21,196
6									
7	Expenses								
8		Rent					$ 475		
9		Utilities					$ 120		
10		Internet/Phone					$ 120		
11		Food		$ 75	4.3		$ 323		
12		Public Transportation		$ 25	4.3		$ 108		
13		Hair/Clothes/Shoes		$ 35	4.3		$ 151		
14		Entertainment		$ 30	4.3		$ 129		
15		Medical/Dental					$ 60		
16		College Loan					$ 150		
17		Vacation Savings					$ 50		
18		Personal Savings					$ 75		
19								$ 1,760	$ 21,114
20									
21								Extra	$ 82
22									

toolbar will help save you time. For example, you can calculate numerous separate equations without using the fx toolbar. If it is necessary to change one number to balance the budget, you need to recalculate every item. However, if the fx toolbar is used, numerous items change instantly without any additional steps. Note that the sample budget in Figure 12-1 does not include any credit card bills or other expenses. If you use a credit card to pay for items, subtract the amount from your checking account so you have enough money to pay off the credit card statement each month. This technique saves having to pay interest on the debt incurred. Also remember to save for vacations and emergencies, so you have a cushion of money in reserve for planned and unplanned expenses. Vacations are more enjoyable when you are not incurring debt while having fun.

The next type of budget to investigate might belong to a member of the 15% of the population (46.2 million people) who lived in poverty in the United States in 2011.[1] Why does an evaluator need to think about this type of budget? The reason is that evaluators work with many types of people, including individuals and families living in poverty. For example, if during the evaluation, individuals are required to participate in two focus groups, the evaluation team needs to budget for potential transportation costs and perhaps childcare during the focus group. If the evaluation is taking place in the community room at the local library of a neighborhood with lower socioeconomic status, it is likely that participants are at or below the poverty level. Therefore, proximity of public transportation is of consideration if the evaluators expect individuals to comply with return visits. Another consideration would be to schedule focus groups to accommodate individuals with limited flexibility due to work schedules. Lastly, evaluators should not jump to the conclusion that individuals who fail to keep appointments are forgetful, disorganized, or not interested in participating; instead, evaluators should remain mindful of exploring the barriers that keep individuals in poverty from attending the focus groups (e.g., employment schedules, lack of transportation, lack of adequate childcare, low literacy). **Figure 12-2** shows a sample budget for a single person living at the federal poverty level. The U.S. federal poverty guidelines are $11,170 for one person and $23,050 for a family of four.[2] Keep in mind that the 2013 federal minimum wage was $7.25 per hour, but many states have increased their minimum wage limits.[3]

FIGURE 12-2 Budget for a single person living at the poverty level.

	H13			f_x	=SUM(G6:G12)				
	A	B	C	D	E	F	G	H	I
1	Income		Hours	Pay/Hour	Weeks			Monthly	Annual
2		Job	25	$ 7.25	4.3		$ 779		
3						17.65%	$ 138	$ 917	$ 11,003
4									
5	Expenses								
6		Rent		$ 95	4.3		$ 409		
7		Food		$ 62	4.3		$ 267		
8		Public Transportation		$ 20	4.3		$ 86		
9		Mobile Phone		$ 10	4.3		$ 43		
10		Clothes		$ 15	4.3		$ 65		
11		Drug Store		$ 4	4.3		$ 17		
12		Savings		$ 7	4.3		$ 30		
13								$ 916	$ 10,991
14									
15								Extra	$ 12
16									

Evaluation and Research Project Budgets

All evaluation projects have a budget. Whether a study is a multimillion dollar grant funded by the National Institutes of Health or a $1000 evaluation in a small community agency, the principal investigator of the evaluation is in charge of tracking the funding and verifying that the money is spent appropriately. Even if the institution has a finance department to track grant funding, it is ultimately the responsibility of the individual conducting the evaluation to provide the appropriate oversight.

It should also be noted that when evaluators apply for grant funding, the budget is a critical component of the grant application. Whether the funding comes from the federal government, a private organization, or a community agency, the funding is highly regulated and frequently audited to prevent fraud and waste. For example, evaluators must calculate grant budgets accurately for each budget category. There are many rules and regulations regarding grant budgets to protect against waste, misuse, and fraud. It is not possible for evaluators to move money from one category to another category (e.g., salaries to travel expenses) without written permission from the funding agency. Further, it is also not possible to alter the number or salary rate of personnel on the grant budget. There are also specific regulations guarding against purchasing equipment and food. For instance, evaluators may not purchase a new laptop without a specific need to use the laptop for data collection in the community.

Lastly, most large institutions and universities have contracts with certain vendors that guarantee the lowest price (e.g., rental car companies, print goods suppliers, airlines). Evaluators are required to use only these vendors, even if there is some inconvenience involved, such as longer flight layovers or less direct routes. It is important to know the regulations for your agency or institution related to the specific rules regarding budget spending. In all situations and circumstances, evaluators are required to abide by the budget regulations at their institutions or else risk censure, fines, and even criminal investigation. When in doubt, find out the policy prior to making the purchase or changing any line of an approved budget.

Before examining an actual budget, let's define three common types of budgets that are used by funding agencies: cost reimbursable, fixed priced, and cost sharing. First, cost-reimbursable budgets are defined as follows: Each time the evaluators spend money for the evaluation, they save detailed receipts and submit the receipts for reimbursement on a regular schedule, such as the first week of each month. With this type of budget, the funding agency knows exactly how their money is being spent each month. Usually, this type of budget provides the evaluators with a small amount of start-up funding to get the evaluation initiated in the first month. The funding agency realizes that evaluators cannot afford to spend several thousand dollars of their own personal or agency's money to initiate a funded evaluation. The start-up money requires receipts as with each of the following months of spending. This type of budget is advantageous when the evaluator is not certain how much it will cost to complete the funded evaluation. If the evaluation exceeds the proposed budget, the funding agency can decide to end the project or continue to provide funding over the original budget.

Second, fixed-price budgets are defined as a final proposed budget for the entire evaluation. In this case, there is no need to collect detailed receipts and there is no monthly accountability to the funding agency. However, there is internal monthly accountability with the evaluation team to ensure that the project is on track with its timeline and budget. With fixed-price budgets, the evaluators must complete the project on time and within budget. Funding agencies paid the agreed-upon budget, so they expect a finished product for their money. In some situations, there are additional penalties and fines written into signed evaluation contracts if the project is not completed on time and as written in the contract.

Third, cost-sharing or cost-matching budgets are defined as when a funding agency states that they will provide a percentage of the money and it is up to the evaluators to find additional money. For example, the local Healthy Start Coalition posts a "Request for Proposals" (RFP) stating that they have $50,000 to contribute to reducing child maltreatment in the tri-county area, but any agency applying for the evaluation must match (or share) the Healthy Start Coalition money with another $50,000. This type of budget allows the original agency to double their funding or share the cost of the evaluation with other agencies. In this example, it is possible for an evaluation team at the local university to partner with several local agencies, such as the YMCA, Child Abuse Council, the Children's Hospital, and Big Brothers Big Sisters. The university evaluation team requests that each agency donate $10,000 toward the good cause of reducing child maltreatment in their tri-county region. Keep in mind that the $10,000 donation may be actual cash or an in-kind donation. An in-kind donation could be office space rent in the YMCA administrative office located where the evaluation will take place. The cost of this office space would be calculated per square foot and priced at the local rent charges to determine the amount of such an in-kind donation. Another type of in-kind donation would be the hospital paying the salary of their medical transcription team to transcribe the data collected by the evaluation team at the focus groups. Each type of in-kind donation is not actual cash, but rather a cost that would be incurred by the evaluation team if the item or service had not been donated in kind. All three types of budgets have advantages and disadvantages for each unique situation

and evaluation project. It is up to the evaluator to be familiar with each type of budget prior to writing and submitting a proposal for the evaluation requested.

Now let's expand this discussion by examining a budget for an evaluation. These budgets include an Excel spreadsheet and a budget justification. When a budget is created for a project, it is not simply a total projected amount of money required to successfully complete the evaluation or study. It is necessary to justify why the projected amount of money is required. The budget justification is a written description that explains the specific expenditures of the proposed budget. Budget justifications allow the institution or organization funding the proposed project to determine if the planned costs are reasonable. **Figure 12-3** shows a sample budget for an evaluation project, and **Box 12-1** shows the budget justification.

In the budget justification in Box 12-1, you will notice that there is an item called indirect costs. Indirect costs are a percentage of the total expenses for an evaluation project that are collected by an institution or agency hosting the project. For example, universities charge evaluators a predetermined rate on all funded research. This amount provides funding to the university to pay expenses used by the project staff but not listed on the research budget (e.g., building utilities and maintenance, office furniture, the cost of general administrative and personnel work). For example, the available funding for the evaluation is listed as $100,000 with 15% indirect costs, or $15,000. If the evaluators submit a budget of $97,500, the 15% indirect costs amount to $14,625 rather than the full $15,000.

Budget Summaries: Profit and Loss Statements

As already noted, budgets serve multiple purposes for evaluators, such as tracking available resources, costs, and payments. Budgets also summarize information. A budget summary is called a profit and loss statement. These statements allow individuals, departments, or large companies to determine at a quick glance if they are gaining or losing money and in which areas (see **Table 12-1**).

COST ANALYSIS

Now that the budgets have been introduced, it is time to explain the concept of cost analysis. Simply stated, cost analysis combines the budgets and costs; in this discussion these will be related to healthcare costs. Although most evaluators are not expected to know the complexities of financial analyses and how they relate to their work, it is important to have a basic understanding of the various types of cost analyses. From the viewpoint of evaluation, some cost analyses are

BOX 12-1 Sample Budget Justification for an Evaluation Project

FIGURE 12-3 Sample budget for an evaluation project.

	A	B	C	D	E	F	G
		Salary	FTE	Subtotal	Percent	Benefits	Total
1	Personnel						
2	Principal Investigator	$ 100,000	0.20	$ 20,000	0.28	$ 5,600.00	$ 25,600.00
3	Director	$ 80,000	1.00	$ 80,000	0.28	$ 22,400.00	$ 102,400.00
4	Team Leader	$ 65,000	1.00	$ 65,000	0.28	$ 18,200.00	$ 83,200.00
5	Adm Assistant	$ 45,000	1.00	$ 45,000	0.28	$ 12,600.00	$ 57,600.00
6	Data Collector	$ 40,000	0.25	$ 10,000	0.28	$ 2,800.00	$ 12,800.00
7	Data Entry Clerk	$ 40,000	0.25	$ 10,000	0.28	$ 2,800.00	$ 12,800.00
8							
9	Biostatistician	$ 175	50				$ 8,750.00
10							
11	Incentives	$ 25	200				$ 5,000.00
12							
13	Mileage	$ 0	200	12			$ 1,176.00
14							
15	Printer	$ 600					$ 600.00
16	Computers	$ 3,000					$ 3,000.00
17	Office Supplies	$ 300		12			$ 3,600.00
18	Paper	$ 200		12			$ 2,400.00
19	Printer Cartridge	$ 75		12			$ 900.00
20	Postage	$ 30		12			$ 360.00
21	Space Lease	$ 1,800		12			$ 21,600.00
22	Telephone/Internet	$ 300		12			$ 3,600.00
23	Utilities	$ 200		12			$ 2,400.00
24						Subtotal	$ 347,786
25					Indirect	$ 0.15	$ 52,168
26						Total	$ 399,954
27							

Used with permission from Microsoft.

Personnel

- Ima Wright, PhD, serves as principal investigator with 0.20 full-time equivalent (FTE) commitment for $20,000 salary and $5600 benefits, for a total of $25,600.
- Alison Richards, PhD, serves as director with 1.00 FTE commitment for $80,000 salary and $22,400 benefits, for a total of $102,400.
- Barbara Villiotti, MA, serves as team leader with 1.00 FTE commitment for $65,000 salary and $18,200 benefits, for a total of $83,200.
- Erica Patterson, BS, serves as administrative assistant with 1.00 FTE for $45,000 salary and $12,600 benefits, for a total of $57,600.

(continues)

BOX 12-1 Sample Budget Justification or an Evaluation Project (Continued)

- Daniel Kohler, BSPH, serves as data collector with 0.25 FTE for $10,000 salary and $2800 benefits, for a total of $12,800.
- Marie Gomez, BSPH, serves as data entry clerk with 0.25 FTE for $10,000 and $2800 benefits, for a total of $12,800.

Consultant

R. C. Blair, PhD, serves as biostatistician consultant with a salary of $175 per hour for 50 hours, for a total fee of $8750.

Incentives

Each of the 200 participants will receive a $25 gift card upon completion of the online survey, for a total for $5000.

Mileage

Mileage is 200 miles per month for 12 months at $0.49 per mile for a total of $1176.

Office

- One printer used for office printing needs is $600.
- Two computers at $1500 each total $3000.
- Miscellaneous office supplies at $300 per month for 12 months total $3600.
- Copy paper and stationery at $200 per month for 12 months are $2400.
- One printer cartridge at $75 per month for 12 months is $900.
- Postage at $30 per month for 12 months is $360.
- Office space lease at $1800 per month for 12 months is $21,600.
- Telephone and Internet charges at $300 per month for 12 months total $3600.
- Utilities at $200 per month for 12 months are $2400.
- Subtotal of expenses: $347,786
- Indirect costs are calculated at 15%: $52,168

Total expenses: $399,954.00

TABLE 12-1 Sample Profit and Loss Statement

Complete Hospital Linen Services	
January 1, 2014 to December 31, 2015	
GROSS INCOME	
Gross sales	$1,100,000
Other income	$300,000
TOTAL GROSS INCOME	$1,400,000
NET INCOME	
Income before taxes	$1,400,000
Personal income taxes	$448,000
TOTAL NET INCOME	$952,000

TABLE 12-1 Sample Profit and Loss Statement (Continued)

Complete Hospital Linen Services	
January 1, 2014 to December 31, 2015	
EXPENSES	
Cost of goods sold	$400,000
Accounting and legal fees	$12,000
Advertising	$58,000
Insurance	$59,000
Maintenance and repairs	$18,000
Supplies	$6,000
Payroll expenses	$24,000
Postage	$2,000
Rent	$65,000
Licenses	$6,000
Taxes	$75,000
Telephone/Internet	$8,000
Travel/transportation/gas	$48,000
Utilities	$19,000
Other	$1,500
TOTAL EXPENSES	$801,500
Subtract Expenses from Net Income	**NET GAIN $150,500**

performed to determine if the program is effective or if the project is providing the "biggest bang for the buck." Cost analysis information is useful when presenting results to various stakeholders. This discussion of cost analysis includes cost benefits, cost effectiveness, cost utility, and cost feasibility, each providing answers to different questions. Let's begin with brief definitions prior to exploring each type of cost analysis in detail (see **Table 12-2**).

Cost-Benefit Analysis

Cost-benefit analysis compares monetary costs among several similar products, programs, or procedures. Cost-benefit analysis is typically used for making short-term decisions. Given limited resources, cost-benefit analysis is used to allocate sparse resources in community organizations (e.g., hospitals, school districts, and police and fire departments). For example, if a brand name nicotine patch offers similar benefits to a generic brand nicotine patch for smoking cessation, the cost-benefit analysis reveals the advantage of purchasing

TABLE 12-2 Summary of Types of Cost Analysis

Type of Cost Analysis	Definition
Cost benefit	Comparison of the monetary costs across several similar programs
Cost effectiveness	Comparison of total costs to total benefits
Cost utility	A type of cost-effectiveness analysis; comparison of benefits gained from different health outcomes (e.g., quality of life)
Cost feasibility	Comparison of project's cost as compared to the attained value and benefits

the generic brand nicotine patch for free distribution at the local community health fair. In other words, evaluators identify costs and benefits associated with products (e.g., environmental impact, shelf life, recyclable qualities), programs, and procedures.

Cost-benefit analyses do not include consideration of the program effectiveness, which is how well the program performs. Although the advantage of cost-benefit analysis is the ability to determine a broad comparison of overall costs across programs, there are several disadvantages. First, it is difficult to determine all of the actual costs and all of the benefits of a program. For example, should safety be measured by less crime, fewer reports of bullying in schools, less family violence, and/or fewer police reports or emergency department admissions from violence? Second, benefits associated with costs may not be seen for years. For example, the positive benefits of improving access to prenatal care may not reduce infant mortality rates for years. Third, the program costs spent this year do not have the same monetary value as when the benefits are realized. In other words, the clinic immunization supplies that cost $20,000 in 2010 might cost $40,000 in 2020. It is difficult to make an accurate cost comparison due to inflation.[4]

In addition, cost benefits are expressed in terms of the common unit of money. Evaluators may explore the positive and negative impact of changing federally subsidized community child care center hours to include Saturdays and to extend the hours from 9:00 a.m. to 5:00 p.m. to 8:00 a.m. to 8:00 p.m. This change would allow low-income parents to work evenings and Saturdays without having to secure safe alternative childcare. The evaluators would use the current daycare expenses and income to calculate the costs per child over 1 month and then calculate the budget if the hours of operation were extended. **Figure 12-4** shows an example

FIGURE 12-4 Monthly expense and income report for community clinic.

	A	B	C	D	E	F	G
1	Expenses			Income			
2	Building				Billable Patient Visits		
3		Utilities				Initial	
4		Maintenance				Intermediate	
5		Security				Extended	
6		Parking			Patient Procedures		
7	Personnel	Physicians				Laboratory	
8		Pharmacists				Office	
9		Nurse Practitioners			Pharmacy		
10		Nurses				Medications	
11		Support Technicians			Clinic Subsidy		
12		Clerks				Federal	
13	Supplies					State	
14		Office Supplies					
15		Medical Supplies					
16		Disposable Supplies					
17	Legal, Accounting, Computer Support						
18			Total				Total
19							
20							
21	Current Budget						
22		Total per month/number of patients			Total per month/number of patients		
23		$500,000/ 500 patients = $1000 per patient			$400,000/ 500 patients = $800 per patient		
24					Clinic Subsidy = $200 per patient		
25		Total	$1000 per patient		Total	$1000 per patient	
26							
27	Extended Hour Budget Projection						
28		Total per month/number of patients			Total per month/number of patients		
29		$800,000/ 900 patients = $888 per patient			$900,000/ 900 patients = $1000 per patient		
30					Clinic Subsidy = $200 per patient		
31		Total	$888 per patient		Total	$1200 per patient	
32					Net Gain: $312 per patient		

of a hypothetical budget for this scenario. However, in this sample, note that the childcare center's expenses for the current hours of operation equal the childcare center's income. In other words, the childcare center "breaks even" on its budget, but does not provide extra money for improvement or expansion. If the hours of operation are extended, the childcare center's income will likely exceed the childcare center's expenses. This occurs because some expenses, such as building and playground maintenance, legal and accounting fees, and computer support, remain the same regardless of hours of operation, because they are flat-rate expenses. The net gain of $312 per child multiplied by 900 children provides an additional $280,800 of income per month. This additional new revenue could be used to upgrade instructional equipment, install electronic monitoring computer software, and provide salary increases for the childcare center personnel. This example illustrates that a cost-benefit analysis allows the childcare center to not only increase its "bottom line," but also find ways to better serve the low-income families in the community. If the childcare center is open longer hours, the working parents have more flexibility in their work hours and less stress trying to secure safe child care during evening and Saturday hours. This change allows the childcare center to invest in new instructional equipment and supplies, increase staff salaries, and most importantly, provide safe child care that will ultimately benefit the entire community.

Another term used for making decisions, such as changing childcare center hours in our example, is called *return on investment (ROI)*. For example, the county commissioners would ask how many months it would take before the childcare center sees the projected extra revenue (return) generated from their investment in hiring and training the extra personnel to staff the extended hours of operation. One last note is to keep in mind that the sample budget (see Figure 12-4) does not calculate the cost savings to the community by improving access to child care for low-income working parents. Other benefits to the community might include higher employment rates due to extended childcare hours, lower child abuse rates because the children are in a safe environment for longer periods of time and not left with siblings or irresponsible adults during evening and Saturday hours, and the children receiving high quality care and instruction leading to improved kindergarten readiness. These long-term benefits would be counted as earned money and part of the ROI.[5]

This discussion includes some of the challenges associated with cost-benefit analysis. First, the most difficult part of cost-benefit analysis in health is calculating equivalencies between two products.[6] For example, when searching for an apartment, individuals evaluate location, distance to work and school, the nearest public transportation, availability of parking, amenities, price per square foot, cost of utilities, and overall satisfaction with floor plan and neighborhood. When selecting a healthcare service, decisions are based on subjective (personality of healthcare provider and communication style) and objective (convenience of location, type of insurance accepted, type of medical specialist required) criteria. Because all healthcare providers are required to have state licensure or board certifications, it is often difficult to determine expertise and skill. Therefore, individuals often rely on word of mouth when choosing healthcare providers—thus making equivalencies, or how a product is measured by different criteria, challenging.

An example of a tradeoff would be an individual selecting an apartment with less living space at a higher cost for an ideal, convenient location. However, in health care, tradeoffs are not limited to selecting one healthcare provider over another. For individuals on a limited budget, an example of a tradeoff could be choosing between an annual mammogram, a dental appointment, or an ophthalmology appointment. Even at the national level, it is difficult to acquire funding to pay for preventive health care, because data trends over several years or decades are required to enable decision makers to determine how preventive services affect health in the future.

Another challenge in healthcare cost-benefit analysis is related to ethics. Because cost-benefit analysis deals with monetary tradeoffs rather than effectiveness, ethical dilemmas enter into decisions. For example, if an individual has enough income to pay $1,000 per month for an apartment, then the apartment search is limited to that budget. If the apartment price exceeds the income, then after a few months, the individual could default on the rent, resulting in eviction or not paying for other important bills or services. This scenario is not the same in health care. If an individual arrives at the emergency department in need of life-saving surgery, the surgery is performed and somehow the cost is paid. If the injured individual does not have health insurance or income to pay the hospital bill, it is written off as bad debt by the hospital. When this scenario occurs over and over in numerous hospitals, the healthcare system begins to question who should and should not receive medical care. For example, ponder the following questions:

1. Should preterm infants weighing less than 1 pound be resuscitated at birth?
2. Is it a good use of resources to allow individuals over the age of 70 years to be eligible for organ transplants?
3. Should the federal government be obligated to pay enormous annual medical expenses for dialysis treatment

for morbidly obese diabetic patients when their kidneys no longer function?

4. Should the federal government pay for lung cancer treatment for individuals with a 20-year or more history of tobacco use?

5. Is palliative care the best choice of health care for individuals over 90 years of age with a cancer diagnosis?

As can be seen in these questions, it is impossible to put a value on human life or to fund every evaluation project that might improve or save a human life. It is less controversial to think in terms of prevention or reducing the risk of acquiring a disease or death.[6]

Cost-Effectiveness Analysis

Cost-effectiveness analysis is a comparison of costs among programs, procedures, or interventions designed to accomplish similar outcomes. However, unlike cost-benefit ratios, cost effectiveness is not expressed in monetary terms. As the name implies, cost effectiveness compares similar interventions in terms of usefulness or effectiveness, such as comparing the effectiveness of providing a bottle of disinfectant spray with instructions to spray the laboratory counter surface once at the end of each 8-hour shift every day versus providing a bottle of disinfectant spray with instructions to spray the laboratory counter surface every 2 hours during each shift. Although both disinfectant sprays show the same disinfectant results in the laboratory, the disinfectant spray used every 8 hours has higher effectiveness. Why? Because it is more likely that lab employees will spray and wipe down their laboratory counter space at the end of their 8-hour shift rather than needing to remember to clear off, spray, and wipe down their work area every 2 hours of their 8-hour shift.

As another example, an environmental manufacturer makes air filter A and air filter B to prevent lung disease caused by fine dust particles and improve indoor air quality in companies that specialize in refurbishing metal car parts, cabinets, and appliances. Each time the air filters are changed, the company needs to shut down for 8 hours to access and change the air filters. Air filter A is effective in removing dust particles from the indoor air ventilation system, but it must be changed every 12 months and costs $3000. Air filter B is equally effective in removing dust particles, must be changed every 3 months, and costs $150. However, the effectiveness of air filter B drops drastically by the 6th month if not changed. The company purchasing air filters is faced with a dilemma. The following list illustrates a few of the many questions that need to be considered by this company:

1. Is the cost of the expensive air filter A worth not having to shut down the company every 3 months?

2. Is it possible to use the less expensive air filter B and only change it three instead of four times per year?

3. Because this type of industry has a large turnover of employees, will using the less expensive air filter B really harm the lungs of the short-term employees?

4. Will the cost of air filter A balance out the cost of shutting down the company every 3 months for changing the less expensive air filters?

Cost-Utility Analysis

Cost-utility analysis is a type of cost-effectiveness analysis that compares quality of life gained by dollars spent used to gain it.[7] To understand cost-utility analysis, it is necessary to understand the terms *quality-adjusted life years (QALY)* and *disability-adjusted life years (DALY)*. As expected, cost-utility analysis is controversial, because it attempts to place value on the health status of human individuals and society. Unlike cost effectiveness, which compares similar benefits or outcomes, cost-utility analysis compares health interventions or procedures with different benefits.

Quality-Adjusted Life Years

Quality-adjusted life years is a calculation combining quantity and quality of health to quantify outcomes based on treatment or other activities that influence health. Evaluators measure QALY by using secondary data from large epidemiological studies and large databases across similar diseases or health conditions to compare and predict life expectancies. QALY measures the cost of producing 1 year of quality living. Quality living data are collected and defined in several ways, including self-report of individuals, medical chart reviews, and caregiver assessment. For example, one 24-year-old person with spinal cord paralysis is involved in paraplegic sporting events and ranks QALY as good, while another 24-year-old person with spinal cord paralysis becomes socially isolated due to depression and ranks QALY as poor. Life circumstances vary as to how individuals view their quality of life. From the evaluators' viewpoint, QALY is a single unit that measures the state of health on a ranked scale from 0 (immediate death) to 100 (perfect health). It is possible for the calculation to yield a negative number when an individual is living indefinitely with poor quality of life.[8]

Cost-utility analysis calculates QALY in years.[9] If it costs $100,000 to gain 1 year of life for an individual with a specific illness, the cost utility is $100,000 per year. With limited healthcare resources, cost-utility analysis compares maximum benefits gained from different health treatments to produce health outcomes. In other words, cost-utility analysis influences whether an individual should or should not be treated for a specific disease.[10] In general, health interventions that yield low QALYs are given fewer scarce resources. Although this type of calculation is appealing to decision makers, cost-utility analysis raises several questions. How is quality of life defined among individuals? Are the calculations valid and measure what is intended to be measured? Are the calculations reliable or repeatable across populations? Is one population adversely affected by the calculation more so than another? For example, is one ethnicity more likely to suffer from a specific disease than another ethnic group? Lastly, what ethical issues are involved in each of the cost-utility calculations?[11]

Disability-Adjusted Life Years

Another type of cost-utility analysis is disability-adjusted life years. DALY measures the years one lives with a disability and years of life lost due to premature death from that disability.[12] When individuals experience a disease or disability due to environmental exposure, natural disaster, or health behavior risks, the term *disability-adjusted life year* is used. One DALY is defined as 1 lost year of "healthy" life. Across a population, the total DALYs measure the gap between no disease and disability. The World Health Organization developed DALY to measure a population's health by comparing nonfatal and fatal outcomes when prioritizing health resources.[12] DALYs are used to calculate the magnitude of disease and health risks globally,[13–15] nationally, and locally. DALY estimates are also used to measure the effectiveness of prevention programs for specific diseases[16] when recommending funding priorities.[17] Although DALY calculations are not always agreed upon by global experts, the measurements provide

a standardized cost-effectiveness analysis of public health interventions in low- and middle-income countries.[18,19]

Even with the limitations, DALYs use standardized disability definitions to compare the health impact of a wide range of medical conditions.[20] If DALYs are the only calculation used, it is possible that factors causing disabilities receive less funding than if several measurements are used. See **Box 12-2** for an example of DALY calculation. As with any social determinant of health, it is necessary to investigate all aspects of the disability including the functional limitations, physical activities, and social interaction.[21]

Cost-Feasibility Analysis

Cost-feasibility analysis is defined as a comparison of the cost required for the project compared to the overall projected value of the project.[22–24] For example, a new 5-year flu vaccine is hypothesized as valuable for a common, but non-life-threatening flu illness; however, the cost is prohibitive for the general population. Evaluators use a SWOT (strengths [advantages], weaknesses [disadvantages], opportunities [prospects for growth], and threats [awareness of internal or external warnings]) analysis to conduct a cost-feasibility study. Gathering data to support each component of the SWOT analysis allows evaluators to report comprehensive findings to the stakeholders and decision makers.[24] SWOT analyses are also used to evaluate current program objectives or to determine future objectives based on results of a previous SWOT analysis.

For a cost-feasibility study, evaluators conduct a SWOT analysis to explore the viability of a current or future project.

BOX 12-2 Example of DALY Calculation

DALY (disability-adjusted life year) = YLL (years of life lost) + YLD (years lost due to disability)

YLL = N (number of deaths) × L (standard life expectancy at age of death in years)

YLD = I (number of incident cases) × DW(disability weight) × L (average duration of the case until remission or death in years)

Example

In the collapse of a mine, 25 miners were killed. In that community, the average life expectancy is 68 years. In addition, 18 miners were injured in the mine collapse. Their disabilities were serious and considered to be 0.6 on a scale of 0 (perfect health) to 9 (dead). Most of the disabled miners lived 8 years with their disabilities.

DALY = (25 deaths × 68 years) + (18 × 0.6 × 8 years)

1786.4 (DALY) = 1700 (YLL) + 86.4 (YLD)

This information is used to alter mine safety policies at the state and national levels.

Data from Grosse SD, Lollar DJ, Campbell VA, Chamie M. Disability and Disability-Adjusted Life Years: Not the Same. *Public Health Rep.* 2009; 124(2):197–202.

For example, if the rural community clinic is considering expanding the pediatric services, evaluators conduct a cost-feasibility study to explore all aspects of the return on the investment. Keep in mind that the costs are not only monetary but are also related to community member satisfaction, the community need for more pediatric care and services, the availability of pediatricians and pediatric nurse practitioners to staff the new services, costs related to converting current space into pediatric examination rooms, and the costs of purchasing pediatric equipment and supplies.

Another way to think about cost feasibility is to answer this question: Is the problem worth solving at a reasonable cost? To answer this question, evaluators must explore four different aspects of feasibility: technical, economic, operational, and organizational. Technical feasibility investigates whether it is possible to solve the problem with existing technology. For example, does the rural clinic have the reliable Internet access needed to obtain laboratory results and medical procedure results from the urban metropolitan hospital? Economic feasibility compares the cost of solving the problem versus the benefits of solving the problem. If the costs are excessive, the benefits are not obtainable. Operational feasibility investigates if the program implementation is compatible with the environment (e.g., physical, political, economic, or administrative). Take, for example, the operational feasibility of implementing pediatric services at the rural clinic. Lastly, organizational feasibility relates to the strategic plan of the organization. If the proposed project is not in alignment with the long-term goals of the organization, then there is no point in moving forward with funding and implementation of the project.

SUMMARY

This chapter began with a detailed description of types of budgets, including personal, evaluation, financial plans, and profit and loss statements. This discussion was followed with an introduction to the various types of cost analysis. Evaluators use cost analysis techniques to determine the most effective and efficient health procedures, treatments, and programs.

CASE STUDY

About 8 years ago, Scott and Andrew opened Good Eats, a small, non-franchised sandwich shop across the street from the front entrance of the community hospital. Good Eats is well known in the community. They purchase their food locally from the farmers' market, community garden, and certified organic dairies. They sponsor an annual 5K and 15K race for the hospital charity foundation plus they hire high school students in the summer to gain experience in food preparation. They offer generous internships to community college students interested in food safety, community gardening, and small business entrepreneur opportunities. On the first Monday evening of the month, they stay open late and offer a free cooking class on using healthy foods on a budget. On the third Saturday morning of each month, they offer free Zumba exercise classes in the parking lot. Good Eats is a valuable partner in the health of this small town.

Because Good Eats is financially successful, Scott and Andrew decided to extend the hours of operation and add more food and drink choices to the menu without compromising on using locally grown fruits and vegetables. For this change, they decided to survey their customers (see **Table 12-3**). They placed a stack of survey postcards on each table and at the take-out cash register. Each customer was given a 5% discount for returning the completed survey postcard at the checkout register.

The survey results overwhelmingly revealed the customers' desire for extended hours, specialty drinks, healthy choices, and ready-made food choices. Because hospital employees and visitors have limited time, the outdoor seating idea was rejected by survey respondents. Scott and Andrew decided to conduct a cost analysis to determine the advantages and disadvantages of going forward with their ideas. First, they considered the ROI by conducting a SWOT analysis.

Strengths:
  Increasing exercise opportunities in the community
  Offering free cooking classes each month to introduce healthy eating
  Offering healthy food choices to hospital employees, visitors, and community members
Weaknesses:
  Longer work hours for Scott and Andrew
  More time away from their families
  Less time to connect with local growers and dairies
  Less time to work with high school and community college students
Opportunities:
  Offer employment for more community citizens
  Encourage option of opening a second Good Eats on the opposite side of town
Threats:
  Risk of growing too fast and taking on too much
  Not recuperating the financial investment used for expansion of meals and hours of operation
  The opening of a similar restaurant by a community outsider

TABLE 12-3 Good Eats Survey

Please circle one response for each question.		
Would you like the hours of operation extended to 6:00 a.m. to 3:00 p.m.?	Yes	No
Would you like to like to have healthy breakfast choices on the menu?	Yes	No
Would you like to have healthy breakfast food available all day?	Yes	No
Which option do you generally use?	Eat-in	Take-out
Which items would you like to see added to the menu:		
Specialty coffee or tea drinks	Yes	No
Fresh fruit blended drinks	Yes	No
Certified organic food choices	Yes	No
Macrobiotic food choices	Yes	No
Vegetarian food choices	Yes	No
Would you purchase ready-made food choices available in a refrigerated case for immediate pick-up?	Yes	No
Would you like the option of placing orders online?		
Would you like to have outdoor seating available?	Yes	No
Any other comments:		

After examining the SWOT analysis, Scott and Andrew decided that they would go forward with obtaining a bank loan for the building expansion. They hired a structural engineer and architect to design the expansion. They decided to close Good Eats for 8 weeks for the construction. After the building permits were obtained, the demolition of the back wall began. The local restaurant health inspector was called to check the first step of the construction. Scott and Andrew were not concerned, because they had not received any restaurant inspection citations in 8 years. The quarterly restaurant inspection involved temperature of refrigerators and ovens for food preparation as well as food dates of expiration, cleanliness of counters, floors, tables, and restrooms. However, the inspection today revealed that the demolished back wall had mold and mildew that extended into the east side wall. With this bad news, Scott and Andrew decided to draw money from their joint business savings account to replace the side wall drywall to remove the mold and mildew. The architect moved the kitchen to the west side and converted the back area into the take-out area.

Now that Good Eats has been open for 12 months after the renovation, Scott and Andrew meet with their accountant to determine if the changes were profitable. See **Figure 12-5** for their annual profit and loss statement.

Given that Scott and Andrew work longer hours and maintain the same salary, they are wondering if they made the correct decision to expand the menu and hours of operation for Good Eats.

FIGURE 12-5 Good eats profit and loss summary.

	A	B	C	D	E	F	G
1	Income		Day	Month		Year	
2	Take-out	$ 2,050	30	$ 61,500	12	$ 738,000	
3	Eat-in	$ 1,475	30	$ 44,250	12	$ 531,000	
4							$ 1,269,000
5							
6	Expenses	Salary	People	Month		Year	
7	Owner Salaries	$ 3,400	2	$ 6,800	12	$ 81,600	
8	Staff (preconstruction)	$ 7,400	4	$ 29,600	12	$ 355,200	
9	New Staff	$ 9,300	4	$ 37,200	12	$ 446,400	$ 883,200
10							
11	Gas/Electricity			$ 387	12	$ 4,644	
12	Telephone/WIFI			$ 376	12	$ 4,512	
13	Water/Sewer			$ 147	12	$ 1,764	
14	Disposable Paper Goods			$ 1,600	12	$ 19,200	
15	Advertising			$ 900	12	$ 10,800	
16	Community Events			$ 450	12	$ 5,400	
17	Equipment Maintenance			$ 670	12	$ 8,040	$ 54,360
18							
19	Fruits/Vegetables			$ 4,600	12	$ 55,200	
20	Breads/Pastas/Pastries			$ 1,900	12	$ 22,800	
21	Dairy/Cheese/Meat			$ 4,700	12	$ 56,400	
22	Beverages			$ 1,300	12	$ 15,600	
23	Condiments/Spices/Oil			$ 870	12	$ 10,440	$ 160,440
24							
25	Sales Taxes		0.06	$ 1,269,000		$ 76,140	
26	Property Tax			$ 320	12	$ 3,840	
27	Payroll Taxes		0.08	$ 883,200		$ 70,656	
28	Employee Health Insurance	$ 130	8	$ 1,040	12	$ 12,480	
29	Loan Payment			$ 980	12	$ 11,760	$ 174,876
30							$ 1,272,876
31							$ (3,876)

Case Study Questions

1. What would you suggest that Scott and Andrew change to increase their profits?
2. Scott and Andrew want to remain closely connected to the community activities. How could they increase their community involvement as well as their profits?
3. Each new staff member works 40 hours per week. Scott and Andrew pay for the health insurance of all eight new staff members. What is the average hourly salary of the staff hired after the construction? (Answer: $13.51 per hour)
4. The preconstruction staff members work 30 hours per week by choice. What is the average salary of the preconstruction staff? (Answer: $14.34 per hour)
5. Since Good Eats lost $3876 over the last year, they went to the bank and asked to reduce their loan payment from $980 to $650 per month. How much money will that save Good Eats? (Answer: $3960)
6. List at least seven ways in which Good Eats is improving the public health of their community?

STUDENT ACTIVITIES

The following is an example of a personal budget. Study the budget and then answer the questions about it.

Brad is 26 years old and works in a small marketing firm in a medium-sized city. This budget reflects his income and expenses for a typical month (see **Table 12-4**).

1. How much money does Brad earn (before taxes) in a:
   Week:
   Month:
   Year:
2. How much money in state and federal taxes is withheld from Brad's paycheck every 2 weeks?
3. Calculate Brad's take-home pay for 1 month.
4. How much discretionary money does Brad have after paying his living expenses from his take-home income?
5. Suppose Brad wants to start saving more money. He considers several amounts. How much money would he need to save each month if he saved 5%, 10%, and 15% of his discretionary money each month?
   5%:
   10%:
   15%:
6. Suppose Brad wants to save the maximum amount of 15% of his discretionary money each month. How much money does Brad then have left over to use

each week for going out, paying for gas for his car, and entertainment?

TABLE 12-4 Brad's Budget

Category	
Income	
Salary $23.00 per hour	40 hours per week
Expenses	
Federal income tax	22%
State income tax	3%
Social Security/Medicare	6.2%
Medical insurance	$64.00 per month
Life insurance	$15.00 per month
401(k) contribution	4%
Savings	?
Rent	$750 per month
Auto payment	$230 per month
Auto insurance	$160 per month
Water	$24 per month
Gas	$60 per month
Electricity	$75 per month
Cable/Internet	$140 per month
Phone/cell phone	$93 per month
Other utilities	$34 per month

Answers

1. How much money does Brad earn (before taxes) in a:
   Week: $920
   Month: $3680
   Year: $47,840
2. How much money in state and federal taxes is withheld from Brad's paycheck every 2 weeks? $574.
3. Calculate Brad's take-home pay for 1 month. $2606.24
4. How much discretionary money does Brad have after paying his living expenses from his take-home income? $1040.24
5. Suppose Brad wants to start saving more money. He considers several amounts. How much money would

he need to save each month if he saved 5%, 10%, and 15% of his discretionary money each month?

5%: $52.01

10%: $104.02

15%: $156.03

6. Suppose Brad wants to save the maximum amount of money each month. How much money does Brad then have left over to use each week for going out, paying for gas for his car, and entertainment? $221.05

REFERENCES

1. De Navas-Walt C, Proctor BD, Smith JC. U.S. Census Bureau. Current Population Reports, P60-243. *Income, Poverty and Health Insurance Coverage in the United States: 2011*. Washington, DC: U.S. Government Printing Office; 2012.

2. Families USA. 2013 Federal Poverty Guidelines. Available at: http://www.familiesusa.org/resources/tools-for-advocates/guides/federal-poverty-guidelines.html. Accessed May 24, 2014.

3. United States Department of Labor. Minimum Wage Laws in the States. Available at: http://www.dol.gov/whd/minwage/america.htm. Accessed February 3, 2013.

4. The Organisation for Economic Co-operation and Development (OECD). OECD Health Data 2012: U.S. Health Care System from an International Perspective. Available at: http://www.oecd.org/unitedstates/HealthSpendingInUSA_HealthData2012.pdf. Accessed June 1, 2014.

5. Rochester Institute of Technology, Department of Outreach Education and Training. Cost Benefit Analysis. Available at: https://www.rit.edu/~w-outrea/training/Module5/M5_CostBenefitAnalysis.pdf. Accessed November 3, 2012.

6. Watkins T. San Jose State University Department of Economics. An Introduction to Cost Benefit Analysis. Available at: http://www.sjsu.edu/faculty/watkins/cba.htm. Accessed November 3, 2012.

7. The World Health Organization. Cost-utility analysis. In: *Introduction to Drug Utilization Research*. Oslo, Norway: The World Health Organization; 2003. Available at: http://apps.who.int/medicinedocs/en/d/Js4876e/5.4.html. Accessed May 24, 2014.

8. Bandolier. QALY. Available at: http://www.medicine.ox.ac.uk/bandolier/booth/glossary/QALY.html. Accessed May 24, 2014.

9. Pettinger T. Cost Utility and Cost Effectiveness Analysis. http://www.economicshelp.org/blog/93/economics/cost-utility-and-cost-effectiveness-analysis/. Accessed September 23, 2013.

10. Vanhook P. Cost-utility analysis: a method of quantifying the value of registered nurses. *Online J Issues Nurs*. 2007;12(3).

11. McGregor M. Cost–utility analysis: use QALYs only with great caution. *CMAJ*. 2003;168(4):433–434.

12. The World Health Organization. Health Statistics and Health Information Systems. Metrics: Disability-Adjusted Life Year. Available at: http://www.who.int/healthinfo/global_burden_disease/metrics_daly/en/. Accessed May 24, 2014.

13. Murray CJ, Acharya AK. Understanding DALYs (disability-adjusted life years). *J Health Econ*. 1997;16(6):703–730.

14. Murray CJL, Lopez AD, eds. *The Global Burden of Disease: A Comprehensive Assessment of Mortality and Disability from Diseases, Injuries, and Risk factors in 1990 and Projected to 2020*. Cambridge, MA: Harvard University Press; 1996.

15. Lopez AD, Mathers CD, Ezzati M, Jamison DT, Murray CJL, eds. *Global Burden of Disease and Risk Factors*. Washington, DC: World Bank; 2006.

16. Lopez AD, Mathers CD, Ezzati M, Jamison DT, Murray CJ. Global and regional burden of disease and risk factors, 2001: systematic analysis of population health data. *Lancet*. 2006;367:1747–1757.

17. Cadilhac DA, Carter RC, Thrift AG, Dewey HM. Why invest in a national public health program for stroke? An example using Australian data to estimate the potential benefits and cost implications. *Health Policy*. 2007;83(2-3):287–294.

18. Gross CP, Anderson GF, Powe NR. The relation between funding by the National Institutes of Health and the burden of disease. *N Engl J Med*. 1999;340(24):1881–1887.

19. Schackman BR, Neukermans CP, Fontain SN, Nolte C, Joseph P, Pape JW, Fitzgerald DW. Cost-effectiveness of rapid syphilis screening in prenatal HIV testing programs in Haiti. *PLos Med*. 2007;4(5):e183.

20. Thacker SB, Stroup DF, Carande-Kulis V, Marks JS, Roy K, Gerberding JL. Measuring the public's health. *Public Health Rep*. 2006;121(1):14–22.

21. Grosse SD, Lollar DJ, Campbell VA, Chamie M. Disability-adjusted life years: not the same. *Public Health Rep*. 2009;124(2):197–202.

22. Young GIM. Feasibility studies. *Appraisal Journal*. 1970;38(3):376–383.

23. Jyoth BN, Babu GR, Krishna IVM. Object oriented and multi-scale image analysis: strengths, weaknesses, opportunities and threats—a review. *J Computer Science*. 2008;4(9):706–712.

24. Hofstrand D. Iowa State University Extension and Outreach. When to Do and How to Use a Feasibility Study. Available at: http://www.extension.iastate.edu/agdm/wholefarm/html/c5-64.html. Accessed May 24, 2014.

Reports and Presentations

CHAPTER OBJECTIVES

By the end of this chapter, students will be able to:

- Discuss the key steps in writing evaluation and technical reports.
- Define the essential elements of a report.
- Summarize how to develop successful oral presentations.
- Discuss the steps used to create simple and concise poster presentations.

KEY TERMS

elements of reports
oral presentations
poster presentations
written reports

INTRODUCTION

After evaluators spend endless hours conducting their evaluation, it is time to present their findings. This chapter provides details on how to create effective written reports, oral presentations, panel discussions, lectures, and poster presentations related to evaluations. Types of written reports are discussed and the developments of each element are defined, including reference styles and overcoming writer's block. Second, effective ways to communicate are reviewed, including oral presentations, ways to prepare useful slide presentations, and powerful rehearsal strategies. Lastly, the chapter concludes with techniques to create winning poster presentations with key bullet points.

TYPES OF WRITTEN REPORTS

It is not unusual for students to experience a feeling of dread when given an assignment to write a report. However, because writing is an essential skill throughout your academic studies as well as in your future professional careers, it is important to learn some basic components of report writing. Prior to discussing types of reports, we divide this section into manageable components in order to make composing the whole report less daunting.

Let's begin with the discussion of types of reports. Keep in mind that even though each type of report is unique, every report should be written clearly and concisely. Evaluation reports present the findings of an evaluation, including best practices, processes, program impact, and long-term outcomes. Evaluation reports may be published in peer-reviewed journals. However, there are evaluation firms that conduct high-quality evaluations whose reports are not always published in peer-reviewed journals. Their evaluation findings are available on the Internet as technical reports or in governmental documents, such as final reports produced for the U.S. Government Accountability Office. Evaluation reports provide the reader with recommendations for future investigations. Another type of report is a technical report that aims to state how the problem was solved or to propose solutions. Technical reports are generally not published in peer-reviewed journals and are written for a specific audience (e.g., stakeholders, board members, nonprofit organizations, funding agency). Technical reports are written using specialized language for an audience of experts, such as computer science software programmers.

After determining the type of report that is appropriate, the next step is to answer a few questions about the purpose of the report.

Who is the audience?

- If the audience is a professor, then it is likely that the professor explained the purpose of the written assignment in class or in the syllabus. If students have additional questions, they should ask for greater clarification from the professor before starting the assignment.
- If the audience members are also stakeholders (e.g., funding agency members, community members, board of directors), then the report should address their concerns.

In all situations, reports should be well organized and written in clear, understandable language. For example, if the report targets computer science engineers implementing an update of a county public health department's electronic medical records software, the report does not need to define the technical terms understood by the computer science engineers. However, if the same report is written for the county health administrators, the technical language is replaced with easy-to-understand terms.

How will the report be used?

- If the report is for a course assignment, the report will be used for a grade. Therefore, the report is written to match the grading rubric provided by the professor.
- If the report is used for seeking additional funding for a community report, the report emphasizes current results plus recommendations and future needs.
- If the report is used to obtain buy-in from stakeholders, then the report focuses on the positive effects of the current activities.

Once the audience and purpose of the report are identified, the writer thinks about these questions:

- What are the specific elements of the report (e.g., number of pages, font, font size, margin allowances, placement of tables and figures, and reference style)?
- What is the explicit message or aim of the report?
- What are the key points you wish to communicate?
- What information that is needed to make your findings understandable should be collected prior to writing the report (e.g., maps, data, graphs, tables, figures)?

After these questions are addressed, it is necessary to outline the report. Begin the outline with basic information. Even the simplest of outlines helps to start the writing process (see **Table 13-1**). More details are added to each segment of

TABLE 13-1 Simple Report Outline

Introduction
Background
Key Points
1.
2.
3.
4.
Recommendations
Conclusion
References

this outline later in this chapter. However, it is best to start with a basic outline rather than add all of the details in the beginning.

As you create the outline, it is useful to think about the readers. The report provides information to meet the needs of the audience. Review **Table 13-2**. In sample 1, the audience is interested in the overall strengths, weaknesses, opportunities, and threats of the clinic. Sample 2 directs the audience to specific areas within the clinic. Both outlines could be either appropriate or inappropriate based on the designated needs of the audience.[1]

ELEMENTS OF THE REPORT

Now that the simple outline is complete, let's begin to delve into the specific elements of the report. For this discussion, the elements expand the basic outline and provide greater detail for the reader. Although most reports have similar sections, if you are writing for a specific journal, you should verify their author guidelines. Author guidelines describe the required components of manuscript and referencing style desired by the agency or publisher requesting the report (see **Table 13-3**).

Now let's explore each element of the report. Under each section, a more detailed outline or description is provided in the discussion.

Title Page

The title page includes the title, author(s), and date of submission. In some situations, the name of the funding agency or report recipient is listed on the title page. The title of the report should describe the scope of the report in a few words. Here are a few examples of titles.

Incomplete description:
  Forms of Violence Directed at Women
Complete description:

TABLE 13-2 Example of Two Basic Report Outlines

Sample 1: Basic Report Outline		Sample 2: Basic Report Outline	
Strengths	Factory Manufacturing and Personnel	Factory Manufacturing and Personnel	Strengths
	Accounting and Finance		Weaknesses
	Plant Maintenance and Grounds		Opportunities
Weaknesses	Factory Manufacturing and Personnel		Threats
	Accounting and Finance	Accounting and Finance	Strengths
	Plant Maintenance and Grounds		Weaknesses
Opportunities	Factory Manufacturing and Personnel		Opportunities
	Accounting and Finance		Threats
	Plant Maintenance and Grounds	Plant Maintenance and Grounds	Strengths
Threats	Factory Manufacturing and Personnel		Weaknesses
	Accounting and Finance		Opportunities
	Plant Maintenance and Grounds		Threats

Data from Virginia Polytechnic Institute and State University. Technical Writing-Progress Reports. Available at: http://wiz.cath.vt.edu/tw/TechnicalWriting/ProgressReports/components4.htm.

Forms of Violence Directed at Women: Success of Support Groups Offered at Residential Facilities for Women and Their Children

Incomplete description:

Ethnic Disparities in Infant Mortality Rates

Complete description:

Ethnic Disparities in Infant Mortality Rates: A Comparison of White, African American, and Hispanic Populations from 2000–2010 in the United States

Incomplete description:

Breastfeeding Rates Among Women in the United States

Complete description:

Knowledge, Attitudes, and Beliefs Related to Breastfeeding for Working Women in the United States: 2000–2010 National Health and Nutrition Examination Survey (NHANES)

Table of Contents

The table of contents provides the reader with a list of the major and minor segments of the report. Because page numbers are provided, it allows the reader to turn to the section that is of most interest. It indicates how the information is organized. All tables and figures are included in the table of contents.

TABLE 13-3 Sample Author Guidelines

Taylor and Francis	http://www.tandf.co.uk/journals/authors/rcrsauth.pdf
Springer Publishing Company	http://www.springerpub.com/content/downloads/Springer_Publishing_Manuscript_Guidelines.pdf
American Psychological Association	http://www.apa.org/pubs/authors/instructions.aspx
American Journal of Public Health	http://ajph.aphapublications.org/userimages/ContentEditor/1318438422261/Instructions_for_Authors.pdf
American Journal of Evaluation	http://www.sagepub.com/journals/Journal201729/manuscriptSubmission
American Journal of Preventative Medicine	http://cdn.elsevier.com/promis_misc/AMEPRE_gfa_dec2013.pdf

Abstract or Executive Summary

Although abstracts or executive summaries are shown first, they are written last. The abstract is a summary of the entire report. Abstracts are provided at the beginning of scientific or academic reporting. They provide a concise summary of complex research. This allows a reader to ascertain the purpose and main findings of the research and decide whether or not they want to continue reading. Abstracts are usually written after all other parts of the report so that the findings and recommendations are reported accurately and in line with how they are reported elsewhere in the report. Always double-check the author guidelines, because abstracts and executive summaries often have length limits. For example, abstracts may range from 50 to 400 words in length. Within the word limit, the author tells the whole story: what the goals and objectives were, how the goals and objectives were evaluated, what the data analysis methods were, how the results aligned with the goals and objectives, and what the recommendations are. In a similar fashion, executive summaries are usually two to three pages and also tell the overall summary of the evaluation report findings.[2] In the report, the abstract or executive summary is placed on a separate page in the report and written as a single paragraph without any indentation. Keep in mind that an abstract or executive summary may be the only portion of the evaluation report read by a general audience. Therefore, it is important that these sections include the most important findings or key points, are clearly written, and are logically organized.

Introduction

An introduction is not a rewritten version of the abstract; rather, the introduction sets the tone of the report (see **Box 13-1**). The introduction is divided into three sections:

1. The statement of the problem provides a brief review of the issues and states the accomplishments completed to date.

2. The purpose of the evaluation briefly describes how this study builds on or adds to the current knowledge.

3. The scope of the evaluation explains the methods used in this research or evaluation.

The extent of specific details in the introduction depends on the audience. For example, a technical report for colleagues needs fewer details and explanation than a quarterly report for a funding agency, such as the National Institutes of Health.

Literature Review or Background

A literature review or background section provides the current knowledge regarding a given topic area, including substantive, theoretical, and methodological findings (see **Box 13-2**). The literature review starts with a broad focus and ends narrowly. Depending on the scope of the topic, the literature review is either comprehensive or selective. The decision between comprehensive or selective is based on the purpose of the report and possible length restrictions. If there is no length restriction as in a thesis or dissertation, a comprehensive review of the literature is used; for example, the historical overview of how public health responded to HIV/AIDS in the United States since the 1980s. A selective review of literature is typical for journal articles. The selective literature review begins with a broad overview of the historical side of the topic and ends with specific targeted literature related to the need for further evaluation of prevention programs. Developing a detailed outline ensures maximum clarity and explains the need for the further evaluations. The outline shows the connection between the known body of knowledge on the topic and its relationship to the proposed program evaluations. A selective

---

BOX 13-1 Outline of an Introduction Section

Introduction
    Purpose of the evaluation
    Goals and objectives
    Scope of the evaluation

BOX 13-2 Outline of a Literature Review Section

Literature review or background
    State limit of the review
        Broad topic: historical background or specific limitations
        Focus topic
        Narrow focus of topic
        Gap in knowledge for the topic
        Transition from review to purpose of reported evaluation

literature review is limited and clearly states those limits for the reader. For example, "This review of the literature is focused on evaluation of HIV/AIDS prevention programs conducted after 2010." Because literature reviews summarize knowledge, direct quotes are sometimes included in this section. Lastly, literature reviews end with a brief summary that serves as a transition to the next component of the report.

Methods

The methods section of a written report shows how an evaluator addressed the goals and objectives of an evaluation (see **Box 13-3**). The methods section is often used to judge the validity of the evaluation. The best way to organize the methods section is to think of a recipe. For example, cookies taste awful if the recipe fails to include the key ingredient of sugar. In the same respect, if this section fails to include enough detail, readers are unable to judge the validity of the findings and duplicate the study. Evaluators duplicate evaluation studies to defend or refute the results. This section, like other sections, must be organized in a logical sequence: what was evaluated, what was found, what interpretations were made, and what judgments were made. Use short informative headings and subheadings. An easy way to remember the components of this section are: who, what, when, where, why, and how.

What is the design of the evaluation?

- If a theory provided the foundation for the evaluation, describe it. Which theory was selected, and why was it selected? If no theory was used, explain why that decision was made.
- How does the design align with the goals and objectives of the evaluation?

> ## BOX 13-3 Outline of a Methods Section
>
> Methods
>   Institutional review board approval process
>   Study design
>   Sampling
>   Setting
>   Pilot test
>   Data collection

- Identify the design and describe why it was selected. Did the design include a pretest and posttest?

Who are the participants? How will the sample be selected?

- Describe the inclusion and exclusion criteria for participants.
- Identify why the inclusion and exclusion criteria were used.
- Describe how the participants were recruited.
- How many participants were needed for the evaluation? How many participants actually participated in the evaluation? Describe why the number of participants was not reached.
- How many participants were lost to follow-up in the study? Why?

Where did the evaluation take place?

- Why was this setting selected for the evaluation?
- What made the chosen site ideal or unique for this evaluation?
- If there were multiple sites, how and why were the sites chosen?
- How were the data collected?

Quantitative data collection:

- What surveys, questionnaires, or instruments were used to collect data?
- How were the instruments collected: mailed, in person, or online?
- How were the data entered for analysis?
- Were some surveys tested with double entry to verify accuracy?
- Were any tests conducted to verify reliability and validity?

Qualitative data collection:

- What types of data were collected: interviews, focus groups, or existing documents?
- Describe the interview/focus group guidelines.

Prior to describing the methods used, evaluators must acknowledge that institutional review board approval was obtained prior to conducting any portion of the evaluation.

Results

The results section describes the findings of the evaluation (see **Box 13-4**). Results are presented concisely. Results tell us the statistics found by quantitative statistical analysis or themes found through qualitative analysis. Generally, if collected, the demographics are presented first, so readers learn

Data analysis
 Statistical methods
 Qualitative methods
Response to goals and objectives
 Description of analysis output
 Tables, graphs, and figures

about the studied population prior to reviewing the results. While a few demographics are typically discussed briefly in the narrative, all demographics are shown in a table format (see **Table 13-4**).

Keep in mind that tables and figures are labeled sequentially throughout the document (e.g., Table 1, Table 2, Figure 1, Table 3, and Figure 2). If the report is divided into chapters, the tables and figures are numbered within each chapter. For example, for Chapter 1 there is Table 1.1 and Table 1.2, for Chapter 2 there is Table 2.1, Table 2.2, Figure 2.1, and Figure 2.2, and so on.

After the demographics, the data used to address the goals and objectives are presented. For example, if a paired samples

t-test was used to determine the difference between pretest surveys and posttest surveys, those results are presented. For example, "Of the 224 high school staff who responded, there was a pretest mean score of 64 and posttest mean score of 97, with a t-test showing a statistically significant difference ($t = 7.08$; $p = 0.03$)." For each objective, the same process is followed throughout the results section. Keep in mind that evaluators do not merely cut and paste the statistical results from the statistical software package into the results section of the report. Evaluators also do not add any additional statistics outside of those that are meant to address the goals and objectives. For example, evaluators notice an interesting correlation in the data analysis while they are conducting the statistics. This interesting correlation is not added to the results section merely because it is a unique finding. If this new finding is indeed unique, it is advised that the evaluator review it further and perhaps report it in the discussion or in another manuscript.

Discussion, Conclusion, Recommendations, and Future Research

The purpose of the discussion section is to compare the results of the current evaluation to a previous evaluation of the same project, the results of similar evaluations, or a previous evaluation published in the literature (see **Box 13-5**). Keep in mind that some agencies require an evaluation of their community programs every 5 years. The results of the current evaluation may defend or refute the results of a previous evaluation, with

TABLE 13-4 Sample of Demographic Data Presented in the Results Section

Description of Demographic Data	Table A. Demographic Data ($n = 224$)	
For demographics, 224 (86%) of the high school staff responded to the survey. For gender, there were 107 (48%) females and 117 (52%) males. For age, there were 78 (35%) clinic workers in the 20–29 age group, 83 (37%) in the 30–39 age group, 43 (20%) in the 40–49 age group, and 20 (8%) in the 50+ age group. As for education, there were 6 (3%) of the high school staff reporting less than a high school degree, 17 (7%) with a high school diploma, 19 (8%) with some college credits, 153 (68%) with a college degree, and 29 (14%) with a graduate degree.	Variable	Number (%)
	Gender	Females: 107 (48%)
		Males: 117 (52%)
	Age	20–29 years: 78 (35%)
		30–39 years: 83 (37%)
		40–49 years: 43 (20%)
		50+ years: 20 (8%)
	Education	< High school: 6 (3%)
		High school: 17 (7%)
		Some college: 19 (8%)
		College degree: 153 (68%)
		Graduate degree: 29 (14%)

evaluators adding what is different about their sample or methods that may have contributed to the differences in the findings. When findings vary from study to study you cannot assume evaluator error or evaluation weakness, but rather the differences could be based on study participants, geographical location, age, culture, income, or education. For example, the participants of the previous evaluation lived in an urban area, while the participants of the current evaluation lived in a remote rural area. This geographical difference could have contributed to the difference in findings. Another example may show that results for one age group of participants are different from another age group for the same intervention.

Limitations are the weaknesses of the evaluation that are reported in the discussion section. Because all evaluations have limitations, it is advised that the final report should reflect any recognized weaknesses. For example, if the results show that only 16% of the participants completed the post-test survey, it should be noted as a weakness. This weakness may be due to an issue with the study design, how the survey was administered, the survey questions themselves, or the number of participants lost during follow-up. Putting this information in the limitations section allows evaluators to improve future evaluations by addressing these issues at the beginning. However, it is up to the evaluator to state what methods were utilized to try to improve the response rate, such as reminder postcards and phone messages. On the other hand, a weakness may not have been noticed until late in the research and could not be corrected.

In the limitations section it is also important to pay attention to the language of the discussion. Even if the project had numerous major limitations, it is critical not to assign blame or make excuses for any aspect or weakness of the evaluation. Focus on presenting possible solutions to establish trust

rather than doubt in the report. The information presented in the report remains neutral and without commendation.

Conclusions are a final brief interpretation of the results. Most conclusions are written in a few sentences or paragraphs. Keep in mind that the abstract or executive summary and the conclusion are the most frequently read segments of reports. The information in the conclusion should be presented in order of importance. The conclusion does not include any speculation, but rather only the evidence supported by the results of the current study. Recommendations follow the conclusion and present direct suggestions or action items for the decision makers reading the report. If an evaluation team has a list of suggestions, the recommendations may be presented in bullet points (see **Box 13-6**).

Future evaluation is the final section of the narrative portion of the report. This section states specifically what further evaluations the evaluators recommend. For example, if two published evaluation studies had similar results and the current study refuted those results, evaluators suggest conducting a similar evaluation to confirm the newly found information. For example, if three evaluations reported that engaging urban high school students in community service

---

BOX 13-7 Outline of References and Appendices

References
Appendices

BOX 13-8 Useful Websites for Referencing Styles

The *Publication Manual of the American Psychological Association* (or simply "APA") is most commonly used to cite sources within the social sciences. The following website provides a brief summary of this style:
http://owl.english.purdue.edu/owl/resource/560/01/.
The *MLA Style Manual and Guide to Scholarly Writing* (or simply "MLA"—the Modern Language Association) is most commonly used to write papers and cite sources within the liberal arts and humanities. The following website provides a brief summary of this style:
http://owl.english.purdue.edu/owl/resource/747/01/.
The *Chicago Manual of Style* (or simple "Chicago") covers a variety of topics from manuscript preparation and publication to grammar, usage, and documentation and is most commonly used in literature, history, and the arts. The following website provides a brief summary of this style:
http://owl.english.purdue.edu/owl/resource/717/01/.
The *AMA Manual of Style* (or simple "AMA"—the American Medical Association) is most commonly used to cite sources within medicine. The following website provides a brief summary of this style: http://medlib.bu.edu/facts/faq2.cfm/content/citationsama.cfm.

---

activities showed an increase in grade point averages and positive social networks but the same evaluation is repeated with rural high school students and finds that community service does not change grade point average or positive social networking, the evaluators engaging rural high school students would recommend repeating the evaluation with another group of rural high school students to refute or verify their first results.

References and Appendices

See **Box 13-7** for a simple outline of this section. There are numerous types of reference styles. It is important to follow the style indicated in the author guidelines of the journal to which you are submitting your report. If there are no author guidelines, which is the case with technical reports, then evaluators may select one of the commonly accepted styles. However, whichever style is chosen, it is important to use it consistently throughout the report. This attention to detail is important for the quality of the overall report. See **Box 13-8** for a list of reference styles.

Appendices appear at the end of the report. The information placed in the appendix is usually not essential to explaining your findings, but it still supports your analysis. The appendices are placed in order of reference in the narrative and labeled with letters. For example, the narrative may refer to Appendix A when discussing a specific document that is too long for placement in the actual report. The appendices are listed as Appendix A, Appendix B, and so on. The page numbering that started with the title page continues through to the end of the appendices.

WRITER'S BLOCK CAUSES AND SOLUTIONS

Sometimes writers experience a condition where they cannot produce any new or creative material. This is called "writer's block." Often this happens when you have been working on the same project for a long period of time, or you are writing something that has some element of technical difficulty. Every writer is likely to experience this phenomenon.

However, many writers have tips and tricks that help them deal with it (see **Table 13-5**).[3]

Presentation of Results

Now that the report is written, it is time to decide how to present the information. There are two basic formats: oral presentations and written presentations. Let's begin with oral presentations.

Oral Presentations

There are numerous situations in which evaluators are asked to present their findings in front of an audience. Here are a few examples of oral presentations:

- The funding agency asks the evaluator to come to a board meeting.
- The evaluators present the results at a local, state, or national conference.

TABLE 13-5 Writer's Block Causes and Solutions

Cause	Solution
If you do not know enough about the topic, you can't write about it.	Go research and read what other people have written about the topic.
You feel that you need to start at the beginning.	Start with an area that you know. For example, if you understand one of three key points, then begin writing at that point.
The blank screen looks intimidating and scary.	Write something; write anything—just begin writing. Nothing is written perfectly on the first try.
Your schedule does not allow you to dedicate 2 hours of time to writing.	Resolve to only write one paragraph each day. It is necessary to fit writing into your life rather than trying to dedicate a specific time.
You lose interest in writing about one topic area.	Leave the unfinished topic and move onto something that is interesting.
You do not think of yourself as a good writer.	The way to get better at writing is to write more. Just like in sports, you need to practice the skill to improve.
You have an outline, but it is not helping.	Spend a little time adding details to the outline. You may recognize that some topics need to be rearranged for greater clarity.
You do not think that what you have written makes sense.	Read that section aloud. The spoken word helps to identify possible flaws in written materials.
You keep thinking that other people will not like what you wrote.	Find a trusted friend or writing coach to critique your work. Be prepared for honest comments. For example, you would not expect to learn how to play golf without a coach. Writing is the same.
You get stuck on one word.	Don't waste time fretting over one word or phrase. Simply type XXX and come back to it later. Type one word and then click on the thesaurus to search for a synonym that might fit.
You are hopelessly stuck.	Take a short break (e.g., go for a walk, get something to drink, make a phone call). If a short break does not solve the problem, save your document and come back to the task in a few hours or the next day.
Your deadline is close and you are about to panic.	This situation is a fatal flaw. No one writes well under stress. Pace yourself. Know your deadline and determine how much of the report needs to be completed each week to make the deadline. This detailed plan allows for planned and unplanned life events. Best of all, a slow, steady writing pace allows you to sleep at night and not panic.

Adapted from Charlie Jane Anders. The 10 Types of Writer's Block (and How to Overcome Them). Available at: http://io9.com/5844988/the-10-types-of-writers-block-and-how-to-overcome-them. Published October 6, 2011.

- The evaluators offer to discuss the evaluation process as a guest lecture in an academic course or in a community setting.

After the type of presentation is determined, the evaluator decides how he or she wishes to prepare the presentation. There are several questions to answer:

- Who is the audience?
- What is the size of the audience?
- What is the location of the presentation (e.g., conference room, classroom, or auditorium)?
- What is the proposed length of the presentation?

- What type of design is appropriate?
  - Will PowerPoint be used?
  - If so, are the computer equipment and projection screen available?

Let's discuss a few examples related to types of presentations.

Example 1

Ms. Irene Williams completed an evaluation for the thrift shop that operates a funding stream for the local homeless shelter. She was asked to present her findings to the auxiliary board so they can agree on whether or not the thrift shop should remain open 7 days per week. Ms. Williams was told that 10–12 individuals would attend the meeting. The auxiliary board meets in the neighborhood library conference room, which is equipped with a laptop, projector, and screen. Because her presentation will be during the regular monthly meeting, it will be one item of several on the agenda. She will have 15 minutes to present the results of the 6-month evaluation project.

Ms. Williams decides that she will create five PowerPoint slides that include a title slide, the purpose of the evaluation, the methods, results, and recommendations. Her PowerPoint slides follow the 5 × 5 rule, which is to have a maximum of five bullet points on each slide and no more than five words per line of each bullet point. She rehearses her presentation a few times to make sure that it stays within 10 minutes so the audience may have 5 minutes to ask questions. She also prepares a one-page handout that summarizes the key points of her presentation.

On the day of the presentation, Ms. Williams dresses in a dark business suit and arrives 45 minutes early. She brought with her two different electronic modes of her presentation in case one mode was not compatible with the library computer equipment. She does not want to be rushed in traffic and wants to have plenty of time to park, find the conference room, and set up the computer prior to individuals entering the room. Because she is well prepared, but not over-rehearsed and tense, her presentation sounds more like a conversation than a script. The audience is comfortable asking a few questions, because Ms. Williams left 5 minutes of the allotted agenda time to clarify her recommendations. Her presentation was a well prepared success.

Example 2

Mr. James Sutton received an email stating that his evaluation abstract was accepted for a national conference. He has never attended a national academic or professional conference, so he is excited. He asks his faculty mentor for advice. His mentor, Dr. Gannon, tells him that the conference is held in two large hotels located directly across the street from each other in Chicago. The break-out room for his presentation is able to host about 50 conference participants, though he does not expect that there will be that many. There will be a panel of speakers with similar evaluation topics; each presenter has 18 minutes to present his or her PowerPoint slides.

Mr. Sutton creates 12 PowerPoint slides using the 5 × 5 rule (see **Figure 13-1**). This type of PowerPoint slide allows the audience to easily read the slide as the presenter explains each point.

FIGURE 13-1 Sample 5 × 5 PowerPoint.

Sample Illness

- Pediatric onset
- Symptoms
  - Fever and upper respiratory congestion
- Transmission
  - Respiratory droplets; coughing
- Treatment
  - Antibiotics
- Recovery
  - 7 to 10 days

Mr. Sutton wants to take no more than 2 minutes explaining each slide. He realizes that the title slide takes only a few seconds to read, while some slides take just a bit more than 2 minutes of explanation. Several weeks before the conference, he meets with Dr. Gannon to practice his presentation. He reads from a formal script because he is so nervous. Dr. Gannon realized that Mr. Sutton was glued to the script and suggested that he reduce his script to a few note cards so he can present the information in a less tense manner. This tip would also help Mr. Sutton relax and make better eye contact with the audience during the presentation. At the conference, Mr. Sutton dressed in a dark suit and tie. He felt overdressed, but noticed that the other three members of the panel were also dressed in business suits, which was appropriate. His presentation was informative and exactly 15 minutes. His precise timing left 3 minutes for two audience questions. James used the opportunity before and after the presentation to introduce himself to other presenters.

Tips for Successful Presentations

Let's introduce some tips related to successful presentations. A 2001 Gallup poll found public speaking was the second biggest (40%) fear among adults, just behind snakes (51%), and ahead of heights (36%).[4] This section provides a few tips to help overcome fear of public speaking and to improve the impact of the presentation.

1. Think about the goal of your presentation.
   Ask yourself these questions:

Are you being interviewed for an evaluation consulting contract?

Are you presenting the results of the evaluation?

Are you persuading the audience to make a decision?

Are you collecting data as in a focus group?

Are you demonstrating a product?

2. Determine what you want to say.

Write the key points of the presentation.

Use the standard format:

Tell the audience what you are going to tell them.

Tell them.

Close by telling them what you told them.

Always keep your presentation simple and clear.

3. Write the full script, using the key points as your outline.

Practice each section until you are comfortable and have the key points memorized.

Once each section feels comfortable, practice reading the full script aloud.

If you are stumbling over specific words, change the words. For example, if you stumble with a word such as *phenomenon*, then substitute the word *occurrence*. Find your comfort zone with the written script.

From the full script, if you intend to use PowerPoint slides or handouts, create them after you are comfortable with the script.

4. Reduce your full script to a few 3" × 5" note cards.

After you have your full script memorized, write the key points and transition statements between each key point onto note cards.

Practice with the note cards so you become familiar with looking at the audience and speaking calmly and confidently rather than reading from your script.

Prepare by rehearsing in front of friends.

5. Rehearse in front of people.

Gather a few friends together and practice a few times.

Time your presentation from start to finish.

Avoid starting over when you are practicing; just go through the full presentation.

Ask for their honest opinion of your presentation, including the quality of the PowerPoint slides.

Look at the audience.

Ask your friends to watch your hand gestures and provide feedback.

6. Practice in different settings.

Practice by standing behind a podium or a conference table. For example, you are told that your presentation is scheduled for the auditorium; however, the room may be changed to the cafeteria due to a

water leak in the auditorium. In this case, you have a conference table instead of a podium.

Practice without a conference table or podium; be prepared for all type of settings.

7. Time management.

With adequate time management, you will have minimum duties 48 hours before your presentation; you can relax and practice your note cards one last time.

All sorts of mishaps may occur, so you should save your full script, note cards, PowerPoint slides, and handouts in at least two electronic formats.

Have paper copies of the PowerPoint slides available in case computer equipment has malfunctioned or is not available.

Have extra copies of handouts in case the emailed file was not received.

8. Focus the audience on you.

Begin and end your presentation with a "thank you" and a smile; both techniques help you to relax and get settled for your presentation.

Engage your audience; do not hide behind your slides or handouts.

If you are passionate about the subject, your presentation will flow with ease.

Well-prepared presenters are calm and confident; even if you are nervous on the inside, adequate rehearsing allows you to feel comfortable with your information.

9. Think about what you will do after your presentation.

Be prepared to answer several questions from the audience related to your presentation.

Answer questions to the best of your ability; do not exaggerate the findings or recommendations.

If you don't know the answer to a question, tell them you don't, but that you will find out and get back to them.

10. Networking.

After the presentation, stay in the room for further questions or discussions with individuals.

Be sure to clean up the area around your presentation: remove extra handouts or bottled water from the podium or conference table; there may be another speaker following your panel or presentation.

Have your business cards easily available without digging in your pockets or purse.

Use this valuable time to network with individuals in the audience to possibly make connections for further research, evaluations, or professional collaboration.

Your attire during your presentation is also important. See **Box 13-9** for some tips on how to dress.

Poster Presentations

As with oral presentations, there are numerous situations in which evaluators are asked to present their results in a poster format. Here are a few examples of poster presentations:

- Poster session presented at a formal conference
- Poster session at a seminar or reception with interested individuals mingling and networking
- Posters displayed in a hallway as a rotating display such as in a college lobby

Although posters are used for various venues, how a poster is designed influences whether the material is noticed and read or ignored without more than a glance. The paragraphs that follow provide details on how to create a standout poster. For this section, Microsoft PowerPoint is used for the poster development.

Step 1: Select a Poster Size

Determine the required size of the poster prior to starting the development. Note: It is difficult to change the size after the poster is developed. See **Figure 13-2** to select poster size. First, on the Toolbar, click Design, then Page Setup. Second, select landscape for your slide orientation, then increase the width and height to those of your poster requirements.

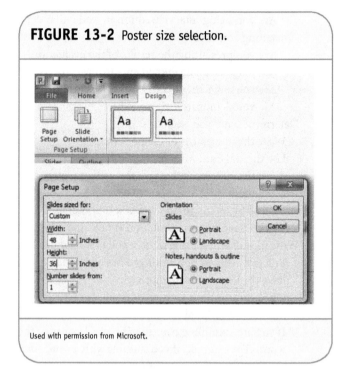

FIGURE 13-2 Poster size selection.

Used with permission from Microsoft.

Step 2: Select a Poster Template

See **Figure 13-3** to select a poster template. First, on the Toolbar, click on Design. Second, select a design. After a design is selected, there are options of colors, fonts, and background

---

BOX 13-9   Rules of Attire: Top-to-Bottom List

Females	Males
Hair: Freshly washed; pinned up and out of face	Hair: Freshly washed and trimmed
Nails: Clean and trimmed with pale polish	Facial hair: Trimmed and neat
Clothing: Dark-colored professional suit	Nails: Clean and trimmed
Blouse: Light color; well-fitting; no button gaps, low neck-lines, no bra straps showing	Clothing: Dark-colored professional suit
Jewelry: Minimal and small; nothing flashy	Shirt: Light color; coordinated tie color; no emblems or sport team ties
Skirt or pants: Well fitting; not too tight or too short; pants length appropriate for shoes	Jewelry: Minimal; nothing flashy or bold
Shoes: Closed toed; no sandals; neutral color; polished; 3-inch or less heels	Pants: Well fitting; not too tight; appropriate length for shoes
Make-up: Minimal; avoid bold, bright colors	Shoes: Polished; black or brown; matching socks

FIGURE 13-3 Selecting a poster template.

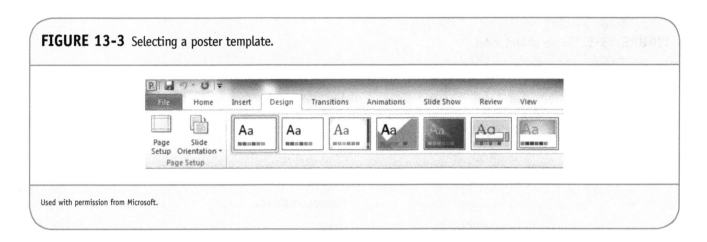

Used with permission from Microsoft.

styles. Test a few combinations prior to making the final selection. Keep in mind that the background needs to be simple and not distract from the information on the poster.

Step 3: Place Information on the Poster

On a plain piece of paper, draw out approximately where each segment of the poster will be placed (see **Figure 13-4**). Once the placement is drafted, type what information will be placed in each segment.

Step 4: Select a Font Style

The ideal font for a poster is simple and plain. In **Figure 13-5**, note how much space the various fonts use. For a poster, it is important to select fonts from column A. Within column A, select a narrow font, such as font 1 or font 3. A narrow font allows more words per line without compromising the clarity. Column B fonts are not appropriate for posters. The font should never distract from the information presented on the poster.

FIGURE 13-4 Information placement.

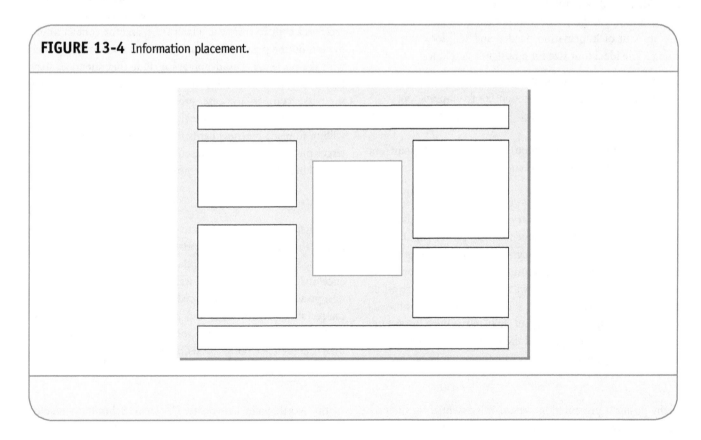

FIGURE 13-5 Sample of font styles.

Column A: Plain, Easy to Read	Column B: Fancy, Harder to Read
1 Information	1 Information
2 Data Analysis	2 Data Analysis
3 Background	3 Background
4 Recommendations	4 Recommendations
5 Conclusion	5 Conclusion

Step 5: Select a Font Size

Font size on a poster is important. Generally, individuals stand about 3 to 4 feet from a poster. If the font is too small, individuals will not stop to read the poster. However, if the font is too large, the poster will not have adequate room for the amount of information needed and will look unprofessional. The ideal font size for a poster is as follows:

- Title: 60–80 point font
- Subheadings for each section: 50- to 60-point font
- Information under each subheading: 40- to 50-point font
- Figures, graphs, and photo captions: 35- to 40-point font
- References: 25- to 30-point font

Step 6: Keep It Simple

The most common mistake is trying to fit too much information on the poster. Each segment of the poster should have plenty of blank space so the segments do not run together. It is useful to have the information flow from one section to the next section. **Figure 13-6** shows the title in a bold box, while the sections are in a light gray for contrast. There are hundreds of ways to configure a poster, but simplicity is most important. It is better to have people read the key points with few details than to have the poster ignored with too much information.

Step 7: Create Talking Points for Your Poster

If the poster is presented in person, it is essential for the presenter to have a 2- to 3-minute speech prepared. Individuals walk around the room, reviewing the posters and stopping to chat with presenters with interesting posters. Presenters should be ready to summarize the key points of the research and to answer questions. There are advantages and disadvantages to having small 8.5" × 11" paper copies of the poster available as a handout. Advantages include that the interested individual receives a copy to review at a later time, and the contact information on the poster allows the person to connect the poster with the presenter. Disadvantages include that attendees may be carrying food or drinks, so they do not have a place to put the paper copy. In any case, presenters should have business cards available at poster presentations. Attendees are more willing to place business cards into their pockets than take a larger piece of paper. The presenter needs to memorize his or her talking points prior to the poster presentation.

SUMMARY

This chapter introduced effective ways to present evaluation results in written and oral formats. First, written reports were discussed, including the essential elements of a report, reference styles, and overcoming writer's block. Second, types of oral presentations were reviewed, including creation of informative slide presentations and powerful rehearsal strategies. Lastly, the chapter concluded with techniques to create informative conference poster presentations with key talking points.

CASE STUDY

In the North State University, Dr. Irene Schmidt, a faculty member in the College of Public Health, was asked by Mr. Peter Blackstone, the Human Resource Director from the

FIGURE 13-6 Simple poster design.

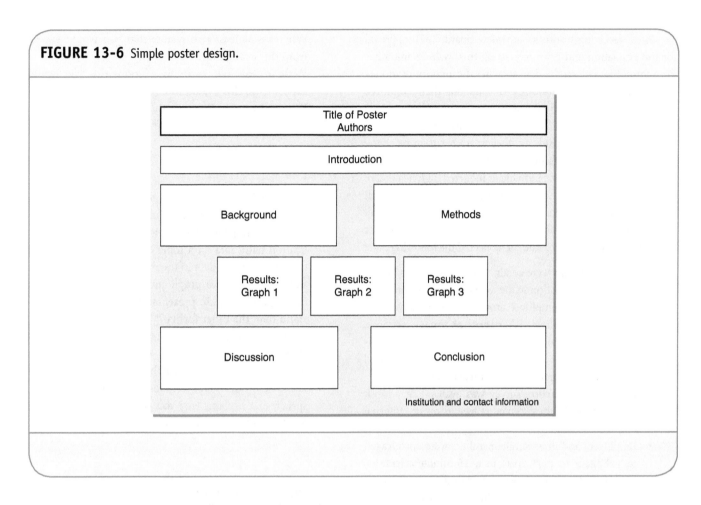

nearby self-insured Greenfield Community Hospital, to conduct a wellness evaluation. A wellness evaluation includes ascertaining the overall current health of employees and determining what health aspects could be improved among the employees. Because the hospital is self-insured, that means that it collects insurance premiums from its approximately 1800 employees. From these collected insurance funds, the hospital is able to pay the medical and hospital costs for the employees. To reduce the Greenfield Community Hospital's healthcare cost, hospital administrators decided to offer a family incentive package to increase the wellness of their employees and their families and thus decrease healthcare costs. Employees and their family members living at home were given the opportunity to be evaluated by the nurse practitioner in the wellness center. Each individual was given recommendations for improving his or her health and wellness over the next 12 months. For example, if an individual was 50 pounds overweight, the recommendation would be to join the hospital's free weekly weight-loss program with the goal of losing at least 25 pounds over the next 12 months. If an individual was a smoker, the recommendation would be to join the hospital's free, ongoing smoking cessation class until he or she

stopped smoking. In addition, if an individual logged 3 hours per week in the hospital fitness center per swipe card verification, for example, he or she would be eligible for incentives.

For employees and their family members with preexisting chronic health conditions that limited their physical activity, the nurse practitioner would recommend nonphysical, but positive, stress-reducing activities, such as attending mindful meditation classes or social support groups. This type of stress reduction was also recommended for busy employees or families in need of more relaxation and stress-management skills.

If the recommended goals for the family members were documented and achieved, the family would receive a $1000 bonus per individual achieving their personal goals up to $10,000. So, for instance, if the husband stopped smoking ($1000) and lost the recommended 25 pounds ($1000) and the wife lost the recommended 35 pounds ($1000), the couple would receive $3000. After the family achieved their goals, they needed to maintain the goals for another 12 months to obtain further incentives. The Greenfield Community Hospital determined that it was less expensive to pay individuals to get and stay healthy than to pay for illness and prescriptions.

After receiving institutional review board (IRB) approval for the evaluation and prior to starting this wellness initiative, Dr. Schmidt was given the data showing the amount of money paid by Greenfield Community Hospital for their employee and family medical and hospital expenses for the previous 12 months. (Note: Dr. Schmidt received aggregated data that showed total expenses paid per category rather than receiving data with employee and family names.) Dr. Schmidt had no reason to know which specific individuals incurred high healthcare expenses. Every 3 months during the evaluation, Dr. Schmidt was given the same financial healthcare pay-out data for all employees and their families. In addition, Dr. Schmidt and her two public health graduate students collected the following data:

- Ten focus groups were conducted to determine satisfaction and participation in the wellness incentive program among various employee groups (administrative staff, nursing/patient care, laboratory, pharmacy services, physical and occupational therapy, food services, environmental, physical plant maintenance, parking and grounds maintenance, and central supply).
- An online satisfaction survey was available at a kiosk in the hospital fitness center as well as on the internal employee website.
- Employees and their family members were encouraged to volunteer to participate in a 15-minute telephone interview about why they accepted or declined the invitation to participate in the wellness incentive program.

Dr. Schmidt and her two public health graduate students worked on this evaluation for 2 years. However, they presented preliminary results every 6 months to the Greenfield Community Hospital Board of Directors.

Case Study Discussion Questions

1. What are some potential limitations of this evaluation?
2. What other types of data should be collected for this evaluation?
3. What are at least two results that you would expect from this evaluation?
4. Write at least two recommendations that you would expect from this evaluation.
5. Where else could the team showcase the results?
6. What would be a possible next phase in this evaluation?

STUDENT ACTIVITIES

1. Using the information presented in the case study, create a poster to explain the findings of the evaluation.
2. Search some peer-reviewed journals and find a publication with data on a topic of interest to you. Using the demographic data in the publication, practice your skills to make a bar graph and pie chart. Explain why one type of graphic presentation is easier to understand than the other format.
3. Using 3" × 5" note cards, outline one section of this chapter and prepare to give a 3-minute presentation without using any other graphic props.
4. Using a copy of your current resume, prepare a 2-minute speech that explains why you are the perfect candidate for the position for which you have applied.

REFERENCES

1. Virginia Polytechnic Institute and State University. Technical Writing-Progress Reports. Available at: http://wiz.cath.vt.edu/tw/TechnicalWriting/ProgressReports/components4.htm. Accessed November 3, 2012.

2. Astia. How to Write an Executive Summary. Available at: http://www.astia.org/resources/How_to_write_an_execsummary.pdf. Accessed May 31, 2014.

3. Anders CJ. The 10 Types of Writer's Block (and How to Overcome Them). IO9. Available at: http://io9.com/5844988/the-10-types-of-writers-block-and-how-to-overcome-them. Published October 6, 2011. Accessed November 3, 2012.

4. Brewer G. Snakes Top List of Americans' Fears. Gallup Poll. Available at: http://www.gallup.com/poll/1891/snakes-top-list-americans-fears.aspx. Published March 19, 2001. Accessed November 3, 2012.

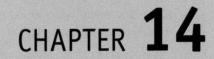

CHAPTER 14

Case Study: Learn, Experience, and Achieve Program (LEAP): Program Planning and Evaluation

YEAR 1: PLANNING

The U.S. Department of Health and Human Services (HHS) Office of Adolescent Health (OAH) posted on their website a request to work on a government grant project. This application process is called request for proposals (RFP). Applications require that each state must select from one of several pre-approved positive youth development (PYD) curricula that includes activities such as after-school clubs, community engagement volunteer projects, and leadership and self-esteem development with the overall goal of increasing standardized test scores and reducing absentee rates. The Georgia State Health Office selected the "Learn, Experience, and Achieve Program" (LEAP) curriculum for use in its grant proposal application because of its focus on youth community engagement. The application required each state to identify its counties with the highest number of at-risk middle school students based on low standardized test scores, low attendance rates, and high levels of reduced-price lunch program eligibility. Of the 78 counties in Georgia, 20 counties were classified as at-risk and having the potential of benefitting from the LEAP curriculum. The federal funding is allocated for 5 years. Year 1 is designated for program planning; Years 2, 3, and 4 for the intervention; and Year 5 for data analyses and reporting.

Several months prior to the submission of the LEAP proposal, the Georgia State Health Office contacted the State University to serve as external evaluators for LEAP. Within the College of Public Health, the evaluation team consisted of five faculty members including the lead writer (Dr. Arden Black), a biostatistician (Dr. Brynn Green), a Positive Youth Development (PYD) expert (Dr. Chris White), and two experienced health educators (Dr. Dharma Brown and Dr. Emery Scarlett) with specific evaluation skills. Because the first names of the co-principal investigators started with A, B, and C, they agreed to be called the ABC team. To write the external evaluation portion of the larger state proposal, the ABC team reviewed the RFP and designed all aspects of the evaluation including the goals and objectives, theoretical framework, study design, curriculum, personnel, budget, target population and sample size, training, and data collection. The external evaluation was submitted to the state health office grant for inclusion in the federal grant.

Goals and Objectives

Goal: By the end of the fourth year, the middle school students involved in LEAP for a minimum of 2 years will show improvement in two of the three academic achievement measurements including higher standardized test scores, lower absentee rates, and higher community-engaged scores.

Objective One: By the end of the fourth year, 100% of the LEAP students will achieve statistically significantly higher standardized test scores than the middle school students who did not participate in LEAP.

Objective Two: By the end of the fourth year, 100% of the LEAP students will achieve statistically significantly lower absentee rates than the middle school students who did not participate in LEAP.

Objective Three: By the end of the fourth year, 100% of the LEAP students will achieve statistically significantly higher community-engagement scores than the middle school students who did not participate in LEAP.

In addition to the goals and objectives, there are process evaluation measures related to fidelity and quality control. Throughout the evaluation, the process measures depend on the current situation. Examples of the process measures are:

- What percentage of weekly reports was submitted on time by each facilitator teaching LEAP in each middle school?
- What percentage of principal, classroom teacher, and parent satisfaction surveys rated LEAP as "very good" or "excellent"?
- What percentage of facilitators was able to complete the 12 LEAP lessons within the allotted number of weeks?
- What percentage of students maintained 95% attendance at weekly LEAP sessions?

Theoretical Framework

After reviewing several models and theories, the ABC team selected Reach Effectiveness Adoption Implementation Maintenance (RE-AIM; see http://www.RE-AIM.org) for the external evaluation framework. This comprehensive framework addresses how an intervention reaches the target population, the effectiveness of the intervention, the adoption at the institutional level, the intervention fidelity, and the sustainability within the community. In addition to the RE-AIM acronym, this framework has five pillars called "the 5 Cs," which are character, competence, caring, connection, and confidence, and are measured throughout the evaluation. **Table 14-1** shows how RE-AIM served as the framework for LEAP.

Curriculum

The LEAP curriculum includes twelve 60-minute required lessons. The purchase price of LEAP by the state health office included training for the facilitators and the ABC team. Each LEAP lesson is introduced in order, because the activities and acquired skills are sequential. The four student-led sections include building trust within the group by getting to know every group member; learning about yourself and sharing your findings with group members; identifying, planning, and completing a community project for a group activity; and building on personal and group success stories for future success:

- Building Trust
  Lesson One: Introduction to LEAP
  Lesson Two: Getting to know each other
  Lesson Three: Trusting others

- Learning About Yourself
  Lesson Four: Telling your story
  Lesson Five: Success stories
  Lesson Six: Lifetime dreams
- Planning the Community Project
  Lesson Seven: Community engagement
  Lesson Eight: Finding time for others
  Lesson Nine: Stress management
- Building on Success
  Lesson Ten: Time management
  Lesson Eleven: Community networking
  Lesson Twelve: Success stories

Target Population and Sample Size

In Georgia, the LEAP target population was middle school students living in one of the 20 counties classified as at-risk. Within the 20 counties, there are a total of 64 after-school programs for 6th, 7th, and 8th grade middle school students. It is estimated that 90% of the middle school students in the participating counties attended the after-school programs offered at their middle schools.

Study Design

This evaluation utilizes a randomized control evaluation with delayed intervention. Because this study is a 5-year intervention, Year 1 involves the program planning phase. Year 2 involves 16 after-school programs followed by adding more after-school programs each year. The delayed intervention is defined as the after-school program that serves as the control group in Year 2, receives LEAP in Year Three, and so on. See **Table 14-2**.

YEAR 1: PROGRAM PLANNING

Year 1 is the planning phase of the evaluation. In Year 2, 16 after-school programs agreed to participate with 8 after-school programs randomized to participate in LEAP and the 8 remaining randomized to serve as a control group. None of the control middle schools will be located in the same counties as the participating middle schools to maintain validity. In each of the following 3 years, 16 after-school programs are added: 8 receiving LEAP and 8 serving as a control group.

Personnel

ABC Evaluation Team Personnel

The evaluation team consisted of the five faculty members including the lead writer, a biostatistician, a PYD expert, and two experienced health educators with specific evaluation skills.

During the planning phase in Year 1, the ABC evaluation team wrote job descriptions, advertised, interviewed

TABLE 14-1 RE-AIM Application to LEAP

RE-AIM Dimension	Level	Objectives	Measures	Instrument
Reach	Student	What percentage of middle school students in the treatment group participated in the after-school program? What percentage of middle school students in the treatment group participated in LEAP during the after-school program?	• Number of eligible students in the after-school programs in the treatment middle schools • Number of middle school students who participated • Gender, age, race/ethnicity, free and reduced-price lunch	• Number of students in the treatment middle schools • LEAP attendance sheets • Self-report survey for participants with items regarding participation, grade, age, race/ethnicity
	Class	What percentage of 6th, 7th, and 8th grade students participated in LEAP?	• Number of middle school students participating in the after-school program	• Excel spreadsheet depicting number of middle school students in the after-school program
	School	What percentage of middle schools with after-school programs in eligible counties opted to participate in the evaluation study?	• Number of eligible counties • Number of middle schools within the counties • Number of middle schools with after-school programs • Number of eligible middle schools that volunteer • Demographics: Size of school, % free and reduced-price lunch, % non-white, teen pregnancy rates for the county, dropout rates for the county, teacher–student ratio, number of schools in the county, statewide school rating, school structure (e.g., regular high school or middle/high school combined), presence or absence of school clinic, ratio of nurse to students, other teen pregnancy prevention programs (yes/no), graduation rates at the school level • Demographics of eligible counties: median income, unemployment rate, current population, race/ethnicity, designated rural/urban county	• Excel spreadsheet depicting number of middle schools within eligible counties • Excel spreadsheet depicting number of participating middle schools within eligible counties • Excel spreadsheet depicting demographics of participating schools • Qualitative semi-structured interviews with principals or other decision maker at eligible but nonparticipating schools

(continues)

TABLE 14-1 RE-AIM Application to LEAP (Continued)

RE-AIM Dimension	Level	Objectives	Measures	Instrument
Efficacy/ Effectiveness	Student	What impact did LEAP have (positive and negative) on program participants?	• Quantitative assessment of 5 Cs and outcome indicators including absentee rates, course failure rates, and suspension rates • Qualitative assessment of participation/non-participation in program	• Self-report survey for students with scales assessing primary outcomes, such as absentee rates, course failure, and school suspension, and secondary outcomes, including the 5 Cs • Objective assessment of school records regarding persistence rates, attendance rates, grades, and school suspension • Focus group guide to explore impacts perceived by youth (both positive and negative) from participating in LEAP, as well as their likes and dislikes of the program
	Parent	What are parents' perceptions regarding the impact of LEAP (positive and negative) on their children?	• Qualitative assessment of parent perception of impact of LEAP on child	• Focus group guide to explore parents' perceptions regarding the impact of LEAP (positive and negative) on their children.
	School	What are school personnel perceptions regarding the impact of LEAP (positive and negative) on program participants?	• Qualitative assessment of school personnel perception of impact of LEAP on students • Quantitative assessment of outcome indicators including course failure rates and suspension rates	• Semi-structured interview guide to explore perceptions of the program and perceived impacts of LEAP on students
Adoption	LEAP facilitators	What percentage of facilitators in eligible counties adopted LEAP? What factors affected decisions to adopt LEAP?	• Volunteer or mandated adoption • Quantitative assessment of factors affecting decision to adopt LEAP	• Self-report survey to explore factors affecting decisions to adopt LEAP
	Schools	What percentage of schools in eligible counties adopted LEAP as part of their curriculum? What factors affected schools' decisions to adopt LEAP within the curriculum?	• Quantitative assessment of factors affecting decision to adopt LEAP	• Self-report survey to explore factors affecting decisions to adopt LEAP

Phase	Group	Research Question	Methods	Data Sources
Implementation	Student	To what extent was LEAP implemented in the after-school program?	• Quantitative assessment among participants regarding perceived climate of LEAP sessions	• Self-report survey for students with scale assessing perceived program climate
	LEAP facilitators	To what extent was LEAP implemented as intended? To what extent was LEAP implemented in the after-school program? What are the barriers to implementation?	• Mixed-methods assessment of LEAP program fidelity • Quantitative assessment of characteristics of the LEAP facilitator • Observation of LEAP sessions	• LEAP curriculum fidelity tool (developed and previously used) • Observational checklist • Self-report survey
Maintenance	Student	What were the long-term effects following the LEAP intervention?	• Quantitative assessment of the 5 Cs and outcome indicators including absentee rates, course failure, and school suspension • Qualitative assessment of participation/non-participation in program	• Self-report survey for students with scales assessing primary outcomes, such as absentee rates, course failure, and school suspension, and secondary outcomes, including the 5 Cs • Objective assessment of school records regarding persistence rates, attendance rates, grades, and school suspension • Focus group guide to explore impacts perceived by youth (both positive and negative) from participating in LEAP, as well as their likes and dislikes of the program
	Parent	What are parents' perceptions regarding the impact of LEAP (positive and negative) on their children?	• Qualitative assessment of parent perception of impact of LEAP on child	• Focus group guide to explore parents' perceptions regarding the impact of LEAP (positive and negative) on their children.
	School	To what extent is LEAP institutionalized in the school?	• Number of participating schools who indicate continued participation post study	• Spreadsheet with information on school, participation, demographics, area of town, percent free and reduced-price lunch served, those agreeing to continue or discontinue implementation of LEAP

The 5 Cs are character, competence, caring, connection, and confidence.

TABLE 14-2 LEAP Study Design

	Year 1	Year 2		Year 3		Year 4		Year 5
	Program planning							
Schools 1–16		Tx One 1–7	Control One 8–16	Follow Tx One 1–7	Control One receives LEAP 8–16	Follow Tx One 1–7	Follow Control One 8–16	
Schools 17–32				Tx Two 17–24	Control Two 25–32	Follow Tx Two 17–24	Control Two receives LEAP 25–32	
Schools 33–48				Tx Three 33–39	Control Three 40–48	Follow Tx Three 33–39	Control Three receives LEAP 40–48	
Schools 49–64						Tx Four 49–55	Control 56–64	
	Ongoing Process > > > > > > > > > > > > > > > > > >							Final Data Analysis

Tx = Treatment

several candidates, and hired the project manager and coordinator. These two individuals supervised the day-to-day operation and supervised the graduate students for the next 5 years. Also, three part-time doctoral graduate students were employed for LEAP.

Because LEAP is planned for implementation in 20 counties, the ABC team divided the state into four regions and hired four region coordinators to oversee the LEAP facilitators in each region. This design reduced the need to make monthly visits to each region.

State Health Office Personnel

The state health office recruited LEAP facilitators within the local county health departments. Although the facilitators teach LEAP in the after-school programs of middle schools, they remained employees of the county health departments. This design helped to ensure stability over the 5-year evaluation.

LEAP Training

The entire ABC evaluation team, regional coordinators, and the county facilitators teaching LEAP were trained by the national LEAP trainers. The training took place in the spring, so facilitators had the summer to learn the curriculum. The 5-day LEAP curriculum training took place at the university because of its central location within the state and its comfortable conference facilities. This type of training was essential to ensure standardization and fidelity of the LEAP

curriculum. Several county facilitators had not yet been hired when the training took place, so their training took placed at a later date at the LEAP headquarters in a nearby state. Each year as additional facilitators were hired, LEAP training was conducted to maintain curriculum fidelity.

Website Development

With advice from the university web designers, the ABC team developed a website for the LEAP evaluation. The website allowed the evaluation to run smoothly and to maintain standardized and up-to-date communication with all personnel, the state health office, regional coordinators, school principals, and facilitators. The website also had a toolbar tab for questions. This tab allowed everyone involved to see the questions and read the responses, which allowed for quick responses from the ABC team and reduced confusion. Through the website, facilitators completed their weekly required data forms related to the curriculum lesson taught, number of students absent and in attendance, activities associated with each lesson and space for comments, and issues of concern. In addition, the website included an overview of the external evaluation; the surveys completed by the middle school principals, after-school program staff, parents, and students; and interview guides. Lastly, the website provided ideas and photos of the various LEAP student community-engaged activities across the state. The website encouraged active posting of testimonials from students. One of the PhD students had the responsibility to monitor the website and remove any unacceptable student postings.

Institutional Review Board

The institutional review board (IRB) monitors the protection of humans or animals involved in any type of research. LEAP required two IRB approvals: one at the state level and one at the university level. After hiring initial personnel, the ABC team submitted the IRB application to the university, while the state health office submitted another IRB application to its institutional review board. IRB applications describe the purpose of the research, the risks and benefits to the human subjects; the oversight procedures; all included documents, such as parental consent forms, student assent forms, survey questions, interview question guides, and satisfaction surveys; sample randomization procedures; data collection; data storage; and data analysis. The state and university IRB approvals were received prior to the initiation of the LEAP research study. The LEAP project manager coordinated with the state health office to obtain IRB approval for each of the 20 county school districts.

School Recruitment

Following IRB approval, the state health office began recruitment of schools within 20 at-risk counties. The process involved contacting county school boards, and then the school board members contacted the principals of middle schools with after-school programs. Principals reviewed the LEAP curriculum and determined whether or not to voluntarily participate. Some declined the opportunity immediately, others waited for additional input, and some accepted the invitation after limited discussion. Even though 20 counties were eligible to participate, only 18 counties agreed to participate over the next few years. Within the participating at-risk counties, 64 middle school principals consented to participate. After the middle school principals signed the memorandum of agreement between their middle school and the state health office, the ABC evaluation team randomly assigned all of the middle schools into experimental schools and control schools. It was essential to ensure that none of the experimental schools were in close proximity to the control school.

YEAR 2: IMPLEMENTATION

Review of Program Planning

After Year 1 of planning and prior to implementation, the ABC team held a half-day internal team meeting to revisit the state health office goals, the RE-AIM theoretical framework, and the LEAP curriculum. The team reviewed inclusion criteria to ensure that identified at-risk counties met the inclusion criteria, including low standardized test scores,

low attendance rates, and high reduced-price lunch program eligibility. This discussion was followed by a summary of how LEAP incorporated the RE-AIM framework. After reviewing the 12-lesson LEAP curriculum, the team was reminded that LEAP focused on involving the middle school students in community engagement activities as a way to improve their academic grades and standardized test scores. In summary, the planning year included approval of the IRB application, design of the randomized control trial design with delayed intervention, hiring staff, randomization of the after-school programs into experimental or control groups, facilitator training for LEAP fidelity, the pilot study, creation of the facilitator website, and creation of process evaluation methods for quality improvement and data analysis for outcome evaluation to address the research questions. LEAP implementation began in September of Year 2. Each facilitator guided the student-led LEAP curriculum 1 day per week in each after-school program. This schedule allowed the facilitators time for lesson planning and report submission during the day.

LEAP Curriculum

LEAP is a student-led curriculum guided by adult facilitators. The curriculum is divided into four sections taught in sequential order with each lesson building on the previous lessons. The four student-led sections include building trust within the group by getting to know every group member; learning about yourself and sharing your findings with group members; identifying, planning, and completing a community project for a group activity; and building on personal and group success stories for future success.

Cultural Competency

Because the curriculum is led by the students, it can be adaptable to any mix of cultural diversity within the student groups. It is up to the facilitator to guide the students toward inclusivity and mutual teamwork. Cultural competency involves awareness of one's own culture and knowledge about different cultures and attitudes toward cultural differences. Cultural competency was an essential consideration throughout the evaluation, starting with writing the grant proposal. The state health office team and the ABC evaluation team remained respectful of the cultural diversity within each county as well as in hiring the facilitators and the development of the survey questions and interview guides.

Development of Data Collection

LEAP required two types of data: qualitative (words) and quantitative (numbers). Qualitative data involved a compilation of the facilitators' weekly reports and interview satisfaction data from facilitators, principals, school staff, parents, and students. Quantitative data consisted of the standardized student pretest and posttest related to the LEAP curriculum and satisfaction surveys. The national LEAP curriculum required the collection of a standardized set of survey questions and the ABC team added more questions to help answer their research questions. Once interview question guidelines and the survey questions were developed and approved by the state health office, these data-collection instruments were added to the IRB application.

Pilot Testing

Prior to conducting data collection, it is essential to pilot-test the interview guides and the survey questions with a comparable audience. The county adjacent to the university location was borderline at-risk and not participating in LEAP, but the two middle school principals agreed to serve as the pilot-test site. Pilot testing allowed the ABC evaluation team to examine whether the materials and curriculum needed any changes prior to implementation with the larger population. During the end of the academic term in Year 1, the ABC evaluation team collected pilot-test data from the school staff, parents, and middle school students attending an after-school program. The pilot data revealed a need to modify a few survey questions and add several additional interview questions. These changes were made and an amendment was sent to the IRB as a supplement to the previously approved application.

Data Collection

During Year 2, the baseline data were collected from the middle school students attending the after-school programs in the treatment schools 1–7 and the control school 8–16. Because the LEAP program is not focused entirely on only 6th-grade students, all middle school students participating in the after-school program were invited to complete the baseline data survey. The control students in the control (schools 8–16) after-school programs completed the pretest survey and the posttest survey in Year 2 and received LEAP in Year 3. The students in after-school programs for schools 17–32 repeated the same process in Year 3 and Year 4. See Table 14-1.

Because the after-school students completed the pretest surveys prior to participating in LEAP, the ABC team hired and trained eight full-time, temporary data collectors to work full-time for pretest data and posttest survey data collection. Four data collection teams were formed and assigned to a region of the state. The project coordinator assigned the graduate students to create a travel box packet for the data-collection team including local county maps, hotel reservations, middle school location, facilitator name, and contact information. As the external evaluators, the ABC team contacted the facilitators to schedule the data collection within the first few weeks of the school year. Prior to the completion of the pretest surveys, facilitators sent home the parental consent forms. Facilitators tracked the number of returned signed parental consent forms. Students not returning the parental consent forms were given a second and, if necessary, a third form to get signed. Facilitators encouraged the students to return the parental consent forms by creating inexpensive incentives, such as travel cups and drink coupons.

Upon arrival, the data-collection teams checked the website to verify the number of parental consent forms posted by the facilitators. Only students with returned parental consent forms and student assent forms completed the pretest survey. The data-collection team instructed the students to fill in response bubbles on Scantron forms. Forms were scanned for ease of data entry. To ensure fidelity, facilitators were not present during data collection. Upon completion of the 12 lessons, the data-collection teams returned to the after-school programs to repeat the process. For control after-school programs, the same process was repeated for acquiring parental consent forms, student assent consent forms, and pretest and posttest surveys (completed on Scantron forms). Control group pretest surveys served as comparative data.

Because the student Scantron forms needed to be matched, the data-collection team taught the students to make their names into a unique code number. This process involved the following steps:

1. The data collectors drew a phone keypad on two large poster boards.

1	2 ABC	3 DEF
4 GHI	5 JKL	6 MNO
7 PQRS	8 TUV	9 WXYZ
	0	

2. They instructed each student to create a unique, 5-digit code using the first letter of their first name, the first letter of their middle name, and the first three letters of their last name. For example, Vijay Ambuj Patel would select 82728 (8 for V, 2 for A, 7 for P, 2 for A, and 8 for T).

3. These unique codes were used to match the pretest and posttest for each student.

4. The data collectors placed all of the pretests, and later all of the posttests, for each after-school program in separate envelopes that were labeled by county, middle school name, and number of students that submitted a pretest or later a posttest.

YEAR 3: EVALUATION

Starting in Year 1 during the planning phase, the ABC evaluation team began the external evaluation process. Throughout the evaluation, the team worked on process and outcome data collection.

Process Evaluation

For the process evaluation, data are collected from the day-to-day implementation activities. The ABC evaluation team held weekly team meetings to ensure the evaluation stayed within budget while meeting state health office goals and timelines for the overall grant. On the LEAP website, the project coordinator posted meeting minutes and tracked emails, phone conversations, and correspondence from county health department personnel, principals, facilitators, data-collection team members, and the graduate students employed on the study. Also on the LEAP website, facilitators posted weekly reports, formats of curriculum delivery, student attendance logs, activities, issues of concern or achievement, and all aspects of the community engagement activity.

Outcome Evaluation

The outcome evaluation addresses the goals and objectives starting with the baseline data. With assistance from the state health office, the ABC evaluation team received baseline aggregate school standardized test scores and school attendance records for the middle school students participating in LEAP as an experimental and control school. The second set of baseline data were the first set of pretest scores from schools 1–16 in Year 2. Pretest surveys provided baseline data about the knowledge, attitudes, and behaviors prior to participation in LEAP and posttest surveys provided post-LEAP data.

Survey response forms were scanned and the data were entered into a computer by matching after-school program pretest surveys with posttest surveys to maintain student anonymity using the unique codes created by the students using the phone keypad technique. Prior to giving data to the ABC team biostatistician, graduate students reviewed the data to identify unusual data caused by the computer misreading the Scantron form. This process is called data cleaning. If the graduate students recognized a misread form, they located the Scantron and verified data against computer-read data. Data cleaning is time-consuming, but necessary for accurate statistical results.

In addition to comparing pretest and posttest survey data, the outcome data included a review of qualitative data gathered from the satisfaction interviews. These interviews were conducted with a small sample of individuals from participating counties. The ABC team conducted the satisfaction interviews.

Data Analysis

Quantitative Data

Dr. Green, biostatistician, did not wait until Year 5 to begin data analysis. By the end of Year 2, the pretest survey numerical data spreadsheets were prepared for analyses. Dr. Green began by merging the data from each after-school program into one database: school standardized test scores, school attendance records, and pretest survey data. At this point, Dr. Green ran frequency data to determine if the data were normally distributed, the percentage of missing data, and how to address the missing data in the analysis. Based on frequency reports, the ABC team determined statistical tests appropriate to address the goals and objectives. **Table 14-3** shows some of the basic statistical tests that were used for this evaluation.

Qualitative Data

While Dr. Green worked on the quantitative data, other ABC team members reviewed the interview transcript data. The interviews were conducted by the ABC evaluation team with the LEAP treatment group school personnel, facilitators, parents, and students. The team coded transcripts and found themes related to represented groups' overall LEAP satisfaction levels. **Table 14-4** shows a sample of some thematic codes found across all types of interviews.

YEAR 5: RESULTS

A summary of quantitative and qualitative data provides results for the 5-year LEAP research. The results are presented as data from facilitators, principals, school staff, parents, and students.

Facilitators

Facilitator data revealed mixed results. After the first year of implementation, five facilitators resigned. Resigning facilitators had overall lower satisfaction scores and frequently submitted late weekly reports. Although rehiring and training were required, the change had positive results. For the

TABLE 14-3 Sample of Statistical Analysis for Pretest Surveys for Participating Students

Variables	Frequency Data	Statistical Tests

Dose response:
    Treatment group participating in LEAP
    Control group not participating in LEAP
	Missing data
	Mean
	Median
	Mode
	Standard deviation
	Skew
		Divide the data into treatment and control groups.

Demographics for each participating student:
    County
    Name of after-school program
    Unique ID code identifier for each student
    Gender
    Race/ethnicity
    Age
    Free/reduced-cost lunch program
    Grade level at time of pretest survey
		Using mean scores and independent t-tests, determine which mean scores are statistically different between the treatment and control groups prior to initiating LEAP.

School data for each participating student:
    Grade point average (GPA) prior to pretest
    Absentee rate prior to pretest survey
		Using the correlation test, determine the association between GPA and absentee rate.

LEAP Subscales:
    Knowledge
    Attitude
    Behavior
		Using mean scores and independent t-tests, determine which LEAP subscale mean scores are statistically different between the treatment and control groups prior to initiating LEAP.

remaining years, facilitators remained stable, enthusiastic, and committed to LEAP's success. Facilitators had positive comments about the LEAP training and ease of submitting weekly reports to the evaluation website. They appreciated the close liaison between the state health office and the ABC team for the evaluation. Facilitators enjoyed the flexibility of moving between sites. Facilitators praised the student-led process, but felt the curriculum activities restricted their creativity. All facilitators shared positive comments about engaging middle school students in community activities, but some facilitators found community engagement activities challenging for small after-school programs.

TABLE 14-4 Sample of Interview Major and Minor Thematic Codes

Major Codes	Minor Codes

Satisfaction	Satisfaction with LEAP being offered in the after-school program:
	    Students enjoy participating in the structured LEAP activities.
	    Students like getting to know students from other grades.
	    LEAP involvement reduces homework tutoring in the after-school program and transfers the tutoring to parents after dinner.

Community engagement	Students like the opportunity to help others in the community. Parents like working with their children on the community engagement projects. Parents dislike giving up Saturdays for community engagement.
Knowledge, attitude, and behavior	Students enjoy that the LEAP activities and projects are "real" rather than merely reading about LEAP out of a textbook. Parents, teachers, and principals see a positive attitude permeating the whole school.

Students

LEAP data revealed student ($n = 1792$) demographic data matched the state demographics of approximately 58% White, 22% Hispanic, 12% Black, 8% Asian, 4% Native American, and 6% multi-ethnic. Fifty-three percent of participants were females and 47% were males, with a mean age of 14.4 years upon entry into LEAP in 8th grade.

In response to goals and objectives, the comparison of middle school students participating in LEAP to students not participating in LEAP showed no change in standardized test scores ($p = 0.07$), but showed a decrease in absentee rates ($p = 0.02$). Community engagement scores increased significantly among the LEAP students ($p = 0.03$).

Multi-level statistical modeling was used to determine the LEAP dose-response effect. At the end of the first year of implementation (Year 2), students completed the first posttest survey. At the end of the second year (Year 3), 18% of these students were lost to follow-up and did not complete the second posttest survey. The modeling found the majority of the students lost to follow-up lived in large counties. This finding was attributed to lack of county economic stability and transient movement of families. In smaller counties, the second posttest revealed a positive lasting effect of decreased absentee rates, and community engagement scores remained high. By the fourth year of implementation (Year 5), 32% of the middle school students were lost to follow-up across all counties. Overall, 2 years after the students participated in LEAP, their absentee rates returned to baseline data. However, community engagement scores remained statistically higher than baseline scores for 2 years after LEAP participation. Throughout the research, the standardized test scores remained unaffected by LEAP participation.

Students praised every aspect of LEAP during the satisfaction interviews. Students enjoyed getting to know after-school program peers and engaging in the community engagement activities. Survey responses included the following positive comments:

- "I would never have gotten to know her without LEAP. We are now best friends even though we are very different." (6th-grade female student)
- "Doing the activities taught me to learn about people that don't look like you or who don't live in your neighborhood." (7th-grade male student)

Parents

Although it was difficult to recruit parents to participate in interviews, parents ($n = 24$) also offered positive comments about LEAP:

- "Brian actually had something to say when I asked him what he did at school that day. He talked about the LEAP community activities all the time." (Parent of 8th-grade male student)
- "Our family helped the kids at the LEAP carwash. We really enjoyed working on the project that the kids organized by themselves." (Parent of 7th-grade female student)

Principals and School Staff

Interviews and satisfaction surveys were completed by a sample of principals and school staff. The ABC evaluation team designed a 10-question satisfaction survey and posted it on the website. Each facilitator provided the link to their principals and school staff. The online convenience of the satisfaction survey yielded a 57% response rate. Using a 5-point Likert scale, the satisfaction mean scores were 4.6 for principals and 4.7 for school staff. Interviews ($n = 31$) revealed generally positive remarks:

- "I believe that LEAP gave the after-school program a purpose. I noticed that more kids started staying in the after-school program just so they could participate in LEAP. It was positive word of mouth among the kids." (Teacher)
- "I am glad that our after-school program was selected to participate in LEAP. It seemed like a good way to get the kids involved, but I'm not sure the positive effects will last over time. I get tired of programs that come and go without any planned sustainability." (Principal)

Using the randomized controlled trial delayed intervention design; LEAP was implemented in 18 counties in a total of 64 middle schools' after-school programs. External evaluation results revealed middle school students participating in LEAP after-school programs had similar standardized test scores when compared to the nonparticipating LEAP students. The statistically significant results showed that LEAP students had lower absentee rates and higher community engagement scores. The students lost to follow-up were mainly from large counties with unstable economies and thus more transient families. LEAP satisfaction interviews and surveys revealed positive results from principals, school staff, parents, and students with special emphasis on the community engagement portion of the curriculum. The dose-response rate showed the lower absentee rates and higher community engagement scores were sustained for approximately 1 year after LEAP participation. Low sustainability rates led to questions about the cost-benefit utility of LEAP. Further research is needed to determine if the cost per student ratio merits the results gained.

CASE STUDY QUESTIONS

1. What other evaluation theory could have been used for this evaluation?
2. How would you increase the involvement of the middle school classroom teachers in this evaluation?
3. How would you suggest that the middle school students decide on their community engagement projects? Make a list of six possible ideas that they might explore in their community.
4. What other types of statistical tests would you think might be appropriate?
5. How would you suggest that the ABC evaluation team disseminate the results of the LEAP evaluation?

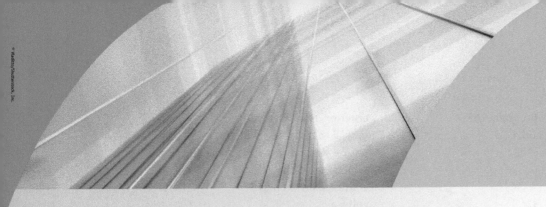

Index

Note: Page numbers followed by *b*, *f*, and *t* indicate material in boxes, figures, and tables respectively.